Advanced MR Imaging in Clinical Practice

Editor

HERSH CHANDARANA

RADIOLOGIC CLINICS OF NORTH AMERICA

www.radiologic.theclinics.com

Consulting Editor
FRANK H. MILLER

May 2015 • Volume 53 • Number 3

ELSEVIER

1600 John F. Kennedy Boulevard • Suite 1800 • Philadelphia, Pennsylvania, 19103-2899

http://www.theclinics.com

RADIOLOGIC CLINICS OF NORTH AMERICA Volume 53, Number 3
May 2015 ISSN 0033-8389, ISBN 13: 978-0-323-37617-4

Editor: John Vassallo (j.vassallo@elsevier.com)
Developmental Editor: Donald Mumford

Radiologic Clinics of North America (ISSN 0033-8389) is published bimonthly by Elsevier Inc., 360 Park Avenue South, New York, NY 10010-1710. Months of issue are January, March, May, July, September, and November. Periodicals postage paid at New York, NY and additional mailing offices. Subscription prices are USD 460 per year for US individuals, USD 709 per year for US institutions, USD 220 per year for US students and residents, USD 535 per year for Canadian individuals, USD 905 per year for Canadian institutions, USD 660 per year for international individuals, USD 905 per year for international institutions, and USD 315 per year for Canadian and foreign students/residents. To receive student and resident rate, orders must be accompanied by name of affiliated institution, date of term and the signature of program/residency coordinatior on institution letterhead. Orders will be billed at individual rate until proof of status is received. Foreign air speed delivery is included in all *Clinics* subscription prices. All prices are subject to change without notice. **POSTMASTER:** Send address changes to *Radiologic Clinics of North America*, Elsevier Health Sciences Division, Subscription Customer Service, 3251 Riverport Lane, Maryland Heights, MO63043. **Customer Service: Telephone: 1-800-654-2452** (U.S. and Canada); **1-314-447-8871** (outside U.S. and Canada). **Fax: 1-314-447-8029. E-mail: journalscustomerservice-usa@ elsevier.com** (for print support); **journalsonlinesupport-usa@elsevier.com** (for online support).

Reprints. For copies of 100 or more of articles in this publication, please contact the Commercial Reprints Department, Elsevier Inc., 360 Park Avenue South, New York, New York 10010-1710. Tel.: +1-212-633-3874; Fax: +1-212-633-3820; E-mail: reprints@elsevier.com.

Radiologic Clinics of North America also published in Greek Paschalidis Medical Publications, Athens, Greece.

Radiologic Clinics of North America is covered in *MEDLINE/PubMed (Index Medicus), EMBASE/Excerpta Medica, Current Contents/Life Sciences, Current Contents/Clinical Medicine, RSNA Index to Imaging Literature, BIOSIS, Science Citation Index,* and *ISI/BIOMED.*

Contributors

CONSULTING EDITOR

FRANK H. MILLER, MD
Chief, Body Imaging Section and Fellowship
Program and GI Radiology; Medical Director
MRI; Professor, Department of Radiology,
Northwestern Memorial Hospital,
Northwestern University, Feinberg School of
Medicine, Chicago, Illinois

EDITOR

HERSH CHANDARANA, MD
Section Chief, Abdominal Imaging,
Department of Radiology, New York University
School of Medicine, New York University
Langone Medical Center, New York, New York

AUTHORS

MUSTAFA R. BASHIR, MD
Director of the Center for Advanced Magnetic
Resonance Research and Development
(CAMRD), Department of Radiology, Duke
University Medical Center, Durham, North
Carolina

JENNY T. BENCARDINO, MD
Department of Radiology, New York University
Hospital for Joint Diseases, New York,
New York

LUBNA BHATTI, MBBS
Department of Radiology, Duke University
Medical Center, Durham, North Carolina

NICHOLAS BHOJWANI, MD
Department of Radiology, University Hospitals
Case Medical Center, Case Western Reserve
University, Cleveland, Ohio

ELIZABETH L. CARPENTER, MD
Department of Radiology, New York University
Hospital for Joint Diseases, New York,
New York

HERSH CHANDARANA, MD
Section Chief, Abdominal Imaging,
Department of Radiology, New York University
School of Medicine, New York University
Langone Medical Center, New York,
New York

BRIAN M. DALE, PhD
Siemens Healthcare, Morrisville, North
Carolina

RICHARD K.G. DO, MD, PhD
Assistant Attending, Department of Radiology,
Memorial Sloan Kettering Cancer Center,
New York, New York

BRENT GRIFFITH, MD
Department of Radiology, Henry Ford Health
System, Detroit, Michigan

AMIT GUPTA, MD
Department of Diagnostic Radiology, Imaging
Institute, Cleveland Clinic, Cleveland, Ohio

JENNY K. HOANG, MBBS
Department of Radiology, Duke University
Medical Center, Durham, North Carolina

RAJAN JAIN, MD
Associate Professor of Radiology, New York
University School of Medicine, New York
University Langone Medical Center, New York,
New York

CHRISTOF KARMONIK, PhD
MRI Core, Houston Methodist Research
Institute, Houston, Texas

ANDREA KIERANS, MD
Department of Radiology, New York
University Langone Medical Center, New York,
New York

IOANNIS KOKTZOGLOU, PhD
Department of Radiology, NorthShore
University HealthSystem, Evanston, Illinois;
Assistant Professor, Department of Radiology,
The University of Chicago Pritzker School of
Medicine, Chicago, Illinois

RUTH P. LIM, MBBS, MMed, MS, FRANZCR
Department of Radiology, Austin Health;
Associate Professor, Departments of
Radiology and Surgery, Faculty of Medicine,
Dentistry and Health Sciences, The University
of Melbourne, Melbourne, Victoria, Australia

KECHENG LIU, PhD, MBA
Magnetic Resonance Imaging, Siemens
Healthcare USA, Malvern, Pennsylvania

LORENZO MANNELLI, MD, PhD
Assistant Attending, Department of Radiology,
Memorial Sloan Kettering Cancer Center,
New York, New York

MARTIN MAURER, MD
Institute of Diagnostic, Interventional and
Pediatric Radiology, Inselspital University
Hospitals Bern, Bern, Switzerland

MATHIAS NITTKA, PhD
Magnetic Resonance Imaging, Siemens AG,
Erlangen, Germany

STEPHANIE NOUGARET, MD
Department of Radiology, Memorial Sloan
Kettering Cancer Center, New York, New York;
Assistant Attending, St Eloi Hospital, CHU
Montpellier, Montpellier, France

NAINESH PARIKH, MD
Department of Radiology, New York University
Langone Medical Center, New York,
New York

SASAN PARTOVI, MD
Department of Radiology, University Hospitals
Case Medical Center, Case Western Reserve
University, Cleveland, Ohio

ANDREW N. PRIMAK, PhD
Computed Tomography, Siemens Healthcare
USA, Malvern, Pennsylvania

JUSTIN M. REAM, MD
Department of Radiology, New York University
School of Medicine, New York University
Langone Medical Center, New York,
New York

MARK R. ROBBIN, MD
Department of Radiology, University Hospitals
Case Medical Center, Case Western Reserve
University, Cleveland, Ohio

ANDREW B. ROSENKRANTZ, MD
Department of Radiology, New York University
School of Medicine, New York University
Langone Medical Center, New York,
New York

AMIT M. SAINDANE, MD
Director, Division of Neuroradiology; Associate
Professor, Department of Radiology and
Imaging Sciences, Emory University Hospital,
Emory University School of Medicine, Atlanta,
Georgia

NAVEEN SUBHAS, MD
Assistant Professor, Department of Diagnostic
Radiology, Imaging Institute, Cleveland Clinic,
Cleveland, Ohio

HEBERT A. VARGAS, MD
Assistant Attending, Department of Radiology,
Memorial Sloan Kettering Cancer Center,
New York, New York

HENDRIK VON TENGG-KOBLIGK, MD
Institute of Diagnostic, Interventional and
Pediatric Radiology, Inselspital University
Hospitals Bern, Bern, Switzerland

Contents

Magnetic resonance neurography (MRN) provides the greatest degree of soft tissue contrast in the evaluation of peripheral nerves. Utilization of MRN relies on (1) peripheral nerve anatomy, (2) the spectrum of pathology, and (3) familiarity with dedicated MR imaging techniques. Although there remain several pitfalls in MRN imaging, awareness of these pitfalls improves imaging quality and limits misinterpretation. Most importantly, maintaining a direct line of communication with the referring clinician allows for the greatest degree of diagnostic accuracy.

An increasing number of joint replacements are being performed in the United States. Patients undergoing these procedures can have various complications. Imaging is one of the primary means of diagnosing these complications. Cross-sectional imaging techniques, such as computed tomography (CT) and MR imaging, are more sensitive than radiographs for evaluating complications. The use of CT and MR imaging in patients with metallic implants is limited by the presence of artifacts. This review discusses the causes of metal artifacts on MR imaging and CT, contributing factors, and conventional and novel methods to reduce the effects of these artifacts on scans.

Multiple nonmorphologic magnetic resonance sequences are available in musculoskeletal imaging that can provide additional information to better characterize and diagnose musculoskeletal disorders and diseases. These sequences include blood-oxygen-level-dependent (BOLD), arterial spin labeling (ASL), diffusion-weighted imaging (DWI), and diffusion-tensor imaging (DTI). BOLD and ASL provide different methods to evaluate skeletal muscle microperfusion. The BOLD signal reflects the ratio between oxyhemoglobin and deoxyhemoglobin. ASL uses selective tagging of inflowing blood spins in a specific region for calculating local perfusion. DWI and DTI provide information about the structural integrity of soft tissue including muscles and fibers as well as pathologies.

Diffusion-weighted imaging (DWI) has become a routine component of clinical MR imaging. Its unique soft tissue contrast mechanism exploits differences in the motion of water molecules in vivo at a biologically meaningful scale. The clinical potential of DWI in lesion detection, characterization, and response assessment has been explored. This review briefly covers basic principles of DWI and introduces advances, specifically for abdominopelvic organs.

Utilization of abdominopelvic MR imaging continues to increase in volume and gain widespread clinical acceptance. Many factors such as diaphragmatic respiratory motion, bulk patient motion, and the need for large volumetric coverage while maintaining clinically feasible scan times have proven challenging for body applications of MRI. However, many advances in MR acquisition, including non-Cartesian T1-weighted and T2-weighted acquisitions, advanced Dixon sequences, and 3-dimensional volumetric T2-weighted imaging have helped to mitigate some of the issues which have hampered abdominopelvic MR. This article will summarize these advances in T1-weighted and T2-weighted imaging, with an emphasis on clinical applications and implementation.

Tremendous advances have been made in abdominopelvic MR imaging, which continue to improve image quality, and make acquisitions faster and robust. We briefly discuss the role of non-Cartesian acquisition schemes as well as dual parallel radiofrequency (RF) transmit systems in the article to further improve image quality of the abdominal MR imaging. Furthermore, the use of hybrid PET/MR systems has the potential to synergistically combine MR imaging with PET acquisition, and the evolving role of hybrid PET/MR imaging is discussed.

PROGRAM OBJECTIVE
The objective of the *Radiologic Clinics of North America* is to keep practicing radiologists and radiology residents up to date with current clinical practice in radiology by providing timely articles reviewing the state of the art in patient care.

TARGET AUDIENCE
Practicing radiologists, radiology residents, and other health care professionals who provide patient care utilizing radiologic findings.

LEARNING OBJECTIVES
Upon completion of this activity, participants will be able to:
1. Review advances in MR imaging in clinical practice.
2. Discuss recent advances in MR hardware and software.
3. Recognize the basic techniques of perfusion imaging in neuro-oncology.

ACCREDITATION
The Elsevier Office of Continuing Medical Education (EOCME) is accredited by the Accreditation Council for Continuing Medical Education (ACCME) to provide continuing medical education for physicians.

The EOCME designates this enduring material for a maximum of 15 *AMA PRA Category 1 Credit*(s)™. Physicians should claim only the credit commensurate with the extent of their participation in the activity.

All other health care professionals requesting continuing education credit for this enduring material will be issued a certificate of participation.

DISCLOSURE OF CONFLICTS OF INTEREST
The EOCME assesses conflict of interest with its instructors, faculty, planners, and other individuals who are in a position to control the content of CME activities. All relevant conflicts of interest that are identified are thoroughly vetted by EOCME for fair balance, scientific objectivity, and patient care recommendations. EOCME is committed to providing its learners with CME activities that promote improvements or quality in healthcare and not a specific proprietary business or a commercial interest.

The planning committee, staff, authors and editors listed below have identified no financial relationships or relationships to products or devices they or their spouse/life partner have with commercial interest related to the content of this CME activity:
Jenny T. Bencardino, MD; Lubna Bhatti, MBBS; Nicholas Bhojwani, MD; Elizabeth L. Carpenter, MD; Anjali Fortna; Brent Griffith, MD; Amit Gupta, MD; Kristen Helm; Jenny K. Hoang, MBBS; Rajan Jain, MD; Christof Karmonik, PhD; Andrea Kierans, MD; Lorenzo Mannelli, MD, PhD; Martin Maurer, MD; Frank H. Miller, MD; Stephanie Nougaret, MD; Nainesh Parikh, MD; Sasan Partovi, MD; Justin M. Ream, MD; Mark R. Robbin, MD; Andrew B. Rosenkrantz, MD; Amit M. Saindane, MD; Karthikeyan Subramaniam; Hebert A. Vargas, MD; John Vassallo; Hendrik von Tengg-Kobligk, MD.

The planning committee, staff, authors and editors listed below have identified financial relationships or relationships to products or devices they or their spouse/life partner have with commercial interest related to the content of this CME activity:
Mustafa R. Bashir, MD has research support from Siemens Corporation.
Hersh Chandarana, MD has research support from Siemens Corporation and a patent on the GRASP technique.
Brian M. Dale, PhD has an employment affiliation with Siemens Corporation.
Richard K.G. Do, MD, PhD is a consultant/advisor for Merck & Co., Inc.
Ioannis Koktzoglou, PhD has research support from Siemens Corporation and the American Heart Association, Inc.
Ruth P. Lim, MBBS, MMed, MS, FRANZCR has research support from the Royal Australian and New Zealand College of Radiology, Diabetes Australia, and Austin Medical Research Foundation.
Kecheng Liu, PhD, MBA has an employment affiliation with Siemens Corporation.
Mathias Nittka, PhD has an employment affiliation with Siemens Corporation.
Andrew N. Primak, PhD has an employment affiliation with Siemens Corporation.
Naveen Subhas, MD has research support from Siemens Corporation.

UNAPPROVED/OFF-LABEL USE DISCLOSURE
The EOCME requires CME faculty to disclose to the participants:
1. When products or procedures being discussed are off-label, unlabelled, experimental, and/or investigational (not US Food and Drug Administration [FDA] approved); and
2. Any limitations on the information presented, such as data that are preliminary or that represent ongoing research, interim analyses, and/or unsupported opinions. Faculty may discuss information about pharmaceutical agents that is outside of FDA-approved labelling. This information is intended solely for CME and is not intended to promote off-label use of these medications. If you have any questions, contact the medical affairs department of the manufacturer for the most recent prescribing information.

TO ENROLL

To enroll in the *Radiologic Clinics of North America* Continuing Medical Education program, call customer service at 1-800-654-2452 or sign up online at http://www.theclinics.com/home/cme. The CME program is available to subscribers for an additional annual fee of USD 315.

METHOD OF PARTICIPATION

In order to claim credit, participants must complete the following:
1. Complete enrolment as indicated above.
2. Read the activity.
3. Complete the CME Test and Evaluation. Participants must achieve a score of 70% on the test. All CME Tests and Evaluations must be completed online.

CME INQUIRIES/SPECIAL NEEDS

For all CME inquiries or special needs, please contact elsevierCME@elsevier.com.

RADIOLOGIC CLINICS OF NORTH AMERICA

THE CLINICS ARE AVAILABLE ONLINE!
Access your subscription at:
www.theclinics.com

Preface
Advances in MR Imaging

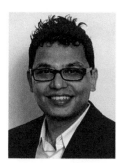

Hersh Chandarana, MD
Editor

MR imaging is a powerful modality, which, in addition to providing excellent morphologic information, enables interrogation of novel contrasts and function. Technical innovations and advances in MR imaging continue to occur at a rapid pace. However, there is a substantial lag time between these advances and clinical utilization as these advances are perceived to be complex and difficult to implement in routine practice.

This issue highlights some of the recent advances in MR imaging, breaks down perceived complexities, and focuses on why and how these techniques and technologies can be deployed in clinical practice. In addition, authors of these articles, who are experts in their respective fields, have provided the readers with a playbook to implement these advances in the clinical setting. My hope is that this issue will excite and encourage readers to implement some of these advances in their own clinical practice.

I am honored to have served as the editor for this issue and wish to thank Dr Frank Miller for this opportunity. I am also thankful to all the authors for their invaluable contributions. I would like to acknowledge the hard work of the Elsevier staff, with special thanks to Donald Mumford and John Vassallo for their administrative and editorial assistance. Special thanks to my family: my wife, Ranjana, and my children, Jai and Aarti, for encouraging me and allowing me the time to devote to this task.

Hersh Chandarana, MD
Section Chief, Abdominal Imaging
Department of Radiology
NYU School of Medicine
NYU Langone Medical Center
660 First Avenue, 3rd Floor
New York, NY 10016, USA

E-mail address:
hersh.chandarana@nyumc.org

Radiol Clin N Am 53 (2015) xi
http://dx.doi.org/10.1016/j.rcl.2015.03.001
0033-8389/15/$ – see front matter © 2015 Published by Elsevier Inc.

Advanced Magnetic Resonance Techniques: 3 T

Lubna Bhatti, MBBS[a], Jenny K. Hoang, MBBS[a], Brian M. Dale, PhD[b], Mustafa R. Bashir, MD[a,*]

KEYWORDS

- High field • 3 T • Field strength

KEY POINTS

- MR imaging at 3 T has become feasible for most clinical applications, and has several advantages and disadvantages compared with 1.5-T MR imaging.
- Advantages of 3-T compared with 1.5-T MR imaging include higher signal/noise ratio, improved contrast enhancement, and stronger susceptibility effects for some applications.
- Disadvantages of 3-T compared with 1.5-T MR imaging include main magnetic field inhomogeneity, radiofrequency field inhomogeneity, and susceptibility-related artifacts.

MR IMAGING PHYSICS AT 3 T

Within the last decade, 3 T MR imaging has evolved from a research modality into a primary clinical imaging technology. With this increased use, there is a need for awareness of the basic physical effects associated with the increased field strength. This article assumes a working knowledge of MR physics at 1.5 T, and focuses primarily on effects that differ or are more pronounced at 3 T.[1]

Relaxation Effects

MR imaging is sensitive to a wide variety of physical effects, and among them the longitudinal relaxation time (T_1) and the transverse relaxation time (T_2) are paramount for clinical diagnosis. T_1 characterizes the amount of time required for the tissue magnetization to regrow after being disrupted; it is longer (slower) at higher field strengths.[1,2] T_2 characterizes the amount of time required for the MR signal to decay after being excited; it has low sensitivity to field strength. T_2^* also characterizes the decay of the MR signal, but includes nonrandom effects, such as dephasing caused by susceptibility changes, as well as the random T_2 effects. T_2^* is generally shorter (faster) at high field strengths.[1,2]

Signal/Noise Ratio

In principle, the amount of fully relaxed longitudinal magnetization depends linearly on field strength, which ideally provides a 2-fold improvement of signal/noise ratio (SNR) at 3 T.[1] However, because T_1 relaxation times are longer at 3 T than at lower field strengths, less magnetization is recovered for the same time to repetition (TR), reducing the anticipated SNR gains to less than the ideal 2-fold increase.[3] In addition, stronger chemical shift effects (discussed later) necessitate the use of higher receiver bandwidth, further reducing SNR gains, particularly for T_1-weighted and non–fat-suppressed imaging.[4] The SNR is still higher at 3 T than at 1.5 T for similar sequences, but often much less than double.

Gadolinium Chelate Contrast Agents

The most common contrast agents used clinically are gadolinium chelate compounds. In clinical

Disclosures: L. Bhatti and J.K. Hoang have no relevant disclosures. B.M. Dale is an employee of Siemens Healthcare. M.R. Bashir receives research support from Siemens Healthcare.
[a] Department of Radiology, Duke University Medical Center, DUMC 3808, Durham, NC 27710, USA; [b] Siemens Healthcare, Morrisville, NC 27560, USA
* Corresponding author.
E-mail address: mustafa.bashir@duke.edu

radiologic.theclinics.com

concentrations, they act primarily as T_1-shortening agents. Despite the contrast agents' reduced relaxivity at 3 T compared with 1.5 T, and because the native tissue T_1 is higher, the T_1 difference between contrast-enhanced and contrast-unenhanced is greater at 3 T.[5,6] Thus, T_1-shortening contrast agents typically perform better at 3 T and result in greater amounts of enhancement.

Spin Labeling

In several applications, such as arterial spin labeling (ASL) or myocardial tissue tagging, it is possible to selectively label certain tissues using specially configured radiofrequency (RF) pulses.[7] One of the main limitations of these techniques is that the labeling decays as a function of T_1.[8,9] Because of the extended T_1 at 3 T, labeling lasts longer and decays more slowly than at 1.5 T.

Chemical Shift

The protons in different chemical species are slightly shielded from the external magnetic field by the neighboring electrons. This shielding depends on a proton's position in the molecule and causes a shift of resonance frequency that is proportional to the field strength.[1] In MR imaging, this leads to 2 primary effects. Chemical shift of the first kind is a spatial misregistration of spins (both in the readout and in slice select directions) from any molecule other than water. Chemical shift of the second kind is a cyclical constructive and destructive interference from different chemical species within the same imaging voxel.[4] Chemical shift of the first kind leads to double the misregistration at 3 T compared with 1.5 T, unless compensated by increased receive bandwidth (for readout shifts) or transmit bandwidth (for slice shifts). Chemical shift of the second kind occurs at twice the frequency (half the echo time [TE]) compared with 1.5 T.

In addition to the artifacts mentioned earlier, the increased chemical shift makes spectrally selective techniques more efficient. Fat suppression and inversion pulses require less time for similar spectral selectivity.[1] Also, spectroscopy benefits from a greater separation and discrimination between neighboring spectral peaks, and spectral modeling techniques typically require less time to acquire. For example, the in-phase TE for a 2-point Dixon sequence is 4.4 milliseconds at 1.5 T, but only 2.2 milliseconds at 3 T.

Radiofrequency Ablation Inhomogeneity

In human tissues, the RF wavelengths at 3 T begin to approach the size of the imaging field of view, which means that the RF fields are noticeably less uniform in the body at 3 T compared with 1.5 T. RF energy propagating through tissues from different directions can interfere destructively, resulting in a characteristic signal dropout often described as dielectric artifact or standing wave artifact.[10] Furthermore, individual coil elements have a less homogeneous sensitivity profile, which can cause increased coil sensitivity artifacts, but it can also improve the spatial discrimination between coil elements in parallel imaging. One often-subtle effect is that inhomogeneous RF transmit fields lead to slight variations in flip angle and tissue contrast across the field of view.[1]

Iron Oxide Contrast Agents and Endogenous Iron

A less common class of contrast agent includes the superparamagnetic iron oxide–based contrast agents (SPIOs, or ultrasmall particles of iron oxide). These agents have much stronger effects on T_2 and T_2^* than the gadolinium chelate agents. Iron also exists naturally within the body, in both healthy and pathologic conditions. On a microscopic level, iron particles induce strong susceptibility (T_2^*) effects that are proportional to field strength, and therefore more pronounced at 3 T than at 1.5 T.[11]

Safety Issues

A magnetic dipole in a uniform magnetic field experiences a torque that is proportional to the square of the field strength.[12] Therefore, there is 4 times more torque on ferromagnetic objects within the magnetic field at isocenter in a 3-T MR imaging system than in a 1.5-T system. In addition, a magnetic dipole in a nonuniform field experiences a net force.[12] The spatial gradient of the main magnetic field is typically higher for 3-T systems than for 1.5-T systems, particularly near the mouth of the bore, which causes an increased net force on ferromagnetic objects in that region.

The higher main magnetic field strength also implies a higher frequency for the RF transmit and receive fields. Specific absorption rate (SAR) is the rate at which power is deposited in the human body, and is approximately 4 times as high at 3 T compared with at 1.5 T, assuming all else is equal.[1] In addition, the higher frequency corresponds with a shorter wavelength, which reduces the characteristic length of an object, such as a wire, that will resonate with the RF field and thereby changes the amount of heat generated.[13] Thus some objects may generate significantly more heat at 3 T than at 1.5 T.

NEUROIMAGING AT 3 T

The care of many patients with diseases of the brain, head and neck, and spine depends on MR imaging for detection and characterization. The advantages that 3-T imaging offers with respect to specific neurologic diseases and to advanced techniques used for neuroimaging are discussed here. In addition, it is important for radiologists to be cognizant of differences in imaging appearances at 1.5 T and 3 T, and of technical considerations when scanning with higher magnetic field strengths.

Conventional Neuroimaging Techniques

The main advantage of increasing the field strength is increased SNR, which theoretically provides improvements in image quality. Therefore, it has been proposed that 3-T MR imaging may offer advantages in the detection of subtle or small findings in the setting of demyelinating plaques, focal epileptogenic lesions, and brain tumors. Researchers who have compared 1.5-T and 3-T systems for these diagnoses have found positive results in favor of 3-T systems.[14–18] However, most of these studies are limited by small sample sizes and/or the bias of comparing scanners with different generations of technology that may favor 3 T.

Wardlaw and colleagues[19] performed a systematic review of studies using both 3 T and 1.5 T for neuroimaging. The review included articles that compared 3 T and 1.5 T for tumors, multiple sclerosis, stroke, epilepsy, and vascular diseases (aneurysms, arteriovenous malformation). There was subjective evidence of increased lesion detection and improved image resolution with 3 T compared with 1.5 T, but there was little evidence of improved diagnostic accuracy. To date, there are few data showing that higher magnetic field strength results in increased diagnostic performance or yield for standard neuroimaging protocols.

Advanced Neuroimaging Techniques

Higher field strength has significant advantages for some advanced techniques in neuroimaging, such as MR spectroscopy (MRS), functional MR (fMR) imaging, brain perfusion imaging, and diffusion tensor imaging (DTI). Other techniques, such as susceptibility-weighted imaging (SWI) and MR angiography (MRA), theoretically have better image quality with higher field strength but, because of advances in 1.5-T scanner technology, there may not be appreciable differences in the clinical setting.

Magnetic resonance spectroscopy

MRS measures the relative quantity of molecules (or metabolites) within a given voxel and is used to characterize disorders. MRS is based on chemical shift, which is the difference in precession frequency for various protons (measured in parts per million) caused by their relative microenvironments. Higher field strength has the dual effect of increasing the chemical shift effect and increasing SNR, which results in better spectral resolution and improved separation of metabolite peaks, especially for low-TE spectroscopy, in which the time to detect signal is short.[19]

Functional magnetic resonance imaging

fMR imaging is used to identify regions in the brain cortex that are functionally active during a task. It is based on the blood oxygenation level–dependent (BOLD) effect, which detects a reduction in deoxyhemoglobin level as increased signal on T_2^*-weighted images. Doubling the magnetic field strength increases the SNR and contrast/noise ratio (CNR) but also increases T_2^* sensitivity (susceptibility effect) 4-fold. Greater susceptibility effects provide increases in activation volumes or can be translated into shorter TEs (and shorter overall imaging times) at 3 T compared with 1.5 T, while maintaining SNR.[20] Shorter imaging times then allow larger coverage volumes, larger numbers of repetitions to increase SNR, or improved temporal resolution.

Brain perfusion imaging

Brain perfusion imaging uses quantitative techniques to identify perfusion defects representing ischemia and to characterize tumors. Perfusion imaging is based on contrast bolus techniques or ASL. Bolus technique for brain imaging is often performed with dynamic susceptibility contrast (DSC) methods, which are based on T_2^* shortening caused by the presence of a contrast agent. As in fMR imaging, increasing field strength increases SNR and T_2^* sensitivity, resulting in considerable improvement in image quality at 3 T, and also allowing shorter TE and improved temporal resolution.

For ASL techniques, the effect of increased magnetic field strength is an increase in SNR as well as lengthening of tissue T_1, allowing more spin label to accumulate. A 2-fold signal gain is readily achievable by performing ASL at 3 T, compared with similar methods at 1.5 T.[7,21]

Diffusion tensor imaging

DTI measures anisotropic diffusion along white matter tracts. DTI describes the magnitude, the degree of anisotropy, and the orientation of diffusion anisotropy, and can be used to derive estimates of white matter connectivity patterns. Imaging is most commonly performed with a spin echo pulse sequence with single-shot echo plan imaging readout. The higher magnetic field strength results in increased SNR that can allow acquisition with smaller voxels or reduce imaging time, although susceptibility and distortion effects caused by main magnetic field inhomogeneity can be significant challenges.

Susceptibility-weighted imaging

SWI is a high-spatial-resolution gradient echo technique that provides sensitive detection of intracranial microhemorrhage, calcification, iron deposition, and small vessels. As in fMR imaging, higher magnetic field strength results in increased SNR and T2* sensitivity, which can be used either to improve image quality or to reduce TE and reduce scan times, while maintaining the same image quality as 1.5 T.

Magnetic resonance angiography

Intracranial MR angiography (MRA) is most often performed with the time of flight (TOF) method, which is a noncontrast technique using a gradient echo sequence that suppresses background signal and enhances flow-related signal to produce angiographic images. At 3 T, longer T_1 relaxation times provide improved background tissue suppression compared with 1.5 T, and therefore improved visibility of the vessels. In addition, increased SNR makes higher spatial resolution possible within reasonable acquisition times.

Special Considerations and Challenges for Neuroimaging

At higher field strengths, the effects of susceptibility-induced geometric distortion and signal loss are increased, and these can negatively

affect imaging in several clinical scenarios. First, distortion may be more noticeable in the region of the skull base, caused by the proximity of air and bone to the brain. Second, spinal and oral hardware cause greater susceptibility artifacts, and it may be preferred to image such patients at 1.5 T. In addition, for head and neck imaging that includes the skull base, susceptibility artifacts may present a problem, especially on fat-saturated techniques. Thus pulse sequences that use fat suppression based on multiecho chemical shift methods, rather than spectrally selective pulses, are preferred for head and neck imaging. In addition, using shorter TEs is useful for reducing distortions at the skull base.

When comparing serial imaging performed on systems with different magnetic field strengths, radiologists should be careful not to interpret differences caused by the field strength as changes caused by disease. A study by Neema and colleagues[14] showed that normal subjects had discrete white matter hyperintensities, periventricular capping, and diffuse posterior white matter hyperintensity that were more numerous or pronounced at 3 T than at 1.5 T (Fig. 1). Similarly, flow-related artifacts in the cerebrospinal fluid at spine imaging tend to be more pronounced at 3 T.

Prolongation of T_1 relaxation times at higher field strength has also been known to reduce the contrast differences between gray and white matter for traditional T_1-weighted sequences of the brain and spine. Therefore, some centers modify T_1-weighted sequences by increasing TR, or replace them with T_1 fluid-attenuated inversion recovery (FLAIR) sequences at 3 T. Signal enhancement in response to contrast media administration can also appear to be increased at 3 T compared with 1.5 T and does not necessarily reflect a change in the disease process (Fig. 2). In addition,

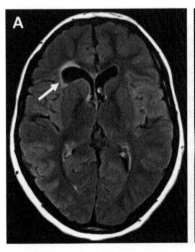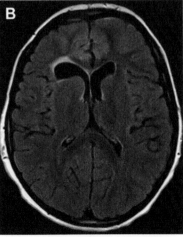

Fig. 1. Fluid attenuation inversion recovery (FLAIR) images from a 10-year-old boy with a history of resected craniopharyngioma obtained at 3 T (*A*) and 1.5 T (*B*). Note the more pronounced appearance of periventricular white matter hyperintensities at 3 T (*white arrow*). Also note higher SNR of the 3-T image, as shown by reduced salt-and-pepper image noise, particularly in the frontal and parietooccipital white matter.

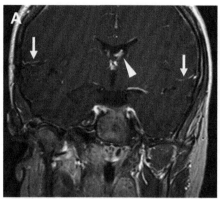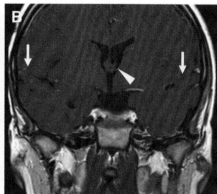

Fig. 2. Thin (3 mm) coronal contrast-enhanced T_1-weighted images from a 10-year-old boy with a history of resected craniopharyngioma obtained at 3 T (*A*) and 1.5 T (*B*). Note more pronounced enhancement of peripheral vessels in the brain at 3 T compared with 1.5 T, especially in the sylvian fissures (*arrows*) and choroid plexus (*arrowhead*).

gradient echo sequences may be preferred to spin echo sequences at 3 T, and spatial saturation bands avoided, in order to maintain SAR below the FDA-mandated limits in brain MR imaging. Avoiding saturation bands may result in greater inflow or motion artifacts, depending on the application.

ABDOMINOPELVIC MR IMAGING AT 3 T

MR imaging is an important technique for evaluating the visceral and luminal organs of the abdomen and pelvis. In the last decade, abdominopelvic MR imaging at 3 T has become a well-established technique. Although there are many important challenges in 3-T imaging, benefits can be realized, especially improved SNR compared with 1.5 T, which can be used to improve image quality or exchanged for higher temporal and spatial resolution. Because there are many clinical applications that can be considered, this article takes a pulse sequence–based approach to describe frequently encountered scenarios at 3-T MR imaging.

Chemical Shift Imaging

Most abdominal MR imaging protocols include a multiecho chemical shift pulse sequence (usually 2 echoes), used to detect fat within solid organs or focal lesions, as well as abnormal susceptibility.[22,23] In addition, multiecho pulse sequences with as many as 6 echoes can be used to obtain quantitative measures of hepatic steatosis.[24–26] The most readily apparent difference between 3-T and 1.5-T imaging with chemical shift sequences is the shorter in-phase and opposed-phase TEs. Although this method requires increased receiver

bandwidth and resultant SNR reductions, it also means that the last echo can be collected at half the time after excitation. For two-dimensional sequences, this shorter data collection time provides the ability to collect more k-space lines per excitation; for three-dimensional sequences, TR can be shortened. In both scenarios, a more rapid acquisition can be achieved and translated into either shorter breath holds or a larger data collection, which can then be used to increase spatial coverage, resolution, and/or SNR.

Dynamic Contrast-enhanced T_1-weighted Imaging

In body imaging, unlike neuroimaging and other applications, equivalent T_1 weighting does not necessarily need to be maintained between 1.5-T and 3-T examinations. Thus parameter optimization is performed based on other requirements, including achieving a rapid acquisition, strong T_1 weighting, and high SNR and CNR. For T_1-weighted imaging, the shortest TR possible is generally chosen to provide fast imaging and strong T_1 weighting. The flip angle is chosen to obtain strong T_1 weighting and high SNR, but must be tempered to avoid excessive SAR.[27,28] Short TE values are chosen to reduce signal loss caused by susceptibility, and choosing TE close to the nominal opposed-phase TE may improve spectrally selective fat suppression. In addition, using short TR and TE values may require higher receiver bandwidth values, which reduces SNR.

The strength of tissue enhancement following intravenous contrast administration depends on a variety of factors. Although contrast agent relaxivity is reduced as field strength increases, increases in tissue T_1 relaxation times cause a net increase in enhancement when pulse sequence parameters are unchanged (Fig. 3).[6,29]

T_2-weighted Imaging and Magnetic Resonance Cholangiopancreatography

In abdominopelvic imaging, T_2-weighted imaging is generally performed with fast-spin echo (FSE) techniques and long echo trains. Because these pulse sequences are insensitive to changes in tissue T_1 and T_2^* relaxation times, and T_2 depends little on field strength, basic parameter values can be maintained between 1.5 T and 3 T. The primary challenges at 3 T are related to SAR and artifacts. Because a large number of high-SAR refocusing pulses is required for FSE imaging, and SAR is proportional to the main magnetic field strength, FSE sequences are highly SAR intensive. SAR can be reduced by increasing TR, lowering the refocusing pulse flip angle systematically, or using variable flip angle pulse sequences that regulate the flip angle of refocusing pulses based on estimates of SAR.[30,31]

In terms of artifacts, T_2-weighted images are especially sensitive to standing wave artifacts and B_1 inhomogeneity, both of which can cause severe SNR reduction overall as well as dark spots in the images.[32,33] Both problems are exacerbated

in large patients and those with ascites (Fig. 4). Furthermore, ascites can cause RF shielding effects, which further reduce SNR. However, specialized techniques, including the use of RF cushions and multichannel transmit coils, can mitigate some of these effects.[34]

MR cholangiopancreatography (MRCP) is a technique used to visualize the biliary and pancreatic ducts. Heavily T_2-weighted sequences are used, and the same strengths and limitations of T_2-weighted sequences in general apply to MRCP. In particular, because the target structures are located in the central abdomen, these sequences are particularly sensitive to the described artifacts. Nonetheless, several studies have shown benefits for 3-T MRCP compared with 1.5 T, in particular with higher SNR, CNR, and improved duct visualization.[35–37]

Diffusion-weighted Imaging

Diffusion-weighted imaging (DWI) has been incorporated into many oncologic imaging protocols. Diffusion weighting is achieved by using a T_2-weighted spin echo pulse sequence with diffusion-encoding gradients on either side of the refocusing pulse, so that spins that are fairly static (diffusion restricted) experience both gradients

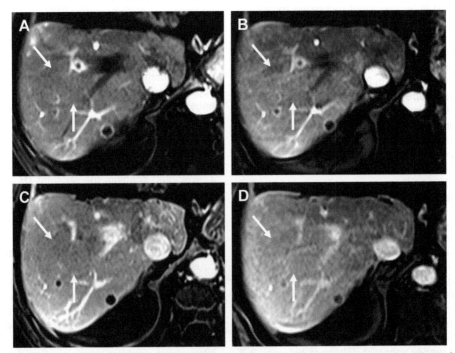

Fig. 3. Arterial phase (*A, B*) and equilibrium phase (*C, D*) images from liver MR imaging examinations obtained in a 79-year-old man with metastatic colon cancer. (*A, C*) Images obtained on a 3-T MR imaging system; (*B, D*) Images obtained on a 1.5-T system. Note improved SNR in the 3-T images, characterized by reduced signal inhomogeneity in normal portions of the liver (*white arrows*) and sharper delineation of the edges of the enhanced vessels.

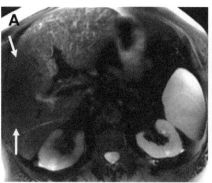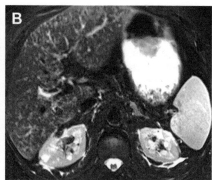

Fig. 4. FSE T_2-weighted images from liver MR imaging examinations obtained in a 71-year-old man with cirrhosis. (A) Image obtained on a 3-T MR imaging system; (B) image obtained on a 1.5 T system. Note substantially greater signal inhomogeneity throughout the 3-T image, likely caused by B_1 inhomogeneity, as well as a large dark spot over the liver caused by RF shielding/standing wave effects (*white arrows, A*).

and contribute greater signal to the image than those that are mobile (nonrestricted). DWI typically uses an echo planar imaging readout in order to provide rapid data collection and motion insensitivity. It is used in oncology primarily based on the concept that malignant tumors tend to be highly cellular, and so they restrict diffusion to a greater degree than normal tissues.[38]

Because the basic pulse sequences for DWI are T_2 weighted, they are sensitive to the same artifacts, including standing wave and RF field inhomogeneity artifacts. In addition, because of their long echo trains and absence of refocusing pulses, DWI sequences are particularly sensitive to susceptibility, and signal loss near the lungs and gas-filled stomach and bowel is often observed. In addition, intrinsic tissue susceptibility can pose a challenge, particularly in the liver.

DWI is considered a key technique in prostate MR imaging, in which it can provide excellent depiction of peripheral zone malignancies. Prostate MR imaging can be challenging in general, because of the small size of the target organ and low achievable SNR, even with local endorectal coils. At 3 T, SNR improvements can be realized so that prostate imaging can be performed with an endorectal coil or with a phased array coil alone, whereas an endorectal coil is considered necessary at 1.5 T.[39] However, even at 3 T, the necessity of an endorectal coil remains controversial.[40] When using an endorectal coil, it can be useful to fill the coil's inflatable balloon with a material other than air (liquid perfluorocarbon or barium) in order to reduce susceptibility and distortion from gas within the balloon.[41]

T_2*-weighted Imaging and Quantification

T_2*-weighted imaging has some applications in abdominopelvic MR imaging, including detecting blood breakdown products as well as uptake of SPIOs in the liver and lymph nodes.[42–44] In general, these applications may benefit from stronger susceptibility effects at 3 T compared with 1.5 T, because strong signal suppression of iron-containing tissues is desired to generate image contrast. However, the SNR of iron-rich tissues may be so low that quantitative measures of T_2* become inaccurate. Therefore, in low-susceptibility situations, quantitative techniques may benefit from stronger susceptibility at high field strengths, but when high susceptibility is expected (for example liver iron quantification in patients with known iron overload) lower field strengths may be desirable. In addition, intravascular signal void artifacts related to susceptibility have been described when using SPIOs for intravascular T_1-weighted imaging.[45] However, it is not clear whether field strength plays an important role in that setting, because T_1-weighted sequences can be designed to be insensitive to susceptibility, and longer tissue T_1 times at high field strength improve contrast medium–related enhancement.

Special Considerations and Challenges for Abdominopelvic MR Imaging

The major advantages of 3-T MR imaging compared with 1.5 T in abdominopelvic MR imaging are in improved SNR, contrast enhancement, and shorter TEs in chemical shift–based imaging. However, RF inhomogeneity caused by dielectric/standing wave effects as well as increased SAR remain major challenges. RF inhomogeneity is particularly pronounced at T_2-weighted imaging and DWI, especially in 2 scenarios. First, MR imaging is frequently used for liver assessment in patients with cirrhosis. These patients also often have ascites, and small amounts of ascites can substantially degrade image quality, whereas large ascites can render MR images nondiagnostic. Second, as the population becomes more overweight and wide-bore imaging more prevalent, RF inhomogeneity effects become pronounced even in patients without ascites. Parallel transmit and RF shimming techniques are in development, which have the potential to substantially reduce these effects.[46-48]

CARDIOVASCULAR MR IMAGING AT 3 T

Cardiovascular magnetic resonance (CVMR) imaging has rapidly evolved as an imaging method of choice for the evaluation of cardiac structure and function in both adult and pediatric populations. In particular, CVMR is widely used for the assessment of myocardial viability, perfusion in ischemic heart disease, and characterization of nonischemic cardiomyopathies. The adoption of 3-T imaging systems for CVMR has been slower than in other areas because of a variety of challenges, including cardiac motion, the proximity of the heart to the lungs and diaphragm, field inhomogeneity, artifacts, longer T_1 relaxation times, and increased SAR. However, CVMR at 3 T also provides several advantages compared with lower field strengths, the most important being increased SNR and CNR, which provide improved spatial and/or temporal resolution. Theoretically, the gain in SNR from 1.5 T to 3 T is a factor of 2 but, as in other applications, the gain is variable and is sequence dependent.[49] Several specific applications are discussed later.

Cine Imaging of Cardiac Function

Cine steady-state free precession (SSFP) imaging is the cornerstone for evaluation of cardiac function, volumes, and myocardial mass.[50-54] At 3 T, high SNR and CNR provide excellent image contrast between the myocardium, blood pool, and fat, thus enabling accurate determination of epicardial and subendocardial borders.[55,56] The most commonly encountered artifact at 3 T with SSFP sequence is the dark band artifact caused by local field inhomogeneity (Fig. 5). Strategies to reduce or shift this artifact away from the imaging region of interest include reducing the TR, local shimming, and adjusting the RF frequency by using a frequency scout sequence.[57,58] Cine gradient echo imaging sequences used frequently in CVMR have also been shown to benefit from the increased CNR at 3 T.[56]

Myocardial Perfusion

Assessment of the extent and location of regional myocardial ischemia by perfusion CVMR is critical in the evaluation of coronary artery disease (CAD). Typically, a rapid multislice perfusion sequence is used to measure changes in myocardial signal intensity during the first pass of an intravenously administered contrast agent bolus. Several studies have shown the high diagnostic accuracy of perfusion CVMR in significant CAD.[59-62] Increased SNR at 3 T can also be exchanged for increased spatial or temporal resolution. In addition, prolonged T_1 relaxation times at 3 T translate into better contrast between perfused and nonperfused myocardium.[63] Several studies have verified an increase in CNR and SNR, and the overall exceptional image quality of perfusion CVMR at 3 T compared with 1.5 T.[55,64,65]

Late Gadolinium Enhancement

Late gadolinium enhancement (LGE) imaging is an important method for the detection of myocardial infarction and viability, and is performed using a T_1-weighted segmented inversion recovery gradient echo pulse sequence. Numerous publications have shown this technique's utility for localizing and quantifying the three-dimensional extent of acute and chronic myocardial infarction.[66-72] Because gadolinium-based contrast agents do not penetrate myocytes with intact membranes, there is little myocardial enhancement following contrast administration. Irreversibly injured myocardium tends to enhance to a greater degree, because of myocyte membrane breakdown and background fibrosis, if chronic. As a result, infarcted myocardium shows delayed wash-in and washout of contrast media and may show higher signal intensity at around 15 minutes after contrast administration, whereas normal myocardium appears dark.[67] The presence of myocardial scar by LGE is a strong predictor of major adverse cardiac outcomes.[73,74] At 3 T, the increase in SNR and CNR improves the delineation of the infarcted myocardial borders, and the longer myocardial T_1 relaxation time increases signal intensity differences between the normal and infarcted (enhanced) myocardium (Fig. 6). Alternatively, the stronger enhancement at 3 T can be used to reduce the dose of administered contrast agent.[75-79] Image acquisition should be triggered to every other cardiac cycle wherever possible at 3 T, in an effort to allow adequate relaxation of longitudinal magnetization between successive inversion pluses, and inversion time must be optimized for the longer T_1 relaxation times at 3 T.[78] The exceptional spatial resolution of CVMR aids in the detection of subendocardial infarcts that can be missed on single-photon emission computed tomography myocardial imaging.[80]

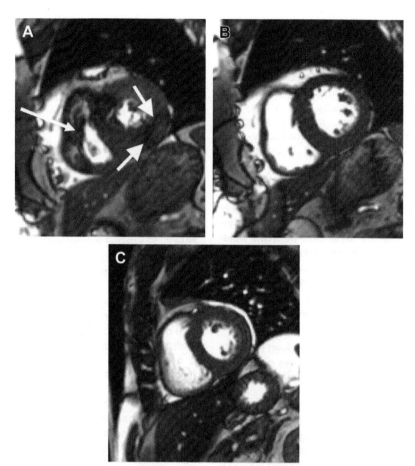

Fig. 5. SSFP images showing dark band artifacts at 3 T passing through the basal right ventricle (*small arrow*) and the inferolateral wall of the left ventricle (*large arrows*) (*A*). These dark bands are caused by center frequency offsets and magnetic field inhomogeneity. After local shimming, running a frequency scout sequence, and reducing TR, the dark band artifacts are confined to the anterior body wall (*B*). At 1.5 T, the cine SSFP sequence is less prone to these artifacts (*C*).

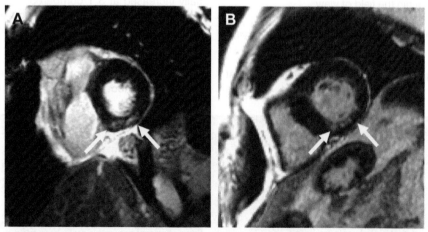

Fig. 6. T_1-weighted segmented inversion recovery gradient echo imaging for late gadolinium enhancement was performed in 2 patients with known history of CAD undergoing revascularization evaluation. Both images show infarcts (*white arrows*) in the inferior wall of the left ventricle (in the right coronary artery territory). Image (*A*) was acquired at 3 T and shows higher SNR and visual contrast enhancement compared with image (*B*), acquired at 1.5 T.

Other Cardiovascular Magnetic Resonance Applications

The increase in SNR and CNR combined with parallel imaging techniques at 3 T, compared with 1.5 T, has been shown to improve image quality for MR coronary angiography with whole-heart coverage.[81,82] In addition, myocardial tagging sequences that show regional contractility show longer tag line persistence at 3 T, because of longer T_1 relaxation times.[55]

The increase in SNR at 3 T also provides improvements in vascular imaging of the aorta, with increases in SNR as high as 50%, and increases in CNR up to 70%.[83] In addition, stronger chemical shift at 3 T increases the frequency separation between water and fat, which can be exploited to improve fat suppression when assessing myocardial fatty infiltration in arrhythmogenic right ventricular dysplasia.

Special Considerations and Challenges for Cardiovascular Magnetic Resonance

Several challenges remain to be resolved in CVMR at 3 T. First, RF field inhomogeneities can cause signal loss and image darkening, particularly in the right ventricular wall; parallel transmit technologies have been shown to reduce this artifact.[84] Ghost artifacts displaced at half the field of view may be accentuated at higher field strengths, particularly with LGE cardiac imaging. Parallel imaging techniques can reduce this type of artifact and additionally shorten acquisition time.[85] High SAR must be carefully managed by modulating pulse sequence flip angles and TRs, and parallel imaging techniques are again beneficial. Local shimming must be performed to reduce the effects of magnetic field inhomogeneity within the field of view.

BREAST MAGNETIC RESONANCE IMAGING AT 3 T

Ultrasonography and mammography are the most common diagnostic imaging tools for the detection of breast cancer but MR imaging has become increasingly important in the detection and delineation of breast cancer. MR imaging is used as an additional diagnostic tool for detection of breast cancer in extremely dense breast tissue, invasive components in ductal carcinoma in situ, occult primary breast cancer in patients presenting with metastatic disease, and multifocal/multicentric spread of invasive lobar carcinoma.[86–89] Malignant breast tumors have greater cellularity than benign lesions and restricted water diffusion, which can be detected by DWI. Several in vivo studies have shown improved characterization of breast lesions at 3 T compared with 1.5 T, using both contrast-enhanced MR imaging and DWI.[90–93] MRS of the breast, combined with DWI at 3 T, has also shown higher specificity and accuracy in differentiating benign from malignant tumors.[94]

Several challenges are frequently encountered in breast MR imaging at 3 T. Because of the small size of the breasts relative to the body and the air cleft between them, it can be difficult to achieve a homogeneous main magnetic field over the field of view. Particularly at 3 T, this can degrade fat suppression, which is essential for T_2-weighted imaging and dynamic contrast-enhanced imaging. The use of inversion recovery techniques and local shimming can be used to address this issue. In addition, B_1 inhomogeneity can cause spatially dependent variations in signal intensity and visible left-right breast asymmetry (**Fig. 7**). Both RF shimming and parallel transmit technology are emerging methods that can reduce the impact of B_1 inhomogeneity.[95] In addition, susceptibility artifacts are substantially increased at 3 T compared with 1.5 T, and in the breast are often seen arising from thoracic chemotherapy ports and surgical or biopsy clips (see **Fig. 7**). Using pulse sequences with short TEs can minimize image degradation, and inversion recovery and chemical shift–based fat suppression methods can be used to counteract

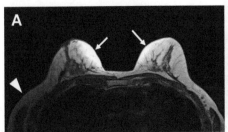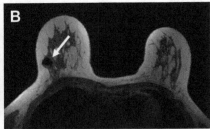

Fig. 7. T_1-weighted precontrast gradient echo images of the bilateral breasts obtained in 2 patients with a history of breast cancer. (A) There are several areas of artifactually increased (*arrows*) or decreased (*arrowhead*) signal in the fat of the second patient, caused by spatially dependent B_1 inhomogeneity. (B) There is substantial susceptibility artifact from a biopsy clip in the right breast of the first patient (*arrow*).

inhomogeneous fat suppression around regions of susceptibility.

Special Considerations and Challenges for Breast MR Imaging

Breast MR imaging at 3 T has become robust. Homogeneity of fat suppression is, under some circumstance, still inferior to 1.5 T; however, this is rarely of clinical significance. In addition, susceptibility-related image degradation from chemotherapy ports is stronger, but rarely significant when optimized protocols are used.

MUSCULOSKELETAL MR IMAGING AT 3 T

MR imaging is the imaging modality of choice for evaluating much of the musculoskeletal system, particularly for abnormalities of the ligaments, tendons, bone marrow, and joints.[96–99] As with other applications, the higher main magnetic field strength can provide increases in SNR and CNR, which can yield either improved SNR in the images or be traded to increase spatial resolution.[100,101]

However, increasing the field strength increases signal loss and distortion caused by susceptibility effects, which is a common problem when attempting to image near joint replacements, spinal fusions, or other metal implants. These challenges have been barriers to widespread adoption of higher field strengths in clinical musculoskeletal imaging practices. Optimized imaging protocols, using the FSE technique with long echo trains and high receiver bandwidths, can be used to mitigate these artifacts. In addition, new pulse sequences using view angle tilting methods and specialized acquisitions/reconstructions are becoming available to suppress metal-related artifacts.[102–104] As these technologies become widely available, 3-T MR imaging may become preferred to 1.5 T for the musculoskeletal system, particularly in SNR-challenged applications in which coils are distant from the target tissues, such as in high-resolution imaging of the hips.[105]

Special Considerations and Challenges for Musculoskeletal MR Imaging

Suppression of artifacts related to metal implants is the primary remaining challenge in musculoskeletal imaging at 3 T and is a major research focus. However, with the technological improvements currently available, the image quality attainable at 3 T is equivalent to or surpasses 1.5 T in many or most applications.

SUMMARY

There are benefits to performing clinical MR imaging studies at 3 T compared with 1.5 T for some applications. Improvements in both SNR and CNR can be used to improve image homogeneity and/or spatial and temporal resolution. Some techniques, such as brain fMR imaging, are considered far superior at 3 T than at 1.5 T. Although several challenges still exist, 3 T has been become well established in clinical MR imaging.

REFERENCES

1. Haacke MB, Thompson M, Venkatesan R. Magnetic resonance imaging: physical principals and sequence design. 1st edition. Hoboken, NJ: Wiley-Liss; 1999.
2. Bottomley PA, Foster TH, Argersinger RE, et al. A review of normal tissue hydrogen NMR relaxation times and relaxation mechanisms from 1-100 MHz: dependence on tissue type, NMR frequency, temperature, species, excision, and age. Med Phys 1984;11(4):425–48.
3. Schindera ST, Merkle EM, Dale BM, et al. Abdominal magnetic resonance imaging at 3.0 T what is the ultimate gain in signal-to-noise ratio? Acad Radiol 2006;13(10):1236–43.
4. Merkle EM, Dale BM, Paulson EK. Abdominal MR imaging at 3T. Magn Reson Imaging Clin N Am 2006;14(1):17–26.
5. Merkle EM, Dale BM, Barboriak DP. Gain in signal-to-noise for first-pass contrast-enhanced abdominal MR angiography at 3 Tesla over standard 1.5 Tesla: prediction with a computer model. Acad Radiol 2007;14(7):795–803.
6. Rohrer M, Bauer H, Mintorovitch J, et al. Comparison of magnetic properties of MRI contrast media solutions at different magnetic field strengths. Invest Radiol 2005;40(11):715–24.
7. Wolf RL, Detre JA. Clinical neuroimaging using arterial spin-labeled perfusion magnetic resonance imaging. Neurotherapeutics 2007;4(3):346–59.
8. Deibler AR, Pollock JM, Kraft RA, et al. Arterial spin-labeling in routine clinical practice, part 1: technique and artifacts. AJNR Am J Neuroradiol 2008;29(7):1228–34.
9. Ibrahim el SH. Myocardial tagging by cardiovascular magnetic resonance: evolution of techniques–pulse sequences, analysis algorithms, and applications. J Cardiovasc Magn Reson 2011;13:36.
10. Soher BJ, Dale BM, Merkle EM. A review of MR physics: 3T versus 1.5T. Magn Reson Imaging Clin N Am 2007;15(3):277–90, v.
11. Haacke MR. Susceptibility weighted imaging in MRI: basic concepts and clinical applications. Hoboken, NJ: John Wiley & Sons; 2011. p. 416.

12. Nitz WR, Schmeets S, Schoenberg S. Torque and attraction. Clinical 3T magnetic resonance. Stuttgart, Germany; 2007. p. 20–21.

13. Dempsey MF, Condon B, Hadley DM. Investigation of the factors responsible for burns during MRI. J Magn Reson Imaging 2001;13(4):627–31.

14. Neema M, Guss ZD, Stankiewicz JM, et al. Normal findings on brain fluid-attenuated inversion recovery MR images at 3T. AJNR Am J Neuroradiol 2009;30(5):911–6.

15. Nobauer-Huhmann IM, Ba-Ssalamah A, Mlynarik V, et al. Magnetic resonance imaging contrast enhancement of brain tumors at 3 tesla versus 1.5 tesla. Invest Radiol 2002;37(3):114–9.

16. Phal PM, Usmanov A, Nesbit GM, et al. Qualitative comparison of 3-T and 1.5-T MRI in the evaluation of epilepsy. AJR Am J Roentgenol 2008;191(3):890–5.

17. Stankiewicz JM, Glanz BI, Healy BC, et al. Brain MRI lesion load at 1.5T and 3T versus clinical status in multiple sclerosis. J Neuroimaging 2011;21(2):e50–6.

18. Wattjes MP, Lutterbey GG, Harzheim M, et al. Higher sensitivity in the detection of inflammatory brain lesions in patients with clinically isolated syndromes suggestive of multiple sclerosis using high field MRI: an intraindividual comparison of 1.5 T with 3.0 T. Eur Radiol 2006;16(9):2067–73.

19. Wardlaw JM, Brindle W, Casado AM, et al. A systematic review of the utility of 1.5 versus 3 Tesla magnetic resonance brain imaging in clinical practice and research. Eur Radiol 2012;22(11):2295–303.

20. Krasnow B, Tamm L, Greicius MD, et al. Comparison of fMRI activation at 3 and 1.5 T during perceptual, cognitive, and affective processing. Neuroimage 2003;18(4):813–26.

21. Yongbi MN, Fera F, Yang Y, et al. Pulsed arterial spin labeling: comparison of multisection baseline and functional MR imaging perfusion signal at 1.5 and 3.0 T: initial results in six subjects. Radiology 2002;222(2):569–75.

22. Bashir MR, Merkle EM, Smith AD, et al. Hepatic MR imaging for in vivo differentiation of steatosis, iron deposition and combined storage disorder: single-ratio in/opposed phase analysis vs. dual-ratio Dixon discrimination. Eur J Radiol 2012;81(2):e101–9.

23. Bashir MR, Zhong X, Dale BM, et al. Automated patient-tailored screening of the liver for diffuse steatosis and iron overload using MRI. AJR Am J Roentgenol 2013;201(3):583–8.

24. Zhong X, Nickel MD, Kannengiesser SA, et al. Liver fat quantification using a multi-step adaptive fitting approach with multi-echo GRE imaging. Magn Reson Med 2014;72(5):1353–65.

25. Yokoo T, Shiehmorteza M, Hamilton G, et al. Estimation of hepatic proton-density fat fraction by using MR imaging at 3.0 T. Radiology 2011;258(3):749–59.

26. Hines CD, Frydrychowicz A, Hamilton G, et al. T(1) independent, T(2) (*) corrected chemical shift based fat-water separation with multi-peak fat spectral modeling is an accurate and precise measure of hepatic steatosis. J Magn Reson Imaging 2011;33(4):873–81.

27. Bashir MR, Husarik DB, Ziemlewicz TJ, et al. Liver MRI in the hepatocyte phase with gadolinium-EOB-DTPA: does increasing the flip angle improve conspicuity and detection rate of hypointense lesions? J Magn Reson Imaging 2012;35(3):611–6.

28. Bashir MR, Merkle EM. Improved liver lesion conspicuity by increasing the flip angle during hepatocyte phase MR imaging. Eur Radiol 2011;21(2):291–4.

29. Sasaki M, Shibata E, Kanbara Y, et al. Enhancement effects and relaxivities of gadolinium-DTPA at 1.5 versus 3 Tesla: a phantom study. Magn Reson Med Sci 2005;4(3):145–9.

30. Takayama Y, Nishie A, Asayama Y, et al. Three-dimensional T2-weighted imaging for liver MRI: clinical values of tissue-specific variable refocusing flip-angle turbo spin echo imaging. J Magn Reson Imaging 2014. [Epub ahead of print].

31. Kim CY, Bashir MR, Heye T, et al. Respiratory-gated noncontrast SPACE MR angiography sequence at 3T for evaluation of the central veins of the chest: a feasibility study. J Magn Reson Imaging 2015;41:67–73.

32. Schick F. Whole-body MRI at high field: technical limits and clinical potential. Eur Radiol 2005;15(5):946–59.

33. Collins CM, Liu W, Schreiber W, et al. Central brightening due to constructive interference with, without, and despite dielectric resonance. J Magn Reson Imaging 2005;21(2):192–6.

34. Franklin KM, Dale BM, Merkle EM. Improvement in B1-inhomogeneity artifacts in the abdomen at 3T MR imaging using a radiofrequency cushion. J Magn Reson Imaging 2008;27(6):1443–7.

35. O'Regan DP, Fitzgerald J, Allsop J, et al. A comparison of MR cholangiopancreatography at 1.5 and 3.0 Tesla. Br J Radiol 2005;78(934):894–8.

36. Isoda H, Kataoka M, Maetani Y, et al. MRCP imaging at 3.0 T vs. 1.5 T: preliminary experience in healthy volunteers. J Magn Reson Imaging 2007;25(5):1000–6.

37. Schindera ST, Miller CM, Ho LM, et al. Magnetic resonance (MR) cholangiography: quantitative and qualitative comparison of 3.0 Tesla with 1.5 Tesla. Invest Radiol 2007;42(6):399–405.

38. Yu X, Lee EY, Lai V, et al. Correlation between tissue metabolism and cellularity assessed by standardized uptake value and apparent diffusion coefficient in peritoneal metastasis. J Magn Reson Imaging 2014;40(1):99–105.

39. Cornfeld DM, Weinreb JC. MR imaging of the prostate: 1.5T versus 3T. Magn Reson Imaging Clin North Am 2007;15(3):433–48, viii.

40. Turkbey B, Merino MJ, Gallardo EC, et al. Comparison of endorectal coil and nonendorectal coil T2W and diffusion-weighted MRI at 3 Tesla for localizing prostate cancer: correlation with whole-mount histopathology. J Magn Reson Imaging 2014;39(6):1443–8.

41. Rosen Y, Bloch BN, Lenkinski RE, et al. 3T MR of the prostate: reducing susceptibility gradients by inflating the endorectal coil with a barium sulfate suspension. Magn Reson Med 2007;57(5):898–904.

42. Aguirre DA, Behling CA, Alpert E, et al. Liver fibrosis: noninvasive diagnosis with double contrast material-enhanced MR imaging. Radiology 2006;239(2):425–37.

43. Motomura K, Izumi T, Tateishi S, et al. Correlation between the area of high-signal intensity on SPIO-enhanced MR imaging and the pathologic size of sentinel node metastases in breast cancer patients with positive sentinel nodes. BMC Med Imaging 2013;13:32.

44. Rockall AG, Sohaib SA, Harisinghani MG, et al. Diagnostic performance of nanoparticle-enhanced magnetic resonance imaging in the diagnosis of lymph node metastases in patients with endometrial and cervical cancer. J Clin Oncol 2005;23(12):2813–21.

45. Fananapazir G, Marin D, Suhocki PV, et al. Vascular artifact mimicking thrombosis on MR Imaging using ferumoxytol as a contrast agent in abdominal vascular assessment. J Vasc Interv Radiol 2014;25(6):969–76.

46. Sbrizzi A, Hoogduin H, Lagendijk JJ, et al. Fast design of local N-gram-specific absorption rate-optimized radiofrequency pulses for parallel transmit systems. Magn Reson Med 2012;67(3):824–34.

47. Truong TK, Darnell D, Song AW. Integrated RF/shim coil array for parallel reception and localized B shimming in the human brain. Neuroimage 2014;103C:235–40.

48. Nehrke K, Versluis MJ, Webb A, et al. Volumetric B1 (+) mapping of the brain at 7T using DREAM. Magn Reson Med 2014;71(1):246–56.

49. Fischbach F, Muller M, Bruhn H. Magnetic resonance imaging of the cranial nerves in the posterior fossa: a comparative study of t2-weighted spin-echo sequences at 1.5 and 3.0 tesla. Acta Radiol 2008;49(3):358–63.

50. Alfakih K, Plein S, Thiele H, et al. Normal human left and right ventricular dimensions for MRI as assessed by turbo gradient echo and steady-state free precession imaging sequences. J Magn Reson Imaging 2003;17(3):323–9.

51. Bellenger NG, Davies LC, Francis JM, et al. Reduction in sample size for studies of remodeling in heart failure by the use of cardiovascular magnetic resonance. J Cardiovasc Magn Reson 2000;2(4):271–8.

52. Grothues F, Moon JC, Bellenger NG, et al. Interstudy reproducibility of right ventricular volumes, function, and mass with cardiovascular magnetic resonance. Am Heart J 2004;147(2):218–23.

53. Grothues F, Smith GC, Moon JC, et al. Comparison of interstudy reproducibility of cardiovascular magnetic resonance with two-dimensional echocardiography in normal subjects and in patients with heart failure or left ventricular hypertrophy. Am J Cardiol 2002;90(1):29–34.

54. Lorenz CH, Walker ES, Morgan VL, et al. Normal human right and left ventricular mass, systolic function, and gender differences by cine magnetic resonance imaging. J Cardiovasc Magn Reson 1999;1(1):7–21.

55. Gutberlet M, Noeske R, Schwinge K, et al. Comprehensive cardiac magnetic resonance imaging at 3.0 Tesla: feasibility and implications for clinical applications. Invest Radiol 2006;41(2):154–67.

56. Tyler DJ, Hudsmith LE, Petersen SE, et al. Cardiac cine MR-imaging at 3T: FLASH vs SSFP. J Cardiovasc Magn Reson 2006;8(5):709–15.

57. Deshpande VS, Shea SM, Li D. Artifact reduction in true-FISP imaging of the coronary arteries by adjusting imaging frequency. Magn Reson Med 2003;49(5):803–9.

58. Schar M, Kozerke S, Fischer SE, et al. Cardiac SSFP imaging at 3 Tesla. Magn Reson Med 2004;51(4):799–806.

59. Giang TH, Nanz D, Coulden R, et al. Detection of coronary artery disease by magnetic resonance myocardial perfusion imaging with various contrast medium doses: first European multi-centre experience. Eur Heart J 2004;25(18):1657–65.

60. Klem I, Heitner JF, Shah DJ, et al. Improved detection of coronary artery disease by stress perfusion cardiovascular magnetic resonance with the use of delayed enhancement infarction imaging. J Am Coll Cardiol 2006;47(8):1630–8.

61. Nagel E, Klein C, Paetsch I, et al. Magnetic resonance perfusion measurements for the noninvasive detection of coronary artery disease. Circulation 2003;108(4):432–7.

62. Wolff SD, Schwitter J, Coulden R, et al. Myocardial first-pass perfusion magnetic resonance imaging: a multicenter dose-ranging study. Circulation 2004;110(6):732–7.

63. Fenchel M, Kramer U, Nael K, et al. Cardiac magnetic resonance imaging at 3.0 T. Top Magn Reson Imaging 2007;18(2):95–104.

64. Araoz PA, Glockner JF, McGee KP, et al. 3 Tesla MR imaging provides improved contrast in first-pass myocardial perfusion imaging over a range of gadolinium doses. J Cardiovasc Magn Reson 2005; 7(3):559–64.

65. Cheng AS, Pegg TJ, Karamitsos TD, et al. Cardiovascular magnetic resonance perfusion imaging at 3-tesla for the detection of coronary artery disease: a comparison with 1.5-tesla. J Am Coll Cardiol 2007;49(25):2440–9.

66. Choi KM, Kim RJ, Gubernikoff G, et al. Transmural extent of acute myocardial infarction predicts long-term improvement in contractile function. Circulation 2001;104(10):1101–7.

67. Kim RJ, Fieno DS, Parrish TB, et al. Relationship of MRI delayed contrast enhancement to irreversible injury, infarct age, and contractile function. Circulation 1999;100(19):1992–2002.

68. Kim RJ, Wu E, Rafael A, et al. The use of contrast-enhanced magnetic resonance imaging to identify reversible myocardial dysfunction. N Engl J Med 2000;343(20):1445–53.

69. Mahrholdt H, Wagner A, Holly TA, et al. Reproducibility of chronic infarct size measurement by contrast-enhanced magnetic resonance imaging. Circulation 2002;106(18):2322–7.

70. Mahrholdt H, Wagner A, Parker M, et al. Relationship of contractile function to transmural extent of infarction in patients with chronic coronary artery disease. J Am Coll Cardiol 2003;42(3):505–12.

71. Rehwald WG, Fieno DS, Chen EL, et al. Myocardial magnetic resonance imaging contrast agent concentrations after reversible and irreversible ischemic injury. Circulation 2002;105(2):224–9.

72. Wu E, Judd RM, Vargas JD, et al. Visualisation of presence, location, and transmural extent of healed Q-wave and non-Q-wave myocardial infarction. Lancet 2001;357(9249):21–8.

73. Kwong RY, Chan AK, Brown KA, et al. Impact of unrecognized myocardial scar detected by cardiac magnetic resonance imaging on event-free survival in patients presenting with signs or symptoms of coronary artery disease. Circulation 2006;113(23):2733–43.

74. Wu KC, Weiss RG, Thiemann DR, et al. Late gadolinium enhancement by cardiovascular magnetic resonance heralds an adverse prognosis in nonischemic cardiomyopathy. J Am Coll Cardiol 2008; 51(25):2414–21.

75. Cheng AS, Robson MD, Neubauer S, et al. Irreversible myocardial injury: assessment with cardiovascular delayed-enhancement MR imaging and comparison of 1.5 and 3.0 T–initial experience. Radiology 2007;242(3):735–42.

76. Cochet A, Lalande A, Walker PM, et al. Comparison of the extent of delayed-enhancement cardiac magnetic resonance imaging with and without phase-sensitive reconstruction at 3.0 T. Invest Radiol 2007;42(6):372–6.

77. Huber A, Bauner K, Wintersperger BJ, et al. Phase-sensitive inversion recovery (PSIR) single-shot TrueFISP for assessment of myocardial infarction at 3 tesla. Invest Radiol 2006;41(2):148–53.

78. Kim RJ, Shah DJ, Judd RM. How we perform delayed enhancement imaging. J Cardiovasc Magn Reson 2003;5(3):505–14.

79. Klumpp B, Fenchel M, Hoevelborn T, et al. Assessment of myocardial viability using delayed enhancement magnetic resonance imaging at 3.0 Tesla. Invest Radiol 2006;41(9):661–7.

80. Wagner A, Mahrholdt H, Holly TA, et al. Contrast-enhanced MRI and routine single photon emission computed tomography (SPECT) perfusion imaging for detection of subendocardial myocardial infarcts: an imaging study. Lancet 2003;361(9355):374–9.

81. Bi X, Li D. Coronary arteries at 3.0 T: contrast-enhanced magnetization-prepared three-dimensional breathhold MR angiography. J Magn Reson Imaging 2005;21(2):133–9.

82. Huber ME, Kozerke S, Pruessmann KP, et al. Sensitivity-encoded coronary MRA at 3T. Magn Reson Med 2004;52(2):221–7.

83. Maroules CD, McColl R, Khera A, et al. Assessment and reproducibility of aortic atherosclerosis magnetic resonance imaging: impact of 3-Tesla field strength and parallel imaging. Invest Radiol 2008;43(9):656–62.

84. Jia H, Wang C, Wang G, et al. Impact of 3.0 T cardiac MR imaging using dual-source parallel radiofrequency transmission with patient-adaptive B1 shimming. PloS One 2013;8(6):e66946.

85. Griswold MA, Jakob PM, Heidemann RM, et al. Generalized autocalibrating partially parallel acquisitions (GRAPPA). Magn Reson Med 2002;47(6): 1202–10.

86. Brem RF, Hoffmeister JW, Rapelyea JA, et al. Impact of breast density on computer-aided detection for breast cancer. AJR Am J Roentgenol 2005; 184(2):439–44.

87. Hwang ES, Kinkel K, Esserman LJ, et al. Magnetic resonance imaging in patients diagnosed with ductal carcinoma-in-situ: value in the diagnosis of residual disease, occult invasion, and multicentricity. Ann Surg Oncol 2003;10(4):381–8.

88. Mandelson MT, Oestreicher N, Porter PL, et al. Breast density as a predictor of mammographic detection: comparison of interval- and screen-detected cancers. J Natl Cancer Inst 2000; 92(13):1081–7.

89. Mann RM, Hoogeveen YL, Blickman JG, et al. MRI compared to conventional diagnostic work-up in

the detection and evaluation of invasive lobular carcinoma of the breast: a review of existing literature. Breast Cancer Res Treat 2008;107(1):1–14.

90. Chen X, Li WL, Zhang YL, et al. Meta-analysis of quantitative diffusion-weighted MR imaging in the differential diagnosis of breast lesions. BMC Cancer 2010;10:693.

91. Marini C, Iacconi C, Giannelli M, et al. Quantitative diffusion-weighted MR imaging in the differential diagnosis of breast lesion. Eur Radiol 2007; 17(10):2646–55.

92. Partridge SC, DeMartini WB, Kurland BF, et al. Quantitative diffusion-weighted imaging as an adjunct to conventional breast MRI for improved positive predictive value. AJR Am J Roentgenol 2009;193(6):1716–22.

93. Tan SL, Rahmat K, Rozalli FI, et al. Differentiation between benign and malignant breast lesions using quantitative diffusion-weighted sequence on 3 T MRI. Clin Radiol 2014;69(1):63–71.

94. Tsougos I, Svolos P, Kousi E, et al. The contribution of diffusion tensor imaging and magnetic resonance spectroscopy for the differentiation of breast lesions at 3T. Acta Radiol 2014;55(1):14–23.

95. Winkler SA, Rutt BK. Practical methods for improving B1+ homogeneity in 3 tesla breast imaging. J Magn Reson Imaging 2014. [Epub ahead of print].

96. Braun HJ, Dragoo JL, Hargreaves BA, et al. Application of advanced magnetic resonance imaging techniques in evaluation of the lower extremity. Radiol Clin North Am 2013;51(3):529–45.

97. Jain NB, Collins J, Newman JS, et al. Reliability of magnetic resonance imaging assessment of rotator cuff: the ROW study. PM R 2014. [Epub ahead of print].

98. Arkun R, Argin M. Pitfalls in MR imaging of musculoskeletal tumors. Semin Musculoskelet Radiol 2014;18(1):63–78.

99. Viana SL, Machado BB, Mendlovitz PS. MRI of subchondral fractures: a review. Skeletal Radiol 2014; 43(11):1515–27.

100. Masi JN, Sell CA, Phan C, et al. Cartilage MR imaging at 3.0 versus that at 1.5 T: preliminary results in a porcine model. Radiology 2005;236(1):140–50.

101. Link TM, Sell CA, Masi JN, et al. 3.0 vs 1.5 T MRI in the detection of focal cartilage pathology–ROC analysis in an experimental model. Osteoarthritis Cartilage 2006;14(1):63–70.

102. Lu W, Pauly KB, Gold GE, et al. SEMAC: slice encoding for metal artifact correction in MRI. Magn Reson Med 2009;62(1):66–76.

103. Koch KM, Brau AC, Chen W, et al. Imaging near metal with a MAVRIC-SEMAC hybrid. Magn Reson Med 2011;65(1):71–82.

104. Hayter CL, Koff MF, Shah P, et al. MRI after arthroplasty: comparison of MAVRIC and conventional fast spin-echo techniques. AJR Am J Roentgenol 2011;197(3):W405–11.

105. Carballido-Gamio J, Link TM, Li X, et al. Feasibility and reproducibility of relaxometry, morphometric, and geometrical measurements of the hip joint with magnetic resonance imaging at 3T. J Magn Reson Imaging 2008;28(1):227–35.

Noncontrast Magnetic Resonance Angiography

Concepts and Clinical Applications

Ruth P. Lim, MBBS, MMed, MS, FRANZCR[a,b,*], Ioannis Koktzoglou, PhD[c,d]

KEYWORDS

- MR angiography • Noncontrast • Nephrogenic systemic fibrosis • Fast spin echo
- Balanced steady-state free precession • Arterial spin labeling • Time of flight • Phase contrast

KEY POINTS

- Noncontrast magnetic resonance angiography (NC-MRA) techniques offer safe, noninvasive imaging, which is of particular importance in patients with impaired renal function, or in whom intravenous access is challenging.
- NC-MRA techniques are classified into 3 main categories, which obtain arterial signal from (1) flow-related enhancement, (2) the phase of magnetic resonance (MR) imaging signal from moving blood, and (3) the MR imaging physical properties of blood, independent of blood flow.
- Selection of the appropriate NC-MRA technique depends on the properties of the vascular bed of interest, the disorder being studied, and an understanding of each technique's specific strengths and weaknesses.

 Video of respiratory navigator inflow inversion recovery magnetic resonance angiography accompanies this article at http://www.radiologic.theclinics.com.

INTRODUCTION

Magnetic resonance (MR) angiography (MRA) is commonly used clinically, allowing noninvasive, accurate, and comprehensive vascular assessment from head to foot, without ionizing radiation. T1-weighted contrast-enhanced MRA (CE-MRA) performed with a gadolinium chelate[1] is the mainstay of thoracoabdominal and peripheral MRA, with large coverage, high spatial resolution, and rapid acquisition. Time of flight (TOF) MRA and phase contrast (PC) MRA are common noncontrast MRA (NC-MRA) techniques used in neurovascular imaging. However, NC-MRA has not historically been widely used in other vascular beds.

With gadolinium identified in 2006 as a potential causative factor in nephrogenic systemic fibrosis (NSF),[2] multiple NC-MRA techniques have been developed. Contrast dose minimization and restrictions on the use of less stable agents in vulnerable patients[3] have decreased NSF incidence. However, NC-MRA techniques avoid all contrast risks, offering a safe alternative in pregnant patients, or in patients in whom intravenous access

Disclosures: Royal Australian and New Zealand College of Radiology research grant, Diabetes Australia research trust grant, Austin Medical Research Foundation grant (R.P. Lim). American Heart Association grant-in-aid (12GRNT12080013), research support from Siemens Healthcare (I. Koktzoglou).
[a] Department of Radiology, Austin Health, 145 Studley Road, Heidelberg, Victoria 3084, Australia; [b] Departments of Radiology and Surgery, Faculty of Medicine, Dentistry and Health Sciences, The University of Melbourne, Parkville, Victoria 3010, Australia; [c] Department of Radiology, NorthShore University HealthSystem, Walgreen Jr. Building, G507, 2650 Ridge Avenue, Evanston, IL 60201, USA; [d] Department of Radiology, The University of Chicago Pritzker School of Medicine, 5841 South Maryland Avenue, Chicago, IL 60637, USA
* Corresponding author. Austin Health, 145 Studley Road, Heidelberg, Victoria 3084, Australia.
E-mail address: ruthplim74@gmail.com

Radiol Clin N Am 53 (2015) 457–476
http://dx.doi.org/10.1016/j.rcl.2014.12.003

cannot be obtained. NC-MRA is also desirable for economic reasons, because gadolinium can add substantially to MR imaging costs in certain countries. The main challenges of NC-MRA are long acquisition time and concerns about technique robustness.

This article reviews basic properties of blood as background to selection and implementation of NC-MRA techniques. Commercially available and upcoming techniques are reviewed, with a summary of existing clinical experience, providing a framework for their incorporation into clinical practice.

PROPERTIES OF BLOOD
T1 and T2 Relaxation Properties

The longitudinal (T1) and spin-spin (T2) relaxation times of blood profoundly influence the MR imaging techniques used to perform noncontrast MRA. The T1 of blood depends on the main magnetic field strength (B0) and is approximately 1200 milliseconds at 1.5 T[4] and 1600 milliseconds at 3.0 T.[5] The T2 of blood depends on its oxygenation level and is approximately 250 milliseconds for well-oxygenated arterial blood. Deoxygenated, venous blood can have a T2 as low as 100 milliseconds.

Blood Flow

Vascular resistance (primarily influenced by vessel caliber), and the pressure gradient between proximal and distal ends of the vessel determine flow, defined as volume per unit time.[6] In normal large vessels, blood flow is laminar, with a parabolic profile such that the fastest velocity is present centrally within the lumen. Other flow variations include plug flow at the origins of visceral vessels, with constant blood flow across the entire luminal diameter; flow separation at vessel bifurcations leading to formation of vortices; and turbulent flow, where flow is chaotic, as seen in diseased vessels just beyond sites of stenosis. With turbulent flow and vortices, there is variation in speed and direction of flow, with potential signal nulling from phase dispersion of blood spins.[7] In arteries, flow is pulsatile, because of their elasticity and high resistance of downstream arterioles. Approximately one-third of arterial blood flow is transmitted during systole and two-thirds during diastole.[6] Vascular resistance affects arterial waveforms across the body, with persistent forward flow in diastole in low-resistance vascular beds such as the internal carotid and renal arteries. In peripheral arteries where vascular resistance is high, a triphasic waveform with flow reversal is present (**Fig. 1**). Venous flow is lower[8] and more constant, only fluctuating with changes in intrathoracic pressure during respiration.

Velocity, distance per unit time, is an important component of flow. Peak systolic velocity (PSV),

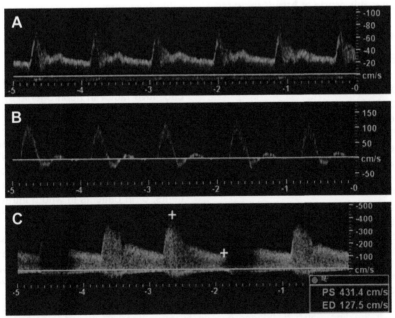

Fig. 1. Duplex Doppler ultrasonography waveforms of (*A*) normal internal carotid artery (ICA), with persistent forward flow throughout the cardiac cycle; (*B*) normal common femoral artery with triphasic waveform, including late systolic flow reversal and forward flow in early diastole; and (*C*) severe (70%–79% by Doppler criteria) ICA stenosis, with increased peak systolic (PS) and end-diastolic (ED) velocities, and spectral broadening indicating turbulent flow.

maximal blood velocity during the cardiac cycle, is variable, with higher PSV in central systemic arteries (approximately 1 m/s in the normal aorta and carotid arteries); 0.3 to 0.6 m/s in the main pulmonary artery[7]; and lower PSV distally, with velocities of 10 to 20 cm/s in normal infragenual arteries.[9] Temporal delay between cardiac systole and arterial PSV increases with increasing distance from the heart, with normal delays of approximately 150 to 200 milliseconds.[10]

Magnitude and direction of blood flow may be affected in disease. With hemodynamically significant stenosis, markedly increased velocities and turbulent flow may result (see Fig. 1C), or substantially decreased velocities with near occlusion. Turbulent and slow flow is observed within aneurysms or the false lumen in arterial dissection. In arteriovenous malformations and fistulas, low resistance and increased flow can occur in feeding arteries, with arterialization of draining veins.[11]

NONCONTRAST MAGNETIC RESONANCE ANGIOGRAPHY TECHNIQUES

NC-MRA can be performed using several techniques. These techniques can be categorized into approaches that exploit flow-related enhancement, the phase of MR imaging signal from moving blood, and those that exploit the MR imaging physical properties of blood, independent of blood flow, as summarized in Table 1.

Flow-related Enhancement

The quintessential NC-MRA technique that depends on flow-related enhancement is TOF angiography. TOF is performed by applying a gradient-echo sequence with repetitive radiofrequency (RF) pulses to a slice or slab perpendicular to the vascular structures under interrogation. Repeated application of RF pulses saturates the MR imaging signal of stationary background tissue and highlights vascular structures containing blood flowing into the slice or slab (Fig. 2A). TOF MRA can be performed using two-dimensional (2D) or three-dimensional (3D) gradient-echo sequences; Fig. 2B shows the general image appearance for 2D and 3D TOF. Saturation RF pulses are applied downstream of the slice or slab to suppress the appearance of inflowing venous spins. Examples of neurovascular TOF angiograms are shown in Fig. 3.

With TOF MRA, arterial contrast depends on the T1s of arterial blood and background tissue, the RF spacing and flip angle of the gradient-echo sequence, and the velocity of inflowing blood.[12] To better visualize distal vascular anatomy and

maintain more uniform vascular signal throughout the 3D TOF slab thickness, tilt-optimized nonsaturating RF pulses may be used.[13] These specialized RF pulses apply larger flip angles at downstream locations within the slab. With 3D TOF, multiple overlapping thin slabs are acquired to reduce inflow requirements and artifacts at slab boundaries.[14]

Compared with 3D TOF, 2D TOF reduces inflow requirements for optimizing arterial opacification. Nonetheless, 3D TOF can provide submillimeter slice resolution, which is not possible with 2D TOF. Because of the longer T1s, TOF at 3.0 T provides better background tissue suppression than at 1.5 T.[15] Arterial contrast may also be improved with the addition of magnetization transfer contrast.[16,17]

Advantages of TOF include widespread availability on clinical MR imaging systems, simplicity of execution, and image quality for displaying arteries with brisk, continuous, unidirectional flow. Drawbacks of TOF include long acquisition times and suboptimal display of vessels containing slow or highly pulsatile flow. Additional limitations include poor display of tortuous vessels and vessels with in-plane flow, artifacts from respiratory motion and arterial pulsation, and signal loss at severe stenoses.[18]

Inflow and Outflow Techniques

Inflow inversion-recovery magnetic resonance angiography

Inflow inversion recovery (IFIR) is a technique that images the inflow of fully magnetized arterial spins while stationary background tissues have been suppressed by an inversion RF pulse.[19,20] Fig. 4 shows 2 timing diagrams for the IFIR sequence and an image obtained with the technique. The IFIR method applies a slab-selective inversion pulse followed by an inflow time (TI) of several hundred milliseconds. The TI is chosen to provide adequate inflow into the target vascular anatomy and a sufficient degree of background suppression. Imaging then occurs using a rapid readout. Fat is suppressed by chemical shift-selective fat saturation, short-tau inversion recovery, or water-excitation RF pulses. Trade names for IFIR include TimeSLIP, NATIVE TrueFISP, Inhance Inflow IR, and B-TRANCE.

Because angiographic contrast depends on inflow, the IFIR technique performs best for imaging vascular beds containing brisk flow. The imaging readout is either balanced steady-state free precession (bSSFP) or flow-compensated fast spin echo (FSE) to maintain high signal from flowing spins. Inflow requirements are minimized by

Table 1
Summary of noncontrast MRA techniques

Category	MRA Technique	Advantages	Disadvantages	Clinical Applications
Flow-related enhancement	TOF	Widely available Easy to perform	Limited coverage Arterial saturation of slow/in-plane flow T1 hyperintense lesions mimic flow	Neurovascular imaging, especially 3T
	IFIR	Easy to perform Good arterial to background contrast	Decreased coverage with slow flow, low cardiac output	Fast-flow vascular beds; eg, renal and hepatic arteries
	QISS	Robust (arrhythmias, motion) Easy to perform Sensitive to slow flow	Inhomogeneous fat suppression Saturation of in-plane vessels, retrograde flow	Extremity imaging, especially lower extremity MRA
	ASL	Complete suppression of background signal	Long acquisition time Motion sensitive Decreased coverage with slow flow	Neurovascular imaging
Phase dependent	ECG-gated subtractive	Complete suppression of background signal Can tailor to speed of flow in area of interest	Long acquisition time Motion sensitive Challenging to perform (appropriate flow spoiling)	Extremity imaging, including hand and foot MRA
	PC	Flow quantification Complete suppression of background signal with noise masking	Long acquisition times	Neurovascular imaging
Flow independent	bSSFP ± T2 preparation/fat suppression	High arterial signal Fast Readily available	Fat, nonvascular fluid ± veins not suppressed B_0 heterogeneity	Coronary imaging Aortic imaging
	Subtraction-based flow independent	Excellent suppression of background signal	Long acquisition times Sensitive to motion	Extremity and neurovascular imaging including venography

Abbreviations: ASL, arterial spin labeled; bSSFP, balanced steady-state free precession; ECG, electrocardiogram; IFIR, inflow inversion recovery; QISS, quiescent interval single shot.

positioning the upstream edge of the inversion pulse close to the arterial bed under interrogation. Prospective navigator or bellows gating is used to compensate for respiratory motion.

Variations of IFIR first apply a nonselective inversion RF pulse and then a slice-selective inversion pulse to the inflowing blood pool before its entry into the target anatomy. This approach is referred to as outflow MRA. Compared with inflow MRA, outflow MRA can improve the degree of background signal suppression and image quality in some applications.[21] The main strengths of IFIR are its ease of execution and image quality, especially for depicting the renal arteries. The main drawback of IFIR is poor display of vessels containing slow flow.

Quiescent interval single-shot magnetic resonance angiography

Quiescent-inflow single-shot (QISS) angiography is a MRA technique introduced for imaging lower

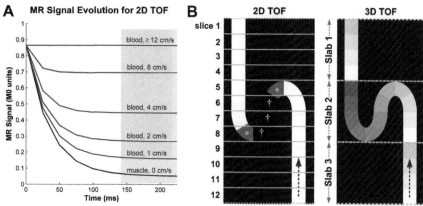

Fig. 2. (*A*) MR imaging signal evolution for two-dimensional (2D) TOF angiography (3-mm slice thickness, 60° flip angle). Application of RF pulses every 25 milliseconds rapidly saturates stationary background tissue, resulting in flow-related enhancement of blood. Maximal signal from inflowing blood occurs for velocities greater than or equal to 12 cm/s, when there is complete replenishment of flow every 25 milliseconds. The shaded region highlights the steady-state signals, which determine image contrast. (*B*) MR signal appearance for 2D and 3D TOF. Dashed horizontal lines show slice/slab boundaries. With 2D TOF, saturation of in-plane (*asterisk*) and retrograde (*daggers*) flow is seen because of the imaging and tracking venous saturation RF pulses. Flow with three-dimensional (3D) TOF is progressively saturated as it flows into the slab.

extremity arteries.[22] As shown in **Fig. 5**, QISS applies (1) an in-plane RF saturation pulse to suppress static tissue; (2) a tracking venous saturation RF pulse to suppress venous signal; (3) a waiting period (or quiescent interval) of ~230 milliseconds to ensure arterial inflow into the imaging slice; (4) chemical shift-selective fat saturation; and (5) a single-shot Cartesian 2D bSSFP readout. ECG gating ensures that the quiescent interval overlaps systole with data acquired in diastole. One slice is acquired every heartbeat. Using 3-mm slices, a peripheral arterial examination from the abdomen to the feet can be completed in less than 10 minutes.

A version of QISS using a highly undersampled radial k-space trajectory can be used to acquire multiple slices within a single heartbeat, shortening scan times by a factor of 2 to 3 (see **Fig. 5**D).[23] Compared with single-slice QISS, the

thickness of the in-plane saturation RF pulse is increased to span all slices that are acquired in each heartbeat. Fat saturation is applied before the bSSFP readout for each acquired slice.

Strengths of QISS MRA include imaging speed and ease of use, with no sequence tailoring required, and the ability to depict slow flow. Drawbacks include suboptimal display of flow parallel to the imaging slice and poor display of retrograde flow. Partial volume averaging in the slice direction can be overcome by acquiring thinner slices, at the expense of acquisition time.

Arterial spin labeled magnetic resonance angiography

Arterial spin labeling (ASL) techniques acquire 2 image sets, which are later subtracted. The 2 image sets are almost identical; they differ only in

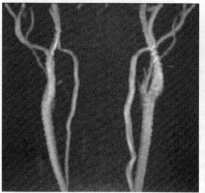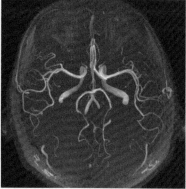

Fig. 3. (*Left*) 2D TOF coronal maximum intensity projection (MIP) depicting the carotid and vertebral arteries. (*Right*) 3D TOF axial MIP displaying the intracranial arteries.

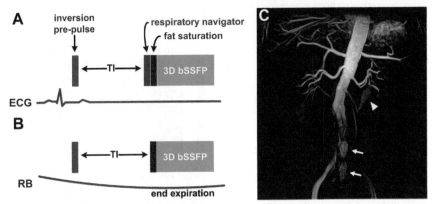

Fig. 4. Timing diagrams for IFIR renal MRA acquired using (*A*) electrocardiogram (ECG) gating and (*B*) respiratory bellows (RB) gating. (*C*) IFIR image of the aorta and renal arteries acquired with the pulse sequence in (*B*). Note visualisation of urine in the left renal pelvis (*arrowhead*) and cerebrospinal fluid (*arrows*) due to their long T1 relaxation times. (*Adapted from* Shonai T, Takahashi T, Ikeguchi H, et al. Improved arterial visibility using short-tau inversion-recovery (STIR) fat suppression in non-contrast-enhanced time-spatial labeling inversion pulse (Time-SLIP) renal MR angiography (MRA). J Magn Reson Imaging 2009;29:1476; with permission from John Wiley and Sons.)

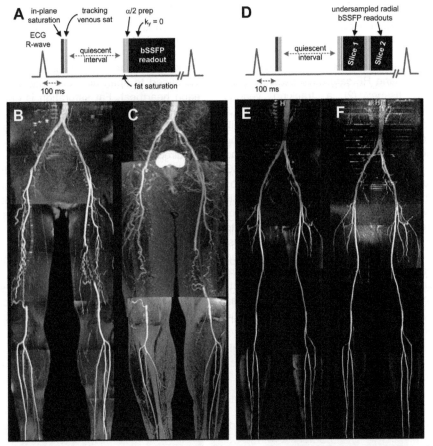

Fig. 5. QISS MRA. (*A*) Pulse sequence timing diagram for single-slice Cartesian QISS. (*B*) QISS angiogram of a patient with peripheral arterial disease; excellent correlation with (*C*) CE-MRA is observed. (*D*) Timing diagram for 2-slice QISS using an undersampled radial k-space trajectory. Comparison of (*E*) single-slice radial QISS (scan time 4.8 minutes) and (*F*) 2-slice radial QISS (scan time 2.4 minutes). (*From* Edelman RR, Sheehan JJ, Dunkle E, et al. Quiescent-interval single-shot unenhanced magnetic resonance angiography of peripheral vascular disease: Technical considerations and clinical feasibility. Magn Reson Med 2010;63(4):957, with permission from John Wiley and Sons; and Edelman RR, Giri S, Dunkle E, et al. Quiescent-inflow single-shot magnetic resonance angiography using a highly undersampled radial k-space trajectory. Magn Reson Med 2013;70(6):1664, with permission from John Wiley and Sons.)

the magnetization of inflowing arterial spins. This difference in arterial magnetization is imparted by a process known as labeling. Subtraction of the 2 image sets displays the labeled arterial inflow and suppresses background signal.

Labeling of arterial spins during ASL MRA is usually accomplished by applying inversion RF pulses. This variation of ASL, referred to as pulsed ASL, applies an inversion RF pulse to arterial spins flowing into the target vasculature, followed by a TI time to accommodate inflow, and an imaging readout. The difference between this data set and its counterpart acquired without the labeling RF pulse depicts the labeled arterial anatomy. Diagrams for 2 pulsed ASL approaches, signal targeting with alternating RF (STAR)[24] and flow-alternating inversion recovery (FAIR),[25] are shown in **Fig. 6**A and B.

Other ASL techniques apply a quasicontinuous or pseudocontinuous stream of RF energy to label arterial spins flowing through a thin (~1 cm thick)

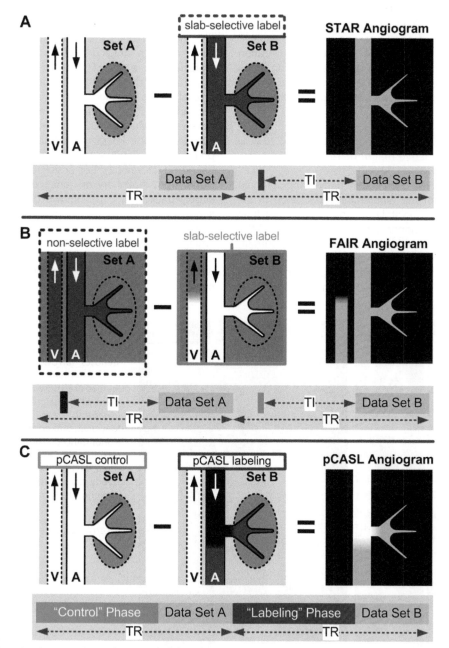

Fig. 6. Three implementations of ASL MRA: (*A*) STAR ASL MRA, (*B*) FAIR ASL MRA, and (*C*) pseudocontinuous ASL (pCASL) MRA. A, artery; TR, repetition time; V, vein.

labeling plane.[26] An implementation of pseudo-continuous ASL (pCASL) is shown in **Fig. 6C.** Compared with pulsed techniques, pCASL can improve the signal/noise ratio (SNR) of vessels near the labeling plane where short inversion times are realized.[27] Pseudocontinuous and pulsed ASL methods may be combined to improve SNR and vascular coverage.[28,29]

High arterial contrast and complete elimination of background signal are the main strengths of ASL MRA. **Fig. 7** shows angiograms obtained with ASL MRA. Extended, multiphase readouts can also be used in conjunction with ASL to display the temporal passage of arterial spins.[30] Drawbacks of ASL MRA include misregistration artifact from subtraction, lengthened scan times caused by acquisition of 2 data sets, and limited anatomic coverage when imaging slow flow.

Subtractive, Phase-dependent Techniques

Gated subtractive magnetic resonance angiography

Other NC-MRA techniques derive angiographic contrast from the differential appearance of arteries between systole and diastole.[31] Fast flow during systole dephases arterial spins during the echo train and renders arteries dark. In contrast, arterial signal is preserved when imaging slow flow in diastole. Subtraction displays the arterial anatomy (**Fig. 8**). The flow sensitivity of these techniques, which use FSE readouts, can be controlled by the length of the echo train, the flip angle of the refocusing RF pulses, supplementary gradient lobes for flow compensation or spoiling, and the orientation of the frequency-encoding axis.[32,33] Commercially available gated subtraction techniques include fresh blood imaging, Non Contrast MRA of ArTerIes and Veins (NATIVE), Sampling Perfection with Application optimized Contrast using different flip angle Evolutions (SPACE), Inhance DeltaFlow, and Triggered Angiography Non-Contrast Enhanced (TRANCE).

With FSE-based gated subtraction MRA, dephasing of arterial spins during systole is accomplished by the imaging readout. However, when imaging with a bSSFP readout that preserves signal from flowing arterial blood, dephasing of arterial spins during systole is achieved by applying a flow-suppressing motion-sensitized driven equilibrium (MSDE) magnetization preparation before the imaging readout. These MSDE preparations spoil signal from arterial blood based on its velocity[34] or acceleration,[35] leaving signal from stationary or nonaccelerating tissue largely unaltered. **Fig. 9** shows one such pulse sequence and associated magnetization preparations. The degree of flow spoiling depends on the timing, strength, and duration of the gradient lobes applied within the MSDE preparation, and when the preparation is applied within the cardiac cycle.

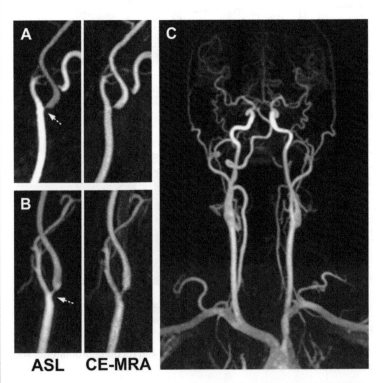

Fig. 7. (A, B) Oblique sagittal ASL MIP angiograms of 2 patients with severe carotid arterial stenoses (arrows); corresponding contrast-enhanced MRA (CE-MRA) images are shown. (C) ASL angiogram of the supra-aortic arteries. (Adapted from Koktzoglou I, Meyer JR, Ankenbrandt WJ, et al. Nonenhanced arterial spin labeled carotid MR angiography using three-dimensional radial balanced steady-state free precession imaging. J Magn Reson Imaging 2014. http://dx.doi.org/10.1002/jmri.24640; with permission of John Wiley and Sons.)

ASL   CE-MRA

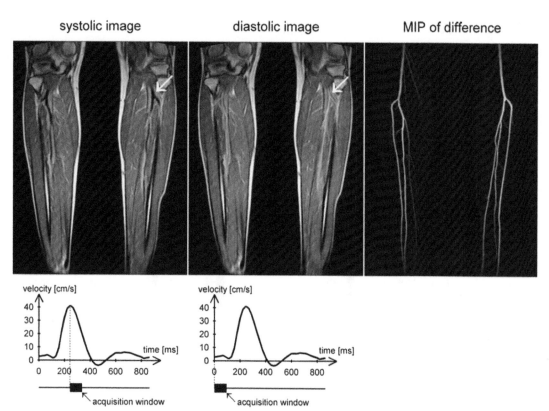

Fig. 8. Gated subtractive FSE-MRA of the calf. Imaging in systole and diastole suppresses and retains arterial signal (*arrows*), respectively. The difference between the two acquisitions yields an angiogram. (*From* Storey P, Atanasova IP, Lim RP, et al. Tailoring the flow sensitivity of fast spin-echo sequences for noncontrast peripheral MR angiography. Magn Reson Med 2010;64(4):1100; with permission from John Wiley and Sons.)

The strength of gated subtractive MRA is the complete suppression of nonvascular background signals. Drawbacks include misregistration artifact from patient motion, operator involvement to synchronize the acquisition to phases of maximal and minimal flow and tune the degree of flow spoiling (ie, to optimize arterial dephasing and minimize venous contamination), and poor display of arteries with slow flow and diminished pulsatility.

Phase contrast magnetic resonance angiography

PC MRA leverages the phase of the MR imaging signal for NC-MRA. In PC MRA, bipolar magnetic field gradients are added to a gradient-echo pulse sequence so that the phase of the MR imaging signal is proportional to the velocity of flowing blood. This flow-encoded data set is then contrasted with a flow-compensated reference data set acquired without bipolar gradients. The difference in the phase of the MR imaging signal between these two data sets yields the flow velocity in the direction of the applied bipolar gradients.

One approach used to generate a 3D PC MR angiogram is shown in **Fig. 10**.[36,37] Flow-encoded data are acquired along 3 orthogonal axes. The complex differences between these data sets and a flow-compensated reference set are then computed. Square-root sum-of-squares combinations of the difference data and application of noise mask (to suppress arbitrary phase values in regions of low SNR) produce the PC angiogram.

Advantages of PC MRA include the ability to quantify arterial flow velocity, and good suppression of nonflowing background signal with the use of noise masking. The emerging technique of four-dimensional PC can display and quantify the velocity of blood flow in 3 spatial dimensions over the cardiac cycle.[38] The main drawback of PC MRA is the long scan time needed to acquire multiple image sets. An important consideration when using PC MRA is the selection of a velocity-encoding sensitivity (VENC) that avoids phase aliasing and maximizes velocity/noise ratio (VNR). A VENC that is too low results in phase aliasing, with regions of high velocity mimicking those of low velocity. In contrast, a VENC that is too high reduces the VNR of slower flow. Other pitfalls of PC MRA include phase imperfections

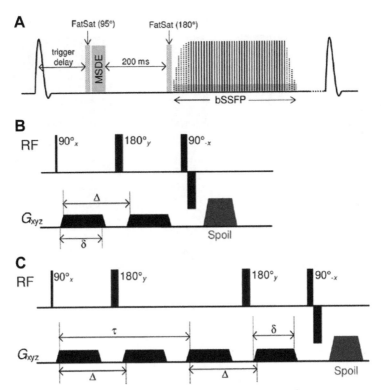

Fig. 9. (*A*) Pulse sequence diagram for gated subtractive bSSFP-based MRA. Arterial flow is dephased in systole during the application of the flow-suppressing MSDE preparation, and bSSFP imaging occurs in diastole. The scan is acquired twice, with gradients in the MSDE preparation turned on (dark artery image) and off (bright artery image). The difference between image sets produces an angiogram. RF and gradient activity for MSDE preparations that dephase arterial flow are based on (*B*) velocity and (*C*) acceleration. (*Reprinted from* Priest AN, Taviani V, Graves MJ, et al. Improved artery-vein separation with acceleration-dependent preparation for non-contrast-enhanced magnetic resonance angiography. Magn Reson Med 2013;72:700; with permission from John Wiley and Sons.)

caused by eddy currents, concomitant gradients, and spatially varying background phase offsets.[39]

Flow-independent Methods

Flow-independent methods derive angiographic contrast by exploiting the T1 and T2 properties of the blood pool. Early reports of flow-independent MRA used spin-echo and gradient-echo readouts.[40,41] However, bSSFP is the prevailing contemporary readout for flow-independent MRA because of its widespread availability, speed, and SNR efficiency for displaying arterial blood. Drawbacks of bSSFP-based MRA include high signal from fat and fluids, which preclude routine use of standard maximum intensity projection (MIP) processing, and dark band artifacts from B0 inhomogeneity. However, fat can be suppressed with chemical shift-selective fat saturation or by exploiting the phase difference between fat and water. Signal from fluids and muscle tissue can be suppressed with inversion-recovery and T2 magnetization preparations, respectively.

Subtraction-based bSSFP techniques may also be used for flow-independent angiography. Compared with nonsubtractive bSSFP acquisitions, subtractive bSSFP techniques provide better suppression of extraneous nonvascular background tissue. A subtractive flow-independent MRA technique is signal targeting alternative RF and flow-independent relaxation enhancement (STARFIRE; **Fig. 11**),[42] which preferentially depicts blood based on its long T1 and T2. Drawbacks of STARFIRE include sensitivity to subtraction artifact from motion, and lengthened scan times caused by the collection of 2 data sets.

CLINICAL APPLICATIONS OF NONCONTRAST MAGNETIC RESONANCE ANGIOGRAPHY

To be successful in clinical practice, MRA techniques need to satisfy several requirements: high vessel-to-background contrast and spatial resolution, and coverage sufficient to accurately assess the vessels of interest. Acceptable scan times are equally important. Different vascular beds

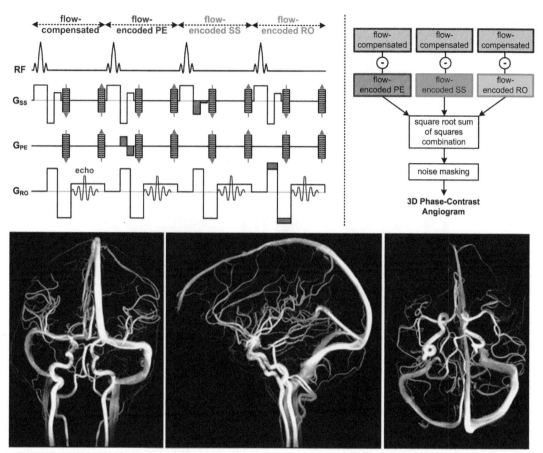

Fig. 10. (*Upper left*) Pulse sequence diagram for 3D Cartesian PC MRA. Flow-encoding bipolar gradients (*orange*) are applied to each axis; a flow-compensated reference acquisition is also acquired. (*Upper right*) Procedure for computing the 3D PC angiogram. (*Bottom*) MIPs of a 3D PC MRA acquired with a radial k-space trajectory. G_{PE}, phase-encoding gradient; G_{RO}, readout gradient; G_{SS}, slice selection gradient; PE, phase encoding; SS, slice selection; RO, readout. (*Reprinted from* Johnson KM, Lum DP, Turski PA, et al. Improved 3D phase contrast MRI with off-resonance corrected dual echo VIPR. Magn Reson Med 2008;60:1333; with permission from John Wiley and Sons.)

require these basic elements to variable degrees. Review of current and potential clinical applications of NC-MRA throughout the body is provided later. Sample parameters for several sequences (Table 2) and advice for optimal imaging in the appropriate vascular beds are also provided.

Neurovascular Imaging

For intracranial imaging, limited volumetric coverage but high spatial resolution are needed. Multidirectional flow can pose challenges that may affect vessel-to-background contrast for flow-dependent techniques. TOF MRA is the main technique used clinically, providing a useful screening and monitoring tool in asymptomatic patients with predisposing factors for cerebral aneurysm, including in polycystic kidney disease.

Previous studies at 1.5 T have shown that TOF MRA is effective in identifying aneurysms larger than 3 mm.[43] Three-tesla systems have enabled voxel volumes as low as 0.08 mm³,[44] improved vessel contrast, and performance comparable with multidetector CT angiogram (CTA) in aneurysm detection.[45]

TOF MRA is a useful monitoring tool in patients treated with endovascular detachable coils,[46,47] but may not perform as well in small (<3 mm) aneurysms.[48] It is less effective after aneurysm clipping with titanium clips, with associated susceptibility artifact precluding accurate assessment for a residual neck or recurrent aneurysm.[49]

Slow or turbulent flow may lead to suboptimal visualization of giant cerebral aneurysms with TOF MRA, and contrast-enhanced MRA may be more accurate for assessment of aneurysms

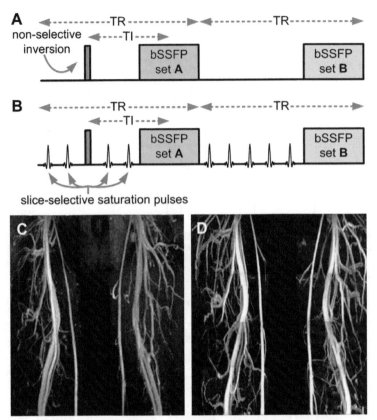

Fig. 11. STARFIRE MRA pulse sequences (*A*) without and (*B*) with additional saturation pulses for venous or arterial suppression. Two data sets are acquired and then subtracted. (*C*) STARFIRE MIP angiogram displaying arteries and veins acquired in a coronal plane with the sequence shown in (*A*). (*D*) STARFIRE MIP venogram acquired with arterial presaturation using axial slabs and the sequence shown in (*B*). (*From* Edelman RR, Koktzoglou I. Unenhanced flow-independent MR venography by using signal targeting alternative radiofrequency and flow-independent relaxation enhancement. Radiology 2009;250(1):241; with permission from the Radiological Society of North America.)

greater than 13 mm in diameter.[50] Methemoglobin in intracranial hemorrhage, which has a short T1, may mimic flow-related enhancement at TOF MRA (**Fig. 12**).

Other intracranial disorders are difficult to image with existing NC-MRA techniques. Cerebral arteriovenous malformations and dural arteriovenous fistulas are less common disorders that require high spatial and temporal resolution to distinguish arterial feeders from draining veins. The gold standard for assessment remains digital subtraction angiography, with time-resolved CE-MRA better able to provide temporal information than NC-MRA. TOF MRA has low sensitive to intracranial stenosis in primary cerebral vasculitis.[51]

Extracranially, spatial resolution requirements are less exacting; however, vessel tortuosity and motion-related artifact from patient swallowing may be problematic. CE-MRA is the preferred method because of superior speed, coverage, and low sensitivity to flow-induced artifacts.[52]

Intracranial magnetic resonance venography (MRV) is important for dural venous sinus thrombosis assessment. In an oblique sagittal plane to minimize in-plane flow saturation, 2D TOF MRA is able to depict flow as low as 2 cm/s[53]; however, a combination of TOF and contrast-enhanced MRV has been advocated for greatest sensitivity.[54] In addition, 3D PC imaging may be used, setting a low threshold velocity encoding of approximately 15 cm/s, but it is slow. Fluid-suppressed STARFIRE[55] and susceptibility-weighted imaging have only been described in healthy volunteers.[56]

Coronary Imaging

Cardiac and respiratory motion are challenges of coronary MRA, with potentially long acquisition times with commercially available, flow-independent, 3D respiratory navigated bSSFP MRA with T2 preparation and fat suppression.

Table 2
Sample parameters for noncontrast MRA sequences

	TOF MRA (3 T)	Flow-independent bSSFP MRA	IFIR MRA	FSE-MRA	QISS MRA
Target arteries	Cerebral	Coronary	Renal	Lower extremity	Lower extremity
Orientation	Axial	Axial	Axial	Coronal	Axial
FOV (mm^3)	200 × 164 × 24	320 × 255 × 120	340 × 244 × 100	450 × 355 × 120	400 × 260 × 144
True spatial resolution (mm)	0.6 × 0.6 × 0.9	1.4 × 1.3 × 1.6	1.3 × 1.3 × 1.4	1.4 × 1.4 × 1.8	1.0 × 1.0 × 3.0
TR	21 ms	3.6 ms	3.9 ms	1–3 cardiac cycles	3.5 ms
TE (ms)	3.4	1.8	1.7	80	1.4
Scan time	5 min	562 cardiac cycles[a]	72 respiratory cycles[b]	80–240 cardiac cycles per station[c]	48 cardiac cycles per station
FA (°)	18	90	90	70–180 (less flow sensitivity at higher FA)	90
Fat suppression	No	Frequency selective	Frequency selective	No	Frequency selective
Cardiac triggering	No	Yes	No	Yes	Yes
Respiratory gating	No	Yes	Yes	No	No
Additional prepulse	Tracking cranial saturation pulse	T2 preparation pulse	Slab-selective inversion pulse (TI 1100–1300 ms)	No	In-plane and tracking caudal saturation pulses
Slabs/stations	4	1	1	3	8–9

Abbreviations: FA, flip angle; FOV, field of view; TE, echo time; TR, repetition time.
[a] Value assumes a navigator efficiency of 40% and 3 readouts to acquire 1 partition.
[b] Value assumes that 1 readout acquires a single partition in full.
[c] Values assume TRs of 1 and 3 cardiac cycles, respectively, and 6/8th partial Fourier in the partition-encoding direction.

Respiratory drift and irregular breathing patterns are particular challenges to successful imaging with this technique. Although multidetector CTA has superior speed and spatial resolution, bSSFP MRA should particularly be considered for young patients in whom ionizing radiation is undesirable. Potential applications include assessment of coronary artery anomalies[57]; Kawasaki disease[58]; and, in adults, coronary artery disease, with reported sensitivity of 88% and specificity of 72% in a multicenter Japanese trial for hemodynamically significant stenosis.[59]

When performing coronary MRA, initial assessment of cardiac motion during the cardiac cycle is essential, and is best performed with standard bright blood cine imaging; in our experience, a 4-chamber view is most useful to evaluate excursion of the right coronary artery during a cardiac cycle. Mid-to-late diastole is usually the least motion-affected portion of the cardiac cycle, but end-systole may be preferable in tachycardic patients. Performing a brief respiratory navigator scout sequence, to assess diaphragmatic position before commencing the volumetric acquisition, is also advised.

Chest Magnetic Resonance Angiography

Chest MRA requires large volumetric coverage as well as respiratory and cardiac motion compensation. The same respiratory navigated bSSFP MRA approach used for coronary imaging can be

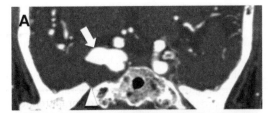

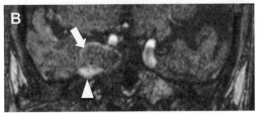

Fig. 12. Giant cerebral right ICA aneurysm. (A) CT angiogram shows clot within the inferior sac, with contrast opacification in the remainder of the aneurysm sac (arrow). (B) TOF MRA in which T1 hyperintense clot mimics flow (arrowhead), with suppression of blood signal within the patent portion of the sac caused by slow, turbulent flow (arrow). (Courtesy of Y. Perchyonok, MBBS, MMed, FRANZCR, Austin Health, Melbourne, Australia.)

applied with a larger field of view to thoracic aorta imaging in an oblique sagittal plane, showing improved depiction of the aortic root compared with nongated CE-MRA.[60] A modified highly accelerated breath-hold bSSFP MRA sequence (Fig. 13) has also been described,[61] with high concordance in measured aortic dimensions with CE-MRA.[62]

Pulmonary MRA is challenging because of low parenchymal proton density, susceptibility effects at air–soft tissue interfaces, and very short T2*.[63] Two-dimensional bSSFP imaging has been assessed for pulmonary embolus detection, with reported sensitivity and specificity of 83% and 100% respectively.[64] IFIR or cardiac phase-dependent MRA have been described for pulmonary artery imaging (Fig. 14),[65] with potential application in patients with preoperative lung cancer.[66] However, further clinical experience is required.

Abdominal Magnetic Resonance Angiography

The main requirements for abdominal MRA are large volume coverage, and respiratory motion compensation for the upper abdomen. NC-MRA for renal artery stenosis has been well evaluated in the literature, given the potential benefit to patients in the setting of renal impairment. Katoh and colleagues[67] first described an ECG-triggered respiratory navigator IFIR MRA approach with results that were comparable with CE-MRA in a small patient population, with several subsequent studies confirming utility of bSSFP MRA for this application.

Fast flow within the abdominal aorta and renal arteries enables good craniocaudal coverage with sufficient background suppression with currently commercially available respiratory navigator IFIR MRA (Fig. 15, Video 1). A recent study in 23 patients showed sensitivity of 93% and specificity of 88% of the technique compared with DSA.[68] It has also been applied to transplant renal arteries[69] and renal donor work-up[70] with encouraging results. The main concern with IFIR MRA is a potential to overestimate stenosis in low flow states.

NC-MRA has potential application in potential living liver transplant donors or liver tumor preoperative planning. Volumetric T2-weighted fat-suppressed FSE portography has been described in cirrhotic patients, with visualization of venous

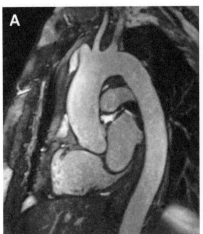

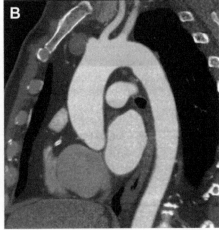

Fig. 13. A 64-year-old man with dilated ascending aorta. (A) Breath-hold flow-independent bSSFP MRA, and (B) gated CTA, showing comparable aortic depiction and maximal aortic dimension of 4.2 cm on both modalities.

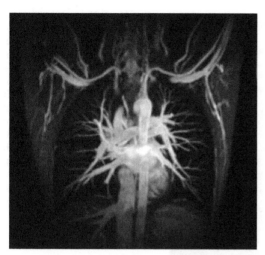

Fig. 14. Pulmonary NC-MRA using 3D half-Fourier FSE with fat suppression and diastolic ECG triggering only. (*From* Miyazaki M, Akahane M. Non-contrast enhanced MR angiography: established techniques. J Magn Reson Imaging 2012;35(1):10; with permission from John Wiley and Sons.)

structures that was comparable with contrast-enhanced imaging.[71] IFIR MRA for hepatic vessel assessment has been described but has yet to be evaluated in a clinical population.[72]

When performing IFIR MRA, appropriate positioning and inversion time of the slab-selective prepulse is paramount. For renal MRA, for which

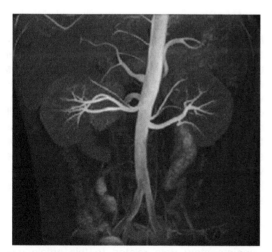

Fig. 15. IFIR MRA coronal MIP image of a 37-year-old healthy volunteer showing clear renal artery depiction. (*From* Wheaton AJ, Miyazaki M. Non-contrast enhanced MR angiography: physical principles. J Magn Reson Imaging 2012;36:298; with permission from John Wiley and Sons; and *Courtesy of* M. Miyazaki, PhD, Toshiba Medical Research Institute, Vernon Hills, IL.)

the technique is most commonly used, the prepulse should be positioned such that it extends slightly caudal to the volume to be imaged, in order to minimize signal from inflowing venous blood. The inversion time should be lengthened for patients in whom flow is suspected to be low, such as for patients with cardiac failure, in order to maximize arterial inflow (at the expense of greater recovery of background signal). Patient education or coaching during the volume acquisition to maintain a regular breathing rate or pattern is also suggested to maximize navigator efficiency.

Peripheral Magnetic Resonance Angiography

For extremity MRA, although flow is predominantly unidirectional (craniocaudal), small caliber vessels and slower arterial flow with increasing distance from the heart can be problematic.

Of the recently described techniques, only FSE-based gated subtraction MRA is commercially available (see **Fig. 8**). Variable performance for evaluation of peripheral arterial disease (PAD) has been reported. As a subtraction-based technique, its sensitivity to motion has affected its robustness, with 2 studies in particular reporting up to 42% to 47% of imaged segments as nondiagnostic, largely because of motion.[73,74] However, if motion can be minimized, high sensitivity and specificity can be achieved.[75,76] Operator experience also has some impact on appropriate parameter selection.[77] A variable refocusing flip angle approach has been described, with greater flow sensitivity that has potential application in distal extremity imaging[78]; however, clinical experience is limited.

QISS MRA (see **Fig. 5**) has been shown to be robust, with good sensitivity (85%–97%) and high specificity (95%–98%) compared with CE-MRA for hemodynamically significant stenosis in PAD at 1.5 T[76,79] and 3 T.[80] It has also specifically been evaluated in diabetics, in whom renal impairment commonly coexists, with 87% to 92% sensitivity and 96% to 97% specificity.[81]

bSSFP readout–based gated subtraction techniques are not yet commercially available. Sensitivity of 80% to 82% and specificity 81% to 91% for 2 similar techniques using systolic phase flow-suppressing magnetization preparations to spoil arterial signal has been described for PAD evaluation in the calf.[62,82] Because of intrinsically high SNR and ability to select degree of flow suppression, the technique also has promise for distal extremity imaging, with reported 92% accuracy for pedal artery stenosis in a diabetic cohort compared with CE-MRA (**Fig. 16**).[83]

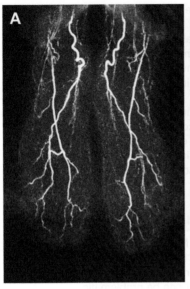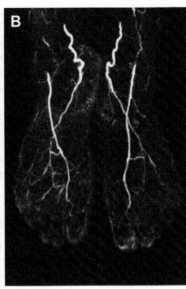

Fig. 16. A 43-year-old diabetic woman with peripheral neuropathy and suspected PAD. Coronal MIP subtraction images from (A) gated subtractive bSSFP MRA with a MSDE preparation; (B) CE-MRA. There is excellent depiction of pedal vessels with gated subtractive bSSFP MRA. (*Courtesy of* X. Liu, MD, Lauterbur Research Center for Biomedical Imaging, Shenzhen, China; and Z. Fan, PhD and D. Li, PhD, Cedars-Sinai Hospital and UCLA, Los Angeles, CA.)

Recently, unenhanced techniques to visualize upper extremity vessels have also been described for vascular access planning in renal failure. A modified, multishot, flow-independent bSSFP technique showed near-complete arterial segmental depiction and superior number of visualized venous segments compared with CE-MRA/MRV in 15 patients on hemodialysis.[84]

Patient comfort is vital when implementing any of the gated techniques described earlier for peripheral arterial assessment, because of the effects of motion on image quality. Padding and limb immobilization are recommended for extremity imaging to minimize motion, and are particularly important for the subtraction-based volumetric techniques, which are vulnerable to misregistration artifact. For FSE-MRA, appropriate selection of the trigger delay for the systolic acquisition is important, based on PC or cine bright blood scout imaging, because the technique depends on differences between diastolic and systolic flow. Selection of parameters to enhance these differences requires operator experience and understanding of parameters influencing degree of flow-related dephasing. As a guideline, lower refocusing flip angles (eg, 90°) and flow spoiling gradients can be used to maximize systolic dephasing in more distal vessels where flow is slow, and higher flip angles and flow compensation gradients can be used to minimize diastolic dephasing in more proximal vessels where flow is greater.

FUTURE DIRECTIONS

Despite the existing breadth and variety of current NC-MRA techniques, additional advancements in applications and pulse sequence design are likely to be made. Software advances implementing undersampled and non-Cartesian k-space trajectories along with compressed sensing are likely to shorten acquisition times, improve spatial-temporal resolution, and enhance clinical robustness. Hardware advances, such as high-density surface coils, multiple RF transmitters, and ultrahigh-field systems (>3 T) are poised to improve SNR, parallel imaging performance, and overall image quality.

SUMMARY

Many NC-MRA techniques are now commercially available or actively being evaluated for clinical use, with clinically acceptable acquisition times and improved robustness. They provide a noninvasive option in situations in which there are concerns regarding renal impairment or difficult intravenous access, or as a radiation-free alternative to CTA and catheter angiography. Technique selection depends on the properties of the vascular bed of interest, the disorder being studied, and an understanding of each technique's strengths and weaknesses.

SUPPLEMENTARY DATA

Supplementary data related to this article can be found online at http://dx.doi.org/10.1016/j.rcl.2014.12.003.

REFERENCES

1. Prince MR. Gadolinium-enhanced MR aortography. Radiology 1994;191(1):155–64.

2. Grobner T. Gadolinium–a specific trigger for the development of nephrogenic fibrosing dermopathy and nephrogenic systemic fibrosis? Nephrol Dial Transplant 2006;21(4):1104–8.

3. Thomsen HS, Morcos SK, Almen T, et al. Nephrogenic systemic fibrosis and gadolinium-based contrast media: updated ESUR Contrast Medium Safety Committee guidelines. Eur Radiol 2013; 23(2):307–18.

4. Greenman RL, Shirosky JE, Mulkern RV, et al. Double inversion black-blood fast spin-echo imaging of the human heart: a comparison between 1.5T and 3.0T. J Magn Reson Imaging 2003;17(6):648–55.

5. Lu H, Clingman C, Golay X, et al. Determining the longitudinal relaxation time (T1) of blood at 3.0 Tesla. Magn Reson Med 2004;52(3):679–82.

6. Sherwood L. The vasculature and blood pressure. Human physiology: from cells to systems. 1st edition. St Paul (MN): West Publishing Company; 1989. p. 298–341.

7. Lee VS. Cardiovascular MR Imaging: Physical Principles to Practical Protocols. Philadelphia: Lippincott Williams & Wilkins; 2006. p. 185–96.

8. Coffman JD, Lempert JA. Venous flow velocity, venous volume and arterial blood flow. Circulation 1975;52(1):141–5.

9. Fronek A, Coel M, Berstein EF. Quantitative ultrasonographic studies of lower extremity flow velocities in health and disease. Circulation 1976;53(6): 957–60.

10. Miyazaki M, Lee VS. Nonenhanced MR angiography. Radiology 2008;248(1):20–43.

11. Ansari SA, Schnell S, Carroll T, et al. Intracranial 4D flow MRI: toward individualized assessment of arteriovenous malformation hemodynamics and treatment-induced changes. AJNR Am J Neuroradiol 2013;34(10):1922–8.

12. Haacke EM, Masaryk TJ, Wielopolski PA, et al. Optimizing blood vessel contrast in fast three-dimensional MRI. Magn Reson Med 1990;14(2): 202–21.

13. Nagele T, Klose U, Grodd W, et al. Nonlinear excitation profiles for three-dimensional inflow MR angiography. J Magn Reson Imaging 1995;5(4): 416–20.

14. Blatter DD, Bahr AL, Parker DL, et al. Cervical carotid MR angiography with multiple overlapping thin-slab acquisition: comparison with conventional angiography. AJR Am J Roentgenol 1993;161(6): 1269–77.

15. Al-Kwifi O, Emery DJ, Wilman AH. Vessel contrast at three Tesla in time-of-flight magnetic resonance angiography of the intracranial and carotid arteries. Magn Reson Imaging 2002;20(2):181–7.

16. Pike GB, Hu BS, Glover GH, et al. Magnetization transfer time-of-flight magnetic resonance angiography. Magn Reson Med 1992;25(2):372–9.

17. Edelman RR, Ahn SS, Chien D, et al. Improved time-of-flight MR angiography of the brain with magnetization transfer contrast. Radiology 1992;184(2): 395–9.

18. Nederkoorn PJ, van der Graaf Y, Eikelboom BC, et al. Time-of-flight MR angiography of carotid artery stenosis: does a flow void represent severe stenosis? AJNR Am J Neuroradiol 2002;23(10):1779–84.

19. Wyttenbach R, Braghetti A, Wyss M, et al. Renal artery assessment with nonenhanced steady-state free precession versus contrast-enhanced MR angiography. Radiology 2007;245(1):186–95.

20. Glockner JF, Takahashi N, Kawashima A, et al. Noncontrast renal artery MRA using an inflow inversion recovery steady state free precession technique (Inhance): comparison with 3D contrast-enhanced MRA. J Magn Reson Imaging 2010;31(6):1411–8.

21. Furuta A, Isoda H, Yamashita R, et al. Non-contrast-enhanced MR portography with balanced steady-state free-precession sequence and time-spatial labeling inversion pulses: comparison of imaging with flow-in and flow-out methods. J Magn Reson Imaging 2013;40:583–7.

22. Edelman RR, Sheehan JJ, Dunkle E, et al. Quiescent-interval single-shot unenhanced magnetic resonance angiography of peripheral vascular disease: technical considerations and clinical feasibility. Magn Reson Med 2010;63(4):951–8.

23. Edelman RR, Giri S, Dunkle E, et al. Quiescent-inflow single-shot magnetic resonance angiography using a highly undersampled radial k-space trajectory. Magn Reson Med 2013;70(6):1662–8.

24. Edelman RR, Siewert B, Adamis M, et al. Signal targeting with alternating radiofrequency (STAR) sequences: application to MR angiography. Magn Reson Med 1994;31(2):233–8.

25. Kim SG. Quantification of relative cerebral blood flow change by flow-sensitive alternating inversion recovery (FAIR) technique: application to functional mapping. Magn Reson Med 1995;34(3):293–301.

26. Dai W, Garcia D, de Bazelaire C, et al. Continuous flow-driven inversion for arterial spin labeling using pulsed radio frequency and gradient fields. Magn Reson Med 2008;60(6):1488–97.

27. Koktzoglou I, Gupta N, Edelman RR. Nonenhanced extracranial carotid MR angiography using arterial spin labeling: improved performance with pseudo-continuous tagging. J Magn Reson Imaging 2011; 34(2):384–94.

28. Wu H, Block WF, Turski PA, et al. Noncontrast-enhanced three-dimensional (3D) intracranial MR angiography using pseudocontinuous arterial spin labeling and accelerated 3D radial acquisition. Magn Reson Med 2013;69(3):708–15.

29. Koktzoglou I, Meyer JR, Ankenbrandt WJ, et al. Nonenhanced arterial spin labeled carotid MR angiography using three-dimensional radial balanced

steady-state free precession imaging. J Magn Reson Imaging 2014. [Epub ahead of print].

30. Bi X, Weale P, Schmitt P, et al. Non-contrast-enhanced four-dimensional (4D) intracranial MR angiography: a feasibility study. Magn Reson Med 2010;63(3):835–41.

31. Wedeen VJ, Meuli RA, Edelman RR, et al. Projective imaging of pulsatile flow with magnetic resonance. Science 1985;230(4728):946–8.

32. Miyazaki M, Takai H, Sugiura S, et al. Peripheral MR angiography: separation of arteries from veins with flow-spoiled gradient pulses in electrocardiography-triggered three-dimensional half-Fourier fast spin-echo imaging. Radiology 2003;227(3):890–6.

33. Storey P, Atanasova IP, Lim RP, et al. Tailoring the flow sensitivity of fast spin-echo sequences for non-contrast peripheral MR angiography. Magn Reson Med 2010;64(4):1098–108.

34. Fan Z, Sheehan J, Bi X, et al. 3D noncontrast MR angiography of the distal lower extremities using flow-sensitive dephasing (FSD)-prepared balanced SSFP. Magn Reson Med 2009;62(6):1523–32.

35. Nicholas Priest A, Taviani V, John Graves M, et al. Improved artery-vein separation with acceleration-dependent preparation for non-contrast-enhanced magnetic resonance angiography. Magn Reson Med 2014;72(3):699–706.

36. Dumoulin CL, Souza SP, Walker MF, et al. Three-dimensional phase contrast angiography. Magn Reson Med 1989;9(1):139–49.

37. Hausmann R, Lewin JS, Laub G. Phase-contrast MR angiography with reduced acquisition time: new concepts in sequence design. J Magn Reson Imaging 1991;1(4):415–22.

38. Markl M, Frydrychowicz A, Kozerke S, et al. 4D flow MRI. J Magn Reson Imaging 2012;36(5):1015–36.

39. Kilner PJ, Gatehouse PD, Firmin DN. Flow measurement by magnetic resonance: a unique asset worth optimising. J Cardiovasc Magn Reson 2007;9(4):723–8.

40. Wright GA, Nishimura DG, Macovski A. Flow-independent magnetic resonance projection angiography. Magn Reson Med 1991;17(1):126–40.

41. Brittain JH, Olcott EW, Szuba A, et al. Three-dimensional flow-independent peripheral angiography. Magn Reson Med 1997;38(3):343–54.

42. Edelman RR, Koktzoglou I. Unenhanced flow-independent MR venography by using signal targeting alternative radiofrequency and flow-independent relaxation enhancement. Radiology 2009;250(1):236–45.

43. Huston J 3rd, Nichols DA, Luetmer PH, et al. Blinded prospective evaluation of sensitivity of MR angiography to known intracranial aneurysms: importance of aneurysm size. AJNR Am J Neuroradiol 1994;15(9):1607–14.

44. Gaa J, Weidauer S, Requardt M, et al. Comparison of intracranial 3D-ToF-MRA with and without parallel acquisition techniques at 1.5T and 3.0T: preliminary results. Acta Radiol 2004;45(3):327–32.

45. Hiratsuka Y, Miki H, Kiriyama I, et al. Diagnosis of unruptured intracranial aneurysms: 3T MR angiography versus 64-channel multi-detector row CT angiography. Magn Reson Med Sci 2008;7(4):169–78.

46. Ferre JC, Carsin-Nicol B, Morandi X, et al. Time-of-flight MR angiography at 3T versus digital subtraction angiography in the imaging follow-up of 51 intracranial aneurysms treated with coils. Eur J Radiol 2009;72(3):365–9.

47. Kwee TC, Kwee RM. MR angiography in the follow-up of intracranial aneurysms treated with Guglielmi detachable coils: systematic review and meta-analysis. Neuroradiology 2007;49(9):703–13.

48. Deutschmann HA, Augustin M, Simbrunner J, et al. Diagnostic accuracy of 3D time-of-flight MR angiography compared with digital subtraction angiography for follow-up of coiled intracranial aneurysms: influence of aneurysm size. AJNR Am J Neuroradiol 2007;28(4):628–34.

49. Grieve JP, Stacey R, Moore E, et al. Artefact on MRA following aneurysm clipping: an in vitro study and prospective comparison with conventional angiography. Neuroradiology 1999;41(9):680–6.

50. Cirillo M, Scomazzoni F, Cirillo L, et al. Comparison of 3D TOF-MRA and 3D CE-MRA at 3T for imaging of intracranial aneurysms. Eur J Radiol 2013;82(12):e853–9.

51. Cosottini M, Canovetti S, Pesaresi I, et al. 3-T magnetic resonance angiography in primary angiitis of the central nervous system. J Comput Assist Tomogr 2013;37(4):493–8.

52. Huang BY, Castillo M. Neurovascular imaging at 1.5 tesla versus 3.0 tesla. Magn Reson Imaging Clin N Am 2009;17(1):29–46.

53. Pui MH. Cerebral MR venography. Clin Imaging 2004;28(2):85–9.

54. Chen HM, Chen CC, Tsai FY, et al. Cerebral sinovenous thrombosis. Neuroimaging diagnosis and clinical management. Interv Neuroradiol 2008;14(Suppl 2):35–40.

55. Edelman RR, Koktzoglou I, Ankenbrandt WJ, et al. Cerebral venography using fluid-suppressed STAR-FIRE. Magn Reson Med 2009;62(2):538–43.

56. Boeckh-Behrens T, Lutz J, Lummel N, et al. Susceptibility-weighted angiography (SWAN) of cerebral veins and arteries compared to TOF-MRA. Eur J Radiol 2012;81(6):1238–45.

57. Ishii M, Sato Y, Matsumoto N, et al. Acute myocardial infarction in a patient with anomalous origin of the right coronary artery: depiction at whole-heart coronary magnetic resonance angiography and delayed-enhanced imaging. Int J Cardiol 2008;131(1):e22–4.

58. Greil GF, Stuber M, Botnar RM, et al. Coronary magnetic resonance angiography in adolescents and young adults with Kawasaki disease. Circulation 2002;105(8):908–11.

59. Kato S, Kitagawa K, Ishida N, et al. Assessment of coronary artery disease using magnetic resonance coronary angiography: a national multicenter trial. J Am Coll Cardiol 2010;56(12):983–91.

60. Francois CJ, Tuite D, Deshpande V, et al. Unenhanced MR angiography of the thoracic aorta: initial clinical evaluation. AJR Am J Roentgenol 2008; 190(4):902–6.

61. Xu J, McGorty KA, Lim RP, et al. Single breathhold noncontrast thoracic MRA using highly accelerated parallel imaging with a 32-element coil array. J Magn Reson Imaging 2012;35(4):963–8.

62. Lim RP, Fan Z, Chatterji M, et al. Comparison of non-enhanced MR angiographic subtraction techniques for infragenual arteries at 1.5 T: a preliminary study. Radiology 2013;267(1):293–304.

63. Stock KW, Chen Q, Hatabu H, et al. Magnetic resonance T2* measurements of the normal human lung in vivo with ultra-short echo times. Magn Reson Imaging 1999;17(7):997–1000.

64. Kluge A, Muller C, Hansel J, et al. Real-time MR with TrueFISP for the detection of acute pulmonary embolism: initial clinical experience. Eur Radiol 2004; 14(4):709–18.

65. Miyazaki M, Akahane M. Non-contrast enhanced MR angiography: established techniques. J Magn Reson Imaging 2012;35(1):1–19.

66. Ohno Y, Nishio M, Koyama H, et al. Journal Club: Comparison of assessment of preoperative pulmonary vasculature in patients with non-small cell lung cancer by non-contrast- and 4D contrast-enhanced 3-T MR angiography and contrast-enhanced 64-MDCT. AJR Am J Roentgenol 2014; 202(3):493–506.

67. Katoh M, Buecker A, Stuber M, et al. Free-breathing renal MR angiography with steady-state free-precession (SSFP) and slab-selective spin inversion: initial results. Kidney Int 2004;66(3): 1272–8.

68. Parienty I, Rostoker G, Jouniaux F, et al. Renal artery stenosis evaluation in chronic kidney disease patients: nonenhanced time-spatial labeling inversion-pulse three-dimensional MR angiography with regulated breathing versus DSA. Radiology 2011;259(2):592–601.

69. Lanzman RS, Voiculescu A, Walther C, et al. ECG-gated nonenhanced 3D steady-state free precession MR angiography in assessment of transplant renal arteries: comparison with DSA. Radiology 2009;252(3):914–21.

70. Laurence I, Ariff B, Quest RA, et al. Is there a role for free breathing non-contrast steady-state free precession renal MRA imaging for assessing live donors? A preliminary study. Br J Radiol 2012; 85(1016):e448–54.

71. Song Q, Zeng M, Chen C, et al. Non-contrast-enhanced magnetic resonance angiography using T2-weighted 3-dimensional fat-suppressed turbo spin echo (SPACE): diagnostic performance and comparison with contrast-enhanced magnetic resonance angiography using volume interpolated breath-hold examination in the detection of porto-systemic and portohepatic collaterals. J Comput Assist Tomogr 2012;36(6):675–80.

72. Shimada K, Isoda H, Okada T, et al. Unenhanced MR portography with a half-Fourier fast spin-echo sequence and time-space labeling inversion pulses: preliminary results. AJR Am J Roentgenol 2009; 193(1):106–12.

73. Haneder S, Attenberger UI, Riffel P, et al. Magnetic resonance angiography (MRA) of the calf station at 3.0 T: intraindividual comparison of non-enhanced ECG-gated flow-dependent MRA, continuous table movement MRA and time-resolved MRA. Eur Radiol 2011;21(7):1452–61.

74. Lim RP, Hecht EM, Xu J, et al. 3D nongadolinium-enhanced ECG-gated MRA of the distal lower extremities: preliminary clinical experience. J Magn Reson Imaging 2008;28(1):181–9.

75. Gutzeit A, Sutter R, Froehlich JM, et al. ECG-triggered non-contrast-enhanced MR angiography (TRANCE) versus digital subtraction angiography (DSA) in patients with peripheral arterial occlusive disease of the lower extremities. Eur Radiol 2011; 21(9):1979–87.

76. Ward EV, Galizia MS, Usman A, et al. Comparison of quiescent inflow single-shot and native space for nonenhanced peripheral MR angiography. J Magn Reson Imaging 2013;38(6):1531–8.

77. Storey P, Lim RP, Kim S, et al. Arterial flow characteristics in the presence of vascular disease and implications for fast spin echo-based noncontrast MR angiography. J Magn Reson Imaging 2011;34(6): 1472–9.

78. Lim RP, Storey P, Atanasova IP, et al. Three-dimensional electrocardiographically gated variable flip angle FSE imaging for MR angiography of the hands at 3.0 T: initial experience. Radiology 2009;252(3): 874–81.

79. Hodnett PA, Koktzoglou I, Davarpanah AH, et al. Evaluation of peripheral arterial disease with nonenhanced quiescent-interval single-shot MR angiography. Radiology 2011;260(1):282–93.

80. Amin P, Collins JD, Koktzoglou I, et al. Evaluating peripheral arterial disease with unenhanced quiescent-interval single-shot MR angiography at 3 T. AJR Am J Roentgenol 2014;202(4):886–93.

81. Hodnett PA, Ward EV, Davarpanah AH, et al. Peripheral arterial disease in a symptomatic diabetic population: prospective comparison of rapid unenhanced

MR angiography (MRA) with contrast-enhanced MRA. AJR Am J Roentgenol 2011;197(6):1466–73.

82. Priest AN, Joubert I, Winterbottom AP, et al. Initial clinical evaluation of a non-contrast-enhanced MR angiography method in the distal lower extremities. Magn Reson Med 2013;70(6):1644–52.

83. Liu X, Fan Z, Zhang N, et al. Unenhanced MR angiography of the foot: initial experience of using flow-sensitive dephasing-prepared steady-state free precession in patients with diabetes. Radiology 2014;272(3):885–94.

84. Bode AS, Planken RN, Merkx MA, et al. Feasibility of non-contrast-enhanced magnetic resonance angiography for imaging upper extremity vasculature prior to vascular access creation. Eur J Vasc Endovasc Surg 2012;43(1):88–94.

Recent Advances in Brain and Spine Imaging

Amit M. Saindane, MD

KEYWORDS

- Advanced MR imaging • High-field imaging • Susceptibility weighted imaging • Time-resolved MRA
- MR perfusion • MR spectroscopy • Diffusion tensor imaging • Functional MR imaging

KEY POINTS

- A variety of advanced MR imaging techniques have been incorporated into clinical imaging protocols for routine use, specific applications to particular disease entities, or as problem-solving tools on an ad hoc basis.
- The advent of high-field MR imaging units, coupled with improvements in gradient performance, coil technology, and pulse sequence design, has facilitated growth of routine use of advanced MR imaging techniques in practice.
- Novel methods of enhancing imaging contrast on structural images include techniques such as balanced steady-state free precession, double inversion recovery, susceptibility weighted imaging, and gadolinium cisternography.
- Techniques such as time-resolved MR angiography, cine phase contrast flow quantification, dynamic susceptibility contrast MR perfusion, arterial spin labeled perfusion, proton MR spectroscopy, and diffusion-weighted imaging allow for imaging of specific physiologic phenomena in the brain.
- Presurgical planning has benefitted from the complementary roles of diffusion tensor imaging and blood oxygenation level dependent functional MR imaging techniques.

INTRODUCTION

Because a broad variety of pathologic processes are found in the practice of neuroradiology, and the structures to be imaged are less affected by cardiac and respiratory motion than in other parts of the body, numerous advanced MR imaging techniques have found clinical use in the imaging of the brain and spine. Some techniques have found such widespread utility that they have been incorporated into nearly all imaging protocols; others have found niche applications to answer specific clinical questions, and yet others have been optimally used in combination with other advanced MR imaging techniques. The later sections highlight the various advanced imaging techniques in use in clinical neuroradiology. Because high-field MR imaging along with advances in scanner hardware and pulse sequence design has facilitated adoption of many of the other techniques, the article begins with a discussion of the contribution of high-field imaging. The next several sections review novel methods of generating image contrast and increasing sensitivity to pathology in structural imaging, such as the use of double inversion recovery (DIR) and susceptibility weighted imaging (SWI). Next, a variety of techniques targeting aspects of brain and spine physiology are reviewed, including cine-phase contrast flow quantification, dynamic susceptibility contrast (DSC) perfusion, and proton MR spectroscopy (MRS). Finally, the techniques of diffusion

Disclosures: There are no relevant disclosures or conflicts of interest with regard to this article submission.
Division of Neuroradiology, Department of Radiology and Imaging Sciences, Emory University Hospital, Emory University School of Medicine, BG22, 1364 Clifton Road Northeast, Atlanta, GA 30322, USA
E-mail address: asainda@emory.edu

Radiol Clin N Am 53 (2015) 477–496
http://dx.doi.org/10.1016/j.rcl.2014.12.004

radiologic.theclinics.com

tensor imaging (DTI) and blood oxygenation level dependent (BOLD) functional MR imaging (fMRI) that have found numerous research applications and a few, but critical, clinical applications for pre-surgical planning are reviewed. Each of the techniques discussed are in use extensively in the routine workflow at the author's institution and have contributed to the care of their patients. Typical indications and specific acquisition parameters are described in Table 1.

ADVANCED MR IMAGING TECHNIQUES
High-Field Clinical MR Imaging Imaging

The advent of high-field clinical MR imaging systems (3-4 T) has allowed for better clinical application of several MR imaging techniques that benefit from higher magnetic field strength. These techniques include BOLD fMRI imaging,[1] DTI,[2] and arterial spin labeled (ASL) perfusion.[3] These and other advanced MRI techniques benefit from the increase in signal-to-noise ratio (SNR) as well as spatial resolution that high-field MR imaging can provide, primarily the result of a linear relationship between the magnetic field strength (B_0) and SNR. Applications of parallel imaging, improved pulse sequences, and higher SNR coils have been added to improve image quality. For dynamic techniques, temporal resolution can be increased by sacrificing SNR and spatial resolution. When the additional SNR is instead used to achieve improved spatial and contrast resolution, conventional structural imaging sequences benefit from high field, affording increased sensitivity to disease. For example, studies of multiple sclerosis (MS) have found an increased number and volume of gadolinium-enhancing lesions and increased volume of T2 hyperintense lesions at 3.0 T versus 1.5 T[4] and determined that additional patients fulfilled diagnostic criteria for MS at the higher magnetic field strength.[5] Fig. 1 demonstrates examples of increased sensitivity to MS lesions at 3.0 T in comparison with 1.5 T.

Steady-State Free Precession for High-Resolution Imaging

Balanced steady-state free precession (bSSFP) based MR imaging techniques have found a variety of clinical applications. Utilization has also been facilitated by the introduction of very fast, strong, and precise gradient systems. A feature of bSSFP sequences is their mixed T1 and T2 contrast and very high SNR.[6] Because the T2/T1-weighted contrast is frequently not optimal for detection of brain signal abnormality in neuroradiology, major applications have focused on high spatial and contrast resolution between cerebrospinal fluid

(CSF) and surrounding structures when performed with heavy T2 weighting. For example, an important cause of trigeminal neuralgia is neurovascular compression. In most cases, a crossing arterial vessel causes compression, but venous structures may also result in neurovascular compression. Steady-state free precession sequences such as the 3-dimensional (3D) constructive interference in the steady state (CISS) and fast imaging employing steady-state acquisition (FIESTA) sequence have shown utility in the evaluation of trigeminal neuralgia[7] and hemifacial spasm[8] wherein there is similar neurovascular compression of the facial nerve. Fig. 2 demonstrates utility of a FIESTA sequence for the identification of neurovascular compression in hemifacial spasm. Similarly, bSSFP sequences have found utility in the evaluation of the fluid-filled inner ear structures in the setting of sensorineural hearing loss[9] as well as high-resolution MR myelography for the detection of CSF leaks and postoperative or posttraumatic pseudomeningoceles.[10]

Double Inversion-Recovery Imaging

DIR sequences suppress signals from both the CSF and the white matter (WM), achieving excellent contrast between gray matter (GM) and WM and improving detection of lesions.[11,12] Compared with the T2-fluid-attenuated inversion recovery (FLAIR) sequence, DIR imaging may exhibit improved sensitivity to identify abnormalities with only slightly prolonged T2 values in relation to the WM or GM. In the setting of MS, by suppressing signals from WM and CSF, DIR MR imaging provides superior delineation of GM and increased lesion contrast in both GM and WM. As a result, cortical lesions are more readily detected by DIR imaging than by conventional imaging sequences that are generally poor at detecting and localizing cortical lesions.[13] In the setting of epilepsy, DIR is considered helpful for increased detectability of hippocampal sclerosis[14] and other abnormal signal changes in epilepsy.[15] Fig. 3 demonstrates an application of DIR Sampling Perfection with Application optimized Contrast using different flip angle Evolutions (SPACE) in the evaluation of epileptogenic foci. In the author's practice, the DIR sequence is used exclusively on their presurgical workup for medically refractory epilepsy and has proven useful in the detection of cryptogenic epileptogenic foci.

Automated Segmentation and Volumetric Analysis

A variety of approaches to automated segmentation and volumetric analysis of the brain structures

Table 1
Typical indications and specific acquisition parameters of MR imaging techniques

Technique	Common Indications	Field Strength	Acquisition Parameters
SSFP	Hearing loss Trigeminal neuralgia Hemifacial spasm	1.5 T or 3.0 T	TR/TE = 5.38 ms/TE = 2.39 ms FA = 70° FOV = 180 cm ST = 0.70 mm Base Res = 256 Slices = 80 Time = 3.05 min
DIR	Epilepsy (seizure focus localization)	3.0 T	TR = 7500 ms TE = 326 ms TI = 3000 ms FOV = 230 cm ST = 1.5 mm Base Res = 192 Slices = 128 IPAT = 2 Time = 5.39 min
SWI	Traumatic brain injury	1.5 T or 3.0 T	TR = 45 ms TE = 6.14 ms FA = 12° FOV = 235 cm ST = 2.0 mm Base Res = 256 Slices = 80 Time = 6.10 min
Gadolinium Cisternography (VIBE)	Skull base and spinal CSF leak	1.5 T or 3.0 T	TR = 20.0 ms TE = 3.69 ms FA = 12° FOV = 200 cm ST = 1.0 mm Base Res = 320 Slices = 40 Time = 2.02 min
Time-Resolved MRA	Intracranial and spinal dAVF	1.5 T or 3.0 T	TR = 3.59 ms TE = 1.47 ms FA = 25° FOV = 192 cm ST = 1.0 mm Base Res = 192 Slices = 104 Time = 1.18 min 12 Measurements Sampling region A = 11% Sampling region B = 25%
Cine PC Flow	Chiari 1 malformation Aqueductal patency Third ventriculostomy patency	1.5 T or 3.0 T	TR = 24.0 ms TE = 7.24 ms FA = 15° FOV = 220 cm ST = 5.0 mm Base Res = 256 VENC = 10 Phases = 25 Time = 5.08 min

(continued on next page)

Table 1
(continued)

Technique	Common Indications	Field Strength	Acquisition Parameters
DSC Perfusion	Intracranial mass characterization Tumor progression vs radiation necrosis	1.5 T or 3.0 T	TR = 1400 ms TE = 32 ms FA = 30° FOV = 230 cm ST = 5.0 mm Base Res = 128 Slices = 19 Time = 1.17 min
ASL Perfusion (3D GRASE pCASL)	Sickle cell vasculopathy Cerebrovascular reserve	3.0 T	TR = 4155 ms TE = 29.9 ms FA = 90° FOV = 240 cm ST = 5.0 mm Base Res = 64 Slices = 30 Time = 6.05 mm
Proton MRS (2D CSI)	Intracranial mass characterization Tumor progression vs radiation necrosis	1.5 T or 3.0 T	TR = 1500 ms TE = 144 ms FA = 90° FOV = 160 cm ST = 15 mm Time = 6.05 min
DWI	Imaging of ischemia Intracranial mass characterization	1.5 T or 3.0 T	TR = 4100 ms TE = 91 ms FOV = 230 cm ST = 5.0 mm Base Res = 192 Slices = 25 Averages = 2 IPAT = 2 Time = 1.11 min
DTI	Presurgical planning for brain tumors and AVMs	3.0 T	TR = 8200 ms TE = 93 ms FOV = 230 cm ST = 2.0 mm Base Res = 128 Slices = 60 IPAT = 2 Time = 4.49 min B = 0, 500, 1000
BOLD fMRI	Presurgical planning for brain tumors and AVMs	3.0 T	TR = 3000 ms TE = 30 ms FA = 90° FOV = 240 cm ST = 4.0 mm Base Res = 64 Slices = 35 Time = 3.36 min

Parameters listed are for 3.0-T Siemens Trio MRI Unit.
Abbreviations: ST, slice thickness; TE, echo time; TR, repetition time.

have been used extensively in the literature. In general, these approaches require manual postprocessing steps that can be labor-intensive and time-consuming, making them impractical for clinical use. More recent developments of automated software have been approved by the US Food and Drug Administration (FDA) for clinical use. These tools have been validated and successfully used to detect hippocampal atrophy in Alzheimer disease[16] and are in use in many Alzheimer disease

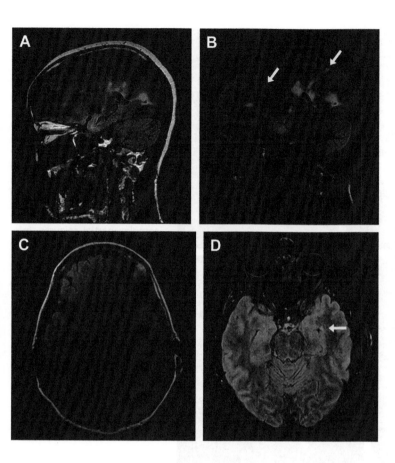

Fig. 1. High-field clinical MR imaging for improved lesion detection. (*A*) 1.5-T MR imaging sagittal T2-FLAIR image showing extensive periventricular lesions characteristic of the known diagnosis of MS. (*B*) 3.0-T MR imaging sagittal T2-FLAIR image with identical in-plane resolution and slice thickness (3 mm) as the study performed at 1.5 T demonstrating greater conspicuity of lesions as well as additional lesions not visible at 1.5 T (*arrows*). (*C*) Different patient being evaluated for MS with axial 1.5-T T2-FLAIR image showing no WM lesions evident. (*D*) At 3.0 T with identical in-plane resolution and slice thickness (3 mm), a characteristic periventricular lesion adjacent to the left temporal horn (*arrow*) is now demonstrated.

clinics. For patients with epilepsy that is refractory to medical therapy, the best option for achieving freedom from seizures is surgical resection of the epileptogenic focus, especially when atrophy of the hippocampus is present.[17] Segmentation and volumetric analysis of the hippocampus have been demonstrated to be a marker for hippocampal atrophy, and studies have found that quantitative MR imaging can improve the detection and laterality of hippocampal atrophy in temporal lobe epilepsy (TLE), with accuracy rates for seizure lateralization of 88% versus the 76% achieved with visual inspection of clinical MR imaging studies.[18] **Fig. 4** demonstrates a clinical application of automated segmentation and hippocampal volumetry to the presurgical evaluation of epilepsy. The software has also been applied to the study of traumatic brain injury (TBI), showing that brain atrophy is more sensitively detected in the setting of TBI than by a radiologist's traditional method of

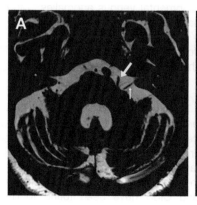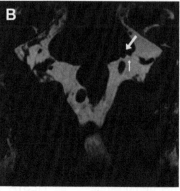

Fig. 2. Steady-state free precession for high-resolution imaging. (*A*) Axial FIESTA image acquired at 0.6-mm isotropic resolution in a patient with left-sided hemifacial spasm shows a vascular loop of the anterior inferior cerebellar artery (AICA) (*arrow*) indenting the root exit zone of the left facial nerve (*small arrow*). (*B*) Coronal reformat of the axial FIESTA acquisition shows the ability to maintain image quality with this high-resolution volumetric acquisition, further illustrating the neurovascular compression involving the left facial nerve (*small arrow*) by the AICA (*arrow*).

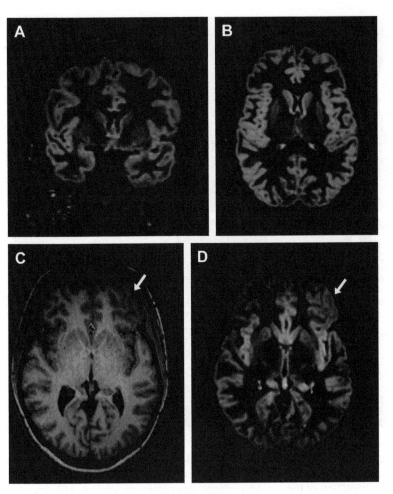

Fig. 3. DIR for detection of cortical dysplasia. (*A, B*) DIR using SPACE. (*A*) Coronal plane of acquisition. (*B*) Axial reformat. Both images show excellent differentiation of the cortical GM and underlying WM without abnormality. (*C*) Axial 3D gradient recalled echo (GRE) T1-weighted image (magnetization prepared rapid acquisition gradient echo, MPRAGE) using 1-mm isotropic resolution in a right-handed woman with chronic medically refractory complex partial seizures. Inferior left frontal cortical dysplasia (*arrow*) was not initially detected on this examination and was missed on prior MR imaging evaluations. (*D*) Axial reformatted coronally acquired DIR SPACE image at 1.5-mm isotropic resolution demonstrating the left inferior frontal cortical dysplasia as abnormal gyration and high T2 signal intensity.

visual inspection.[19] In the author's clinical practice, automated brain segmentation analysis is used in the presurgical workup of medically refractory epilepsy patients as well as workup for patients with dementia. Depending on the indication, normative percentiles of hippocampal volume and degrees of asymmetry are reported.

Susceptibility Weighted Imaging

SWI is a fully velocity-compensated 3D gradient-echo MR imaging technique that exploits the magnetic susceptibility differences of various tissues or materials, such as blood products, iron, and calcification. After the acquisition of images, phase variations in the images due to static magnetic field inhomogeneity are removed and the phase mask is then multiplied with the magnitude data to enhance the depiction of vessels or foci with susceptibility effects.[20] Generated minimal intensity projection images can better demonstrate vascular structures. The SWI technique has been used to increase the conspicuity of detection of

microhemorrhage in the setting of TBI.[21] Fig. 5 demonstrates the use of SWI in this application. In addition to detecting microhemorrhage in the setting of a variety of other conditions, SWI uses paramagnetic deoxyhemoglobin as an intrinsic contrast agent. This application allows for improved depiction of slow-flow venous structures, such as developmental venous anomalies[22] and venous drainage from arteriovenous malformations (AVMs).[23] Clinical use of SWI at the author's institution is for increasing sensitivity to microhemorrhage in the setting of mild TBI.

Gadolinium Cisternography

Contrast cisternography is the imaging of the cerebrospinal system after intrathecal administration of contrast material into the subarachnoid space, typically via lumbar puncture. Although very heavily T2-weighted high-resolution bSSFP sequences such as FIESTA and CISS have been found to be extremely useful as a noninvasive morphologic tool,[9,10] the physiologic information derived from

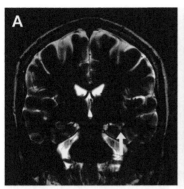 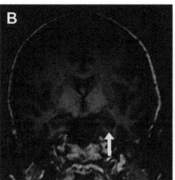 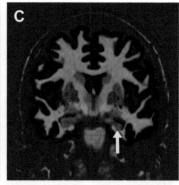

Fig. 4. Automated segmentation and volumetric analysis for mesial temporal sclerosis. (A) Coronal T2-weighted image through the hippocampus shows abnormally high T2 signal and loss of internal architecture within the left hippocampus (arrow). (B) Coronal reformat of a sagittal acquired MPRAGE image shows decreased volume of the left hippocampus (arrow). (C) Automated segmentation of the sagittal MPRAGE using Neuroquant software illustrating a reduced size of the left hippocampus in yellow (arrow) relative to the right. Images showed a calculated hippocampal asymmetry index of 22% in this patient with electrographic seizures from the left temporal lobe and semiology consistent with a left mesial temporal seizure focus.

intrathecal contrast administration (eg, actual demonstration and rapidity of CSF leak) is not obtainable. Intrathecal gadolinium-based contrast agent administration is not FDA-approved, although there is European literature to support its use.[24,25] In a typical imaging protocol, after acquisition of pre-contrast volumetric T1-weighted and heavily T2-weighted MR imaging sequences, 0.5 mL of gadolinium-DTPA is injected into the subarachnoid space via lumbar puncture in the usual sterile fashion. Postcontrast volumetric T1-weighted images are obtained at an early phase, and in some cases, also in a delayed fashion.[26] Gadolinium cisternography has been used to detect cranial CSF leaks in patients presenting with CSF rhinorrhea or otorrhea. In these cases, paranasal sinus

inflammatory mucosal disease and mastoid fluid that may or may not be related to the CSF leak can be a challenge to differentiate and represent a false localizing sign on heavily T2-weighted images. Direct imaging of gadolinium-enhanced CSF leaking through a skull base defect will establish the diagnosis.[25] Fig. 6 demonstrates the use of gadolinium cisternography in this application. A similar application of gadolinium cisternography is identifying spinal CSF leaks in the setting of spontaneous intracranial hypotension.[27] Additional uses include determination of patency of structures such as the cerebral aqueduct and endoscopic third ventriculostomies.[26] At the author's institution, gadolinium cisternography is typically performed in situations where computed tomography (CT) myelography

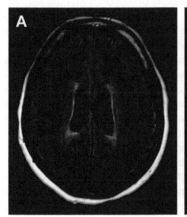 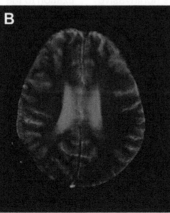 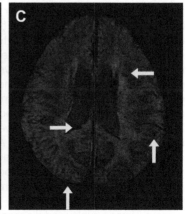

Fig. 5. SWI for TBI. Images from a 52-year-old man who experienced a motor vehicle crash and postconcussive symptoms but had a normal head CT examination. (A) Axial T2-FLAIR image with minimal nonspecific periventricular T2 hyperintensity. (B) Axial conventional T2-GRE image shows no abnormal susceptibility artifact to suggest the presence of microhemorrhage. (C) Axial SWI image shows multiple areas of microhemorrhage (arrows) that were not evident on the GRE image and are consistent with traumatic axonal injury.

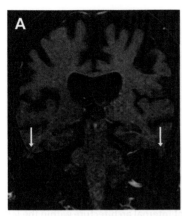
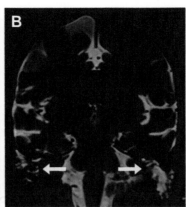
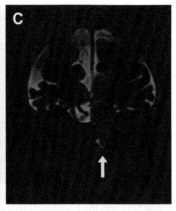

Fig. 6. Gadolinium cisternography for CSF leak localization. (A) Coronal T1-weighted fat-saturated image through the head showing 2 potential areas of skull base defects with brain herniating into the defects (*small arrows*). (B) Same coronal T1-weighted fat-saturated image as in (A) following administration of 1 mL intrathecal gadolinium contrast showing CSF leaks extending into the bilateral mastoid air cells (*arrows*). (C) Additional coronal image showing an occult site of CSF leak into the left sphenoid sinus (*arrow*) and providing an explanation for this patient's CSF rhinorrhea.

and conventional MR imaging sequences fail to unambiguously detect a site of CSF leak. Imaging protocols rely heavily on preintrathecal and postintrathecal gadolinium T1-weighted images, including volumetric fat-saturated images such as volumetric interpolated breath-hold examination (VIBE) as well as conventional fast spin echo T1-weighted fat-saturated images.

Time-Resolved MR Angiography

In conventional bolus-chase MR angiography (MRA), long acquisition times effectively preclude obtaining multiple phases during bolus intravenous gadolinium acquisition. Contrast-enhanced time-resolved MR angiography (CE-TR MRA) techniques have shown great potential as noninvasive approaches to evaluating vascular enhancement in a temporally sensitive manner. Efforts to rapidly image contrast kinetics have benefited from acquisition schemes aimed at accelerated data collection, primarily using parallel received algorithms, novel k-space trajectories, and incorporation of view-sharing techniques.[28] Imaging is typically performed with acquisition of a precontrast mask, a multiple-phase during bolus intravenous gadolinium contrast agent administration. Although standard contrast agents are effective in this indication, protein-bound blood-pool high relaxivity agents such as gadofosveset trisodium (Ablavar) have been demonstrated to result in improved image quality and diagnostic confidence with CE-TR MRA.[29] For clinical neuroradiology applications, CE-TR MRA has been used to evaluate AVMs[30] and dural arteriovenous fistulas (dAVFs)[31] that require both high spatial and temporal

resolution, and also to optimize monitoring of treated intracranial aneurysms.[32] **Figs. 7** and **8** demonstrate the use of CE-TR MRA for intracranial and spinal dAVFs. CE-TR MRA is used extensively at the author's institution for localization for spinal dAVF, and for follow-up of endovascularly treated aneurysms and dAVF. When available, prior imaging that may help localize an abnormality is reviewed before imaging to tailor the field of view (FOV) and specific coverage.

Cine Phase Contrast Flow

Phase contrast (PC) MR imaging generates a differentiation between flowing and stationary nuclei by sensitizing the phase of the transverse magnetization to the velocity of motion. Two data sets are acquired with opposite sensitization, yielding opposite phase for moving nuclei and the same phase for stationary nuclei. The net phase is therefore zero for stationary nuclei and their signal is eliminated; however, flowing spins will move between the 2 flow sensitizations so the net phase after subtraction will not be zero, resulting in residual signal from flowing CSF.[33] Typically, a velocity encoding (VENC) of 5 to 8 cm/s should be selected for CSF imaging. The primary application of this technique has been to the Chiari 1 malformation, a hindbrain malformation characterized by downward displacement of "peglike" cerebellar tonsils below the foramen magnum. Clinical symptoms are thought to be contributed to by alterations in CSF flow at the craniovertebral junction that can be detected on PC flow studies and can help predict outcome after posterior fossa decompression.[34] **Fig. 9** illustrates the PC flow technique as

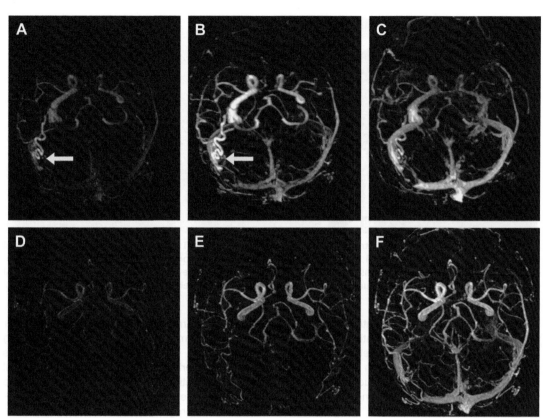

Fig. 7. Intracranial time-resolved MRA for the evaluation of dAVFs. (*A–C*) Successive CE-TR MRA axial maximum intensity projection (MIP) images showing an abnormal fistulous connection between the right occipital artery to the right transverse sinus (*arrow*) in a patient with right-sided pulsatile tinnitus consistent with a Borden type 1 dAVF. (*D–F*) Follow-up CE-TR MRA 1 year after the patient experienced spontaneous resolution of pulsatile tinnitus showing spontaneous resolution of the dAVF.

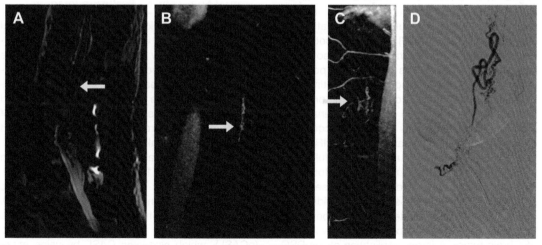

Fig. 8. Spinal time-resolved MRA for the evaluation of dAVF. (*A*) Sagittal T2-weighted image of the lumbar spine showing abnormal flow voids surrounding the conus medullaris and cauda equnia suspicious for a dAVF in this patient after multiple surgeries for low back pain. (*B, C*) Source data and MIP from arterial phase sagittal CE-TR MRA show a dAVF with arterial supply from the right L1 pedicle (not shown). (*D*) Digital subtraction angiogram confirms the presence of a dAVF from the right L1 pedicle.

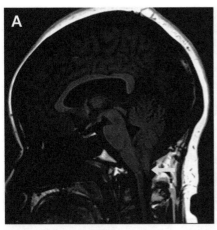
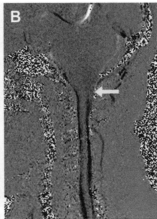
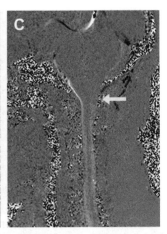

Fig. 9. Cardiac-gated cine phase-contrast CSF flow evaluation. (*A*) Sagittal T1-weighted image showing abnormal peglike cerebellar tonsils extending 1.5 cm below the foramen magnum, consistent with a Chiari 1 malformation. (*B, C*) Sagittal cardiac-gated cine phase contrast phase images through the upper cervical spine showing normal flow ventrally at the foramen magnum but absent flow dorsally (*arrow*) related to the ectopic cerebellar tonsils.

it applies to preoperative evaluation of patients with suspected Chiari 1 malformations. Other applications include determining whether CSF intensity cysts are in communication with the CSF space and for assessing aqueductal and endoscopic third ventriculostomy patency.[35]

Dynamic Susceptibility Contrast Perfusion Imaging

DSC MR perfusion has gained widespread use in clinical practice, primarily applied to intracranial tumors. DSC MR perfusion analysis is generally applied to echo planar T2*-weighted images that are acquired during the injection of a rapid bolus of gadolinium-based contrast agent. The analysis assumes that the contrast agent remains intravascular and estimates measurements of relative cerebral blood volume (rCBV). Although blood-brain barrier breakdown in tumors with leaky neovascularity routinely violates this assumption, postprocessing methods including γ-variate fitting and baseline subtraction can correct, as can preloading with gadolinium-based contrast material from a prior injection, frequently done in an acquisition of dynamic CE perfusion data. The DSC MR perfusion analysis has been found to be useful in the initial workup of intracranial mass lesions, for differentiation of tumor-mimicking processes, for grading of glial neoplasms, and for guiding biopsy.[36,37] Fig. 10 illustrates the DSC perfusion technique as it applies to preoperative evaluation of a brain tumor. A larger application of the DSC MR perfusion technique is for differentiating treatment-related necrosis in the setting of delayed radiation necrosis or pseudoprogression from true tumor progression. Conventional imaging in the setting of treatment-related necrosis might appear similar to tumor progression with increasing enhancement, T2-FLAIR abnormality, and mass effect. DSC perfusion has been shown to be useful in both conditions,[38,39] although there may be substantial overlap in the perfusion findings between tumor progression and pseudoprogression. Fig. 11 shows an example of radiation necrosis on DSC perfusion. DSC perfusion has been implemented as a routine part of the initial characterization of intracranial masses and for follow-up of all treated brain tumors. Postprocessing is performed offline and in conjunction with the conventional imaging sequences.

Arterial Spin-Labeled Perfusion Imaging

ASL perfusion techniques use "labeling" of arterial blood water flowing into a labeling plane with radiofrequency energy and imaging the brain tissue of interest after a predefined delay. During ASL image acquisition, repeated label and control (nonlabeled) images are typically interleaved and perfusion contrast is obtained by subtraction of the label and control datasets. Cerebral blood flow quantification takes into account multiple factors including arterial transit time, magnetization transfer effects, T1, and labeling efficiency. Various approaches to acquiring ASL data have been used, including continuous ASL (CASL), whereby blood water is continuously labeled, pulsed ASL (PASL), and pseudocontinuous ASL (pCASL), which simulates CASL by using many short pulses to achieve better sensitivity.[40] The main application of ASL perfusion is to cerebrovascular disease, including sickle cell vasculopathy in children,[41] and arterial occlusive disease

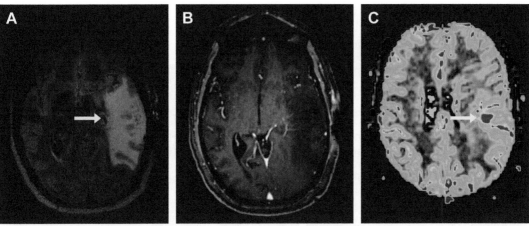

Fig. 10. DSC perfusion for biopsy selection. (*A*) Axial T2-FLAIR image showing an infiltrative tumor involving the left temporal lobe and insula (*arrow*). (*B*) Axial postcontrast T1-weighted image shows hypointense signal of the mass with no contrast enhancement. (*C*) rCBV map demonstrating heterogeneity of perfusion of the tumor with a particular area (*arrow*) demonstrating extremely high rCBV. This area was selectively biopsied revealing gliobastoma.

in adults.[42] The use of ASL perfusion with acetazolamide challenge is an additional method of probing the vascular reactivity and collateral circulation in cerebrovascular disease.[43] **Fig. 12** shows ASL perfusion in the setting of an acetazolamide challenge, which is the primary application of ASL clinically at the author's institution.

Proton MR Spectroscopy

Proton MRS is routinely performed clinically on conventional MR imaging systems at 1.5 T and 3.0 T.[44] MRS plots proton signal intensity against an observation frequency. Shielding of protons influences the position of the peak. Because the frequency changes with field strength, the shift is calculated by dividing the difference in frequency relative to a reference, in parts per million (ppm), allowing for standardization across field strengths. Necessary for successful performance of MRS is adequate shimming to homogenize the magnetic field and adequate water and fat suppression. MRS may be performed as a single voxel spectroscopy or as 2-dimensional (2D) or 3D chemical shift imaging (CSI) and can be performed at a variety of short-echo or long-echo times. The

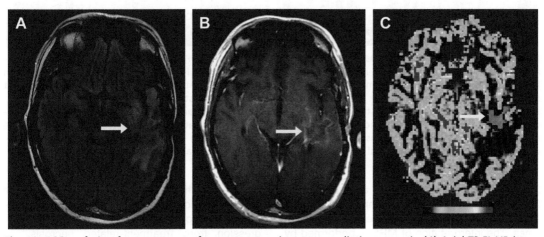

Fig. 11. DSC perfusion for assessment of tumor progression versus radiation necrosis. (*A*) Axial T2-FLAIR image showing abnormal T2 signal in the left insula and temporal lobe in a patient with glioblastoma previously resected and treated with radiation approximately a year before. (*B*) Axial postcontrast T1-weighted image shows minimal peripheral enhancement without a solid enhancing component. (*C*) rCBV map shows hypoperfusion of the enhancing areas supporting the diagnosis of radiation necrosis.

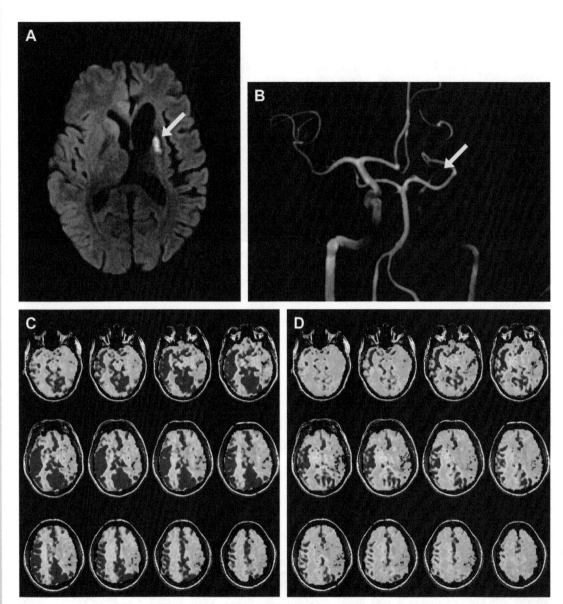

Fig. 12. ASL perfusion for cerebrovascular reserve. A 45-year-old man with high-grade left intracranial middle cerebral artery stenosis. (*A*) Axial DWI image shows recent infarction in the left putamen (*arrow*) superimposed on left hemispheric parenchymal volume loss. (*B*) MIP from 3D time-of-flight MRA shows high-grade proximal left M1 stenosis (*arrow*). (*C*) Pre-Diamox Arterial spin-label perfusion demonstrates normal right hemispheric perfusion with reduced flow throughout the left MCA distribution. (*D*) Post-Diamox Arterial spin-label perfusion demonstrates impaired flow augmentation in the left MCA distribution, indicating that collateral vasculatures for the region are not adequately compensating and that these areas are high risk for infarction. The patient subsequently underwent a left superficial temporal artery to middle cerebral artery bypass procedure.

3 main metabolites of *N*-acetyl aspartate (NAA; 2.0 ppm), creatine (3.0 ppm), and choline (3.3 ppm) are commonly observed at most echo times. The interpretation of MRS is performed by evaluating variations in metabolite ratios, or the appearance of pathologic metabolites such as lactate (1.3 ppm). MRS is used clinically to evaluate diffuse metabolic and hypoxic/ischemic disorders in the pediatric population[45] as well as for interrogation of focal lesions to improve diagnosis, grading, and differentiation of tumor progression from treatment-related necrosis.[46–48] **Figs. 13** and **14** show applications of MRS to de novo and treated primary brain tumors. Proton MRS has been reserved as a problem-solving tool to be used as an adjunct to DSC perfusion

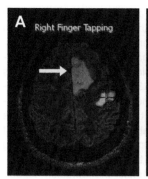
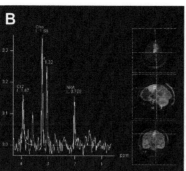
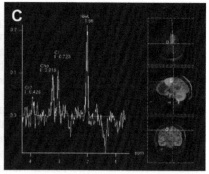

Fig. 13. Proton MRS in a primary brain tumor. (*A*) Axial T2-FLAIR image from an fMRI study showing a T2 hyper-intense mass infiltrating the left frontal lobe including the left supplemental motor area. (*B*) Proton MRS from a multivoxel 2D evaluation shows within the mass that there is elevation of the choline and depression of the NAA peaks. (*C*) Proton MRS in the contralateral normal brain shows a normal metabolite pattern.

for initial characterization of intracranial masses and for challenging cases of treated brain tumors, where it is unclear whether new findings represent tumor progression or treatment-related necrosis. Radiologists are involved in the setup of the technique at the scanner.

Diffusion-Weighted Imaging

DWI is an incredibly important imaging tool in neuroradiology and is used ubiquitously in brain imaging protocols. Diffusion represents the random thermal movement of molecules, and in the brain is determined by a variety of factors including the microarchitecture and temperature. By using appropriate MR imaging sequences that are sensitive to diffusion of water molecules, the different diffusion rates in tissues can be translated into maps of image contrast. Commonly, a T2-weighted echo planar sequence is made sensitive to water diffusion by adding 2 additional diffusion gradients (*b*) symmetrically centered around a 180° refocusing radiofrequency pulse. The second gradient cancels out the phase shift gained by the refocusing pulse. Most frequently, images are acquired with a *b* value of 0 and 1000 s/mm^2; however, because the diffusion gradients are added to a T2-weighted sequence, the signal intensity is determined by both the tissue T2 and the diffusion properties, making the DWI map weighted to both. Maps of diffusion rate are calculated from an analysis of the 2 images with the different *b* values to account for the T2-weighting contribution to the signal. DWI has found extensive clinical use,[49] most importantly in the setting of early ischemia, with DWI showing tissue injury as early as minutes

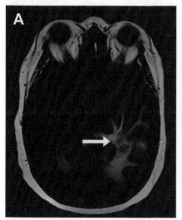
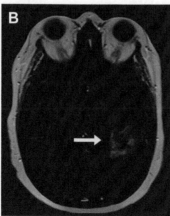
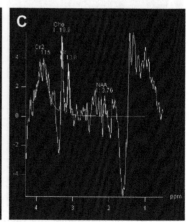

Fig. 14. Proton MRS for the assessment of tumor progression versus radiation necrosis. (*A*) Axial T2-FLAIR image showing abnormal T2 signal in the left insula and temporal lobe in a patient with glioblastoma previously re-sected and treated with radiation approximately 14 months before. (*B*) Axial postcontrast T1-weighted image shows abnormal enhancement of a portion of the T2/FLAIR abnormality. (*C*) Proton MRS spectrum from a multi-voxel 2D evaluation within the enhancing area shows reduction of metabolite peaks without a typical spectrum for tumor, supporting a diagnosis of radiation necrosis.

from onset of ischemia,[50] long before T1-weighted or T2-weighted images show pathologic abnormality, thought to be related to disruption of energy metabolism. A generally predictable time course of appearance on the DWI and apparent diffusion coefficient (ADC) maps is useful for estimating the age of an ischemic injury.[51] Multiple other intracranial applications of DWI have found important clinical uses, with DWI abnormalities noted in the setting differentiating arachnoid cysts from epidermoid tumors,[52] characterizing intra-axial masses as pyogenic abscess or hypercellular tumor,[53] and identification of Creutzfeldt-Jakob disease.[54] Figs. 15 and 16 show applications of DWI to infarction, infection, and hypercellular tumor in the brain. More recently, DWI has found important applications in the spine, including evaluating for spinal cord ischemia, characterization of spinal epidural abscess, and improved detection of metastatic disease and multiple myeloma.[55] Fig. 17 depicts a case that used DWI for diagnosing infarction in the spinal cord.

Diffusion Tensor Imaging

DTI is a form of DWI that assesses physiologic water directionality and motion, providing images of important WM tracts within the central nervous system.[56] Cellular structures such as cell membranes and organelles prevent the random isotropic motion of water molecules and result in anisotropy, causing water molecules to move with directionality. The orientation of WM tracts in the brain causes anisotropy because water diffusion parallel to the axonal fibers is much more likely than perpendicular to the fiber tracts. DTI analyzes the 3D shape of diffusion, characterizing a diffusion ellipsoid by 3 principal diffusivities (eigenvalues, $\lambda 1$, $\lambda 2$, $\lambda 3$) associated with 3 mutually perpendicular principal directions (eigenvectors). The diffusion tensor therefore contains valuable information about the microstructure of brain tissue. At a minimum, 6 diffusion encoding directions are required to solve for the diffusion coefficients that characterize the diffusion tensor. Based on this data, a fractional anisotropy (FA) map can be calculated, defined as the ratio of the anisotropic component of the diffusion tensor to the entire diffusion tensor, varying between 0 and 1. By combining the directional information and magnitude of anisotropic diffusion of individual voxels, the course of WM tracts can be estimated using postprocessing algorithms for tractography. Increasing the number of diffusion-encoding directions allows better resolution of crossing fibers within a voxel. Although many research applications of DTI have been evaluated, the primary use of DTI clinically is in the setting of presurgical planning for resection of primary glial neoplasms. A clear survival benefit has been found for patients who have undergone DTI-assisted tumor resection for the assessment of the pyramidal tracts compared with those without.[57] Frequently, a multimodality approach is used, using DTI, fMRI, and direct intraoperative cortical and subcortical stimulation to identify important functional and

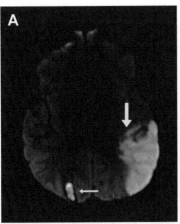 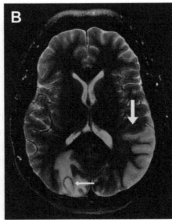 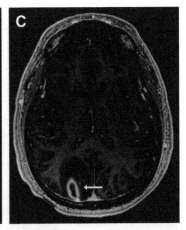

Fig. 15. DWI for intracranial infarction and abscess. (A) Axial DWI image shows a right parietal subcortical round area of restricted diffusion (*small arrow*) as well as a left temporal parietal area of diffusion restriction (*arrow*) involving both GM and WM. (B) Axial T2-weighted image shows a peripheral T2 hypointense rim around the right parietal lesion (*small arrow*) with surrounding edema, and more gyriform T2 hyperintensity on the left. (C) There is peripheral enhancement of the right-sided lesion. The patient had bacterial endocarditis and concurrently developed a cerebral pyogenic abscess in the right parietal lobe and a noninfectious embolic arterial infarction on the left.

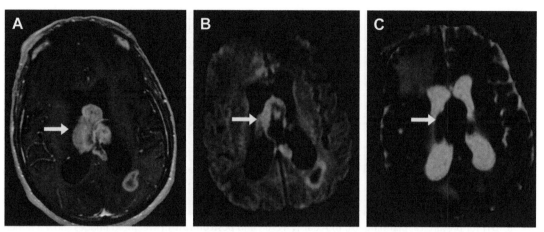

Fig. 16. DWI for hypercellular tumor. (A) Axial postcontrast T1-weighed image shows enhancing masses in the corpus callosum (arrow) and left parietal WM. (B, C) DWI (B) and ADC map (C) show diffusion restriction in the masses that are related to tumor hypercellularity. Stereotactic biopsy revealed lymphoma.

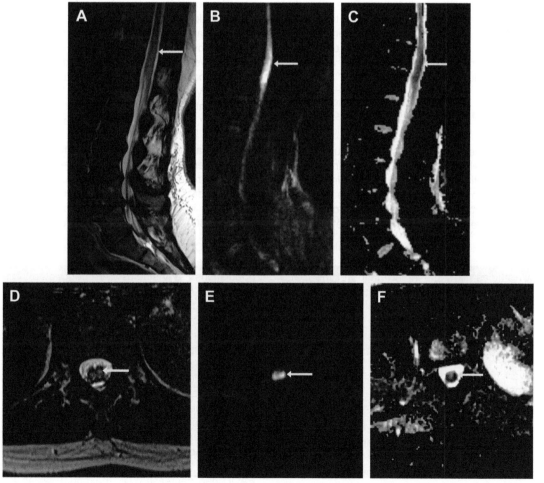

Fig. 17. DWI of the spinal cord. (A, D) Sagittal and axial T2-weighted images through the distal spinal cord and conus medullaris show abnormal increased intramedullary T2 signal in this patient, who experienced sudden onset paraparesis. (B–F) Sagittal and axial DWI (B, E) and ADC map (C, F) show abnormal diffusion restriction consistent with acute spinal cord infarction.

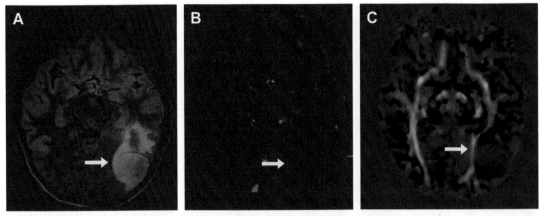

Fig. 18. DTI for presurgical planning. (*A*, *B*) Axial T2-FLAIR and postcontrast T1-weighted images show a nonenhancing T2 hyperintense well-defined mass in the left temporal and occipital lobes (*arrow*). (*C*) DTI axial color FA map shows deviation of the left optic radiation (*arrow*) medially. A gross total resection was performed without resultant visual field deficit.

structural areas near brain tumors. Figs. 18 and 19 show applications of DTI tractography to preoperative planning for primary brain tumor and AVM. At the author's institution, they primarily use DTI for presurgical mapping of brain tumors, and AVMs used in conjunction of fMRI.

Blood Oxygenation-Dependent Functional MR Imaging

fMRI is based on the principle of neurovascular coupling, which assumes that an increase in neuronal activity will cause an increase in blood oxygen consumption and a resultant increase in local cerebral perfusion. This increased blood flow to an activated region alters the ratio between the deoxyhemoglobin and oxyhemoglobin. Because oxyhemoglobin is diamagnetic and deoxyhemoglobin is paramagnetic, the blood oxygenation affects the overall signal in an area. Although the exact physiologic mechanisms explaining this BOLD response are not completely understood, it is generally accepted that changes in the BOLD signal relate to changes in neuronal activity. Commonly, BOLD fMRI uses a paradigm performed in a block design, where a task is performed to activate areas of interest, followed by a period wherein there is an adequate control task, and this process is repeated several times. The resultant data are postprocessed to determine the voxels in the brain that are associated with the task. BOLD fMRI is typically performed with a

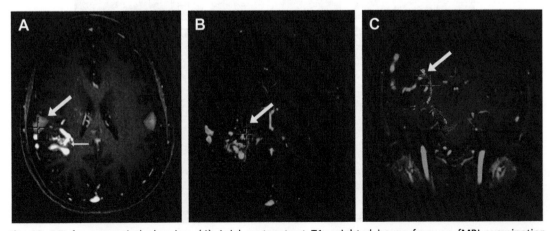

Fig. 19. DTI for presurgical planning. (*A*) Axial postcontrast T1-weighted image from an fMRI examination showing tongue motor activation (*arrow*) lateral to a deep right-sided AVM (*small arrow*). (*B*, *C*) Axial and coronal overlays of tractograms of the corticospinal tracts showing that these fiber tracts lie at the medial border of the AVM (*arrows*).

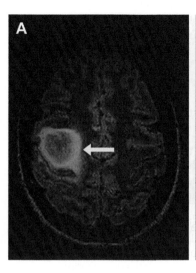
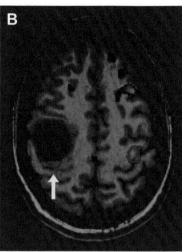

Fig. 20. BOLD fMRI for presurgical motor mapping. (A) Axial T2-FLAIR image of T2 hyperintense mass in the right perirolandic region (arrow). (B) BOLD fMRI with a bilateral finger tapping task shows left-hand motor activation (arrow) is at the posterior border of the mass.

T2*-weighted sequence that makes the technique vulnerable to distortions and artifacts near air-interfaces, such as the paranasal sinuses, and bony interfaces, such as at the skull base.

Although BOLD fMRI has been applied to better understanding basic brain function and a variety of derangements in disease states, the primary clinical application of BOLD fMRI to an individual patient is in presurgical planning to demonstrate areas of eloquent cortex in relation to pathologic abnormality, such as brain tumors. Maximal resection of primary brain tumors can improve survival and the effectiveness of adjuvant therapies if no surgically induced neurologic deficits are generated.[58] The identification of eloquent areas of cortex can be done preoperatively using fMRI or intraoperatively using direct electrical cortical stimulation mapping, which is considered the gold standard. Although accurate, cortical stimulation mapping can be time-consuming, can place

greater stress on the patient intraoperatively, and may require a larger craniotomy. Studies have shown a good concordance between cortical stimulation mapping and fMRI for motor, somatosensory, and visual areas,[59] with language localization using fMRI having less reliable correlation with intraoperative cortical stimulation mapping.[60] Disease-related alterations must be taken into account. For example, high-grade gliomas may attenuate or even lead to paradoxically negative BOLD response,[61] because vessels within brain tumors are typically less responsive than those of the surrounding tissue, and this lack of normal cerebral autoregulation can result in false negative results in the setting of presurgical planning. Other presurgical applications of BOLD fMRI include defining language dominance and predicting verbal outcome after temporal lobe surgery in the setting of medically refractory epilepsy.[62] **Figs. 20–22** show applications of BOLD fMRI to preoperative functional

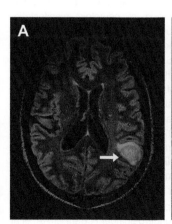
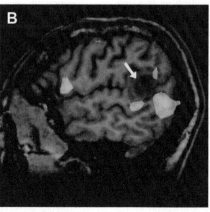

Fig. 21. BOLD fMRI for presurgical language mapping. (A) Axial T2-FLAIR image of T2 hyperintense mass in the left temporal parietal region (arrow). (B) Sagittal MPRAGE with activation map overlay from a sentence completion paradigm shows the mass (arrow) to be in close proximity to Wernicke areas of activation posteriorly. This was determined to be too high a surgical risk for postoperative aphasia if resection were attempted, and the mass was biopsied revealing an infiltrating glioma.

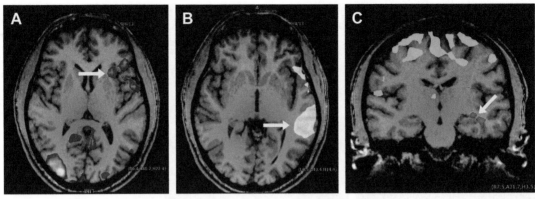

Fig. 22. BOLD fMRI for preoperative language and memory lateralization. (*A, B*) Patient with epilepsy and a suspected right mesial temporal seizure focus. An object naming paradigm (*A*) and a sentence completion paradigm (*B*) both result in strong left-sided language activation (*arrows*). (*C*) A scene memory paradigm shows strong left hippocampal and parahippocampal activation. A Wada examination in this case was performed showing concordance of language and memory lateralization.

localization for primary brain tumor and for language lateralization in epilepsy. At the author's institution, they primarily use fMRI for presurgical mapping of brain tumors and AVMs as well as for language lateralization before epilepsy surgery.

SUMMARY

A variety of advanced MR imaging techniques are used in the imaging of the brain and spine. Some techniques such as DWI have found such widespread utility importance in the routine clinical practice of neuroradiology that they have been incorporated into nearly all brain imaging protocols. Other techniques have benefitted from advances in scanner hardware and software technology and have found specific uses directed at specific pathologic conditions, such as cine phase contrast flow quantification for evaluation of the Chiari 1 malformation, and DIR imaging for the workup of epilepsy. Nevertheless, others have found utility in concert with other advanced techniques, such as the use of DTI and BOLD fMRI in the setting of presurgical planning of patients with brain tumors. Because a variety of pathophysiologic processes affect the brain and spine, and issues with respiratory and cardiac motion are relatively minor in comparison with other parts of the body, newer advanced MR imaging applications will undoubtedly continue to find their way into the routine clinical practice of neuroradiology as they are developed.

REFERENCES

1. Yang Y, Wen H, Mattay VS, et al. Comparison of 3D BOLD functional MRI with spiral acquisition at 1.5 and 4.0 T. Neuroimage 1999;9(4):446–51.

2. Alexander AL, Lee JE, Wu YC, et al. Comparison of diffusion tensor imaging measurements at 3.0 T versus 1.5 T with and without parallel imaging. Neuroimaging Clin N Am 2006;16(2):299–309.

3. Yongbi MN, Fera F, Yang Y, et al. Pulsed arterial spin labeling: comparison of multisection baseline and functional MR imaging perfusion signal at 1.5 and 3 T: initial results in six subjects. Radiology 2002; 222:569–75.

4. Sicotte NL, Voskuhl RR, Bouvier S, et al. Comparison of multiple sclerosis lesions at 1.5 and 3.0 Tesla. Invest Radiol 2003;38:423–7.

5. Wattjes MP, Harzheim M, Kuhl CK, et al. Does high-field MR imaging have an influence on the classification of patients with clinically isolated syndromes according to current diagnostic MR imaging criteria for multiple sclerosis? AJNR Am J Neuroradiol 2006;27:1794–8.

6. Haacke E, Brown R, Thompson M, et al. Magnetic resonance imaging: physical principles and sequence design. New York: Wiley and Sons; 1999.

7. Yoshino N, Akimoto H, Yamada I, et al. Trigeminal neuralgia: evaluation of neuralgic manifestation and site of neurovascular compression with 3D CISS MR imaging and MR angiography. Radiology 2003;228:539–45.

8. Naraghi R, Tanrikulu L, Troescher-Weber R, et al. Classification of neurovascular compression in typical hemifacial spasm: three-dimensional visualization of the facial and the vestibulocochlear nerves. J Neurosurg 2007;107:1154–63.

9. Guirado CR, Martínez P, Roig R, et al. Three-dimensional MR of the inner ear with steady-state free precession. AJNR Am J Neuroradiol 1995;16:1909–13.

10. Ramli N, Cooper A, Jaspan T. High resolution CISS imaging of the spine. Br J Radiol 2001;74:862–73.

11. Turetschek K, Wunderbaldinger P, Bankier AA, et al. Double inversion recovery imaging of the brain:

initial experience and comparison with fluid attenuated inversion recovery imaging. Magn Reson Imaging 1998;16:127–35.

12. Busse RF, Hariharan H, Vu A, et al. Fast spin echo sequences with very long echo trains: design of variable refocusing flip angle schedules and generation of clinical T2 contrast. Magn Reson Med 2006;55: 1030–7.

13. Geurts JJ, Pouwels PJ, Uitdehaag BM, et al. Intracortical lesions in multiple sclerosis: improved detection with 3D double inversion-recovery MR imaging. Radiology 2005;236:254–60.

14. Zhang Q, Li Q, Zhang J, et al. Double inversion recovery magnetic resonance imaging (MRI) in the preoperative evaluation of hippocampal sclerosis: correlation with volumetric measurement and proton magnetic resonance spectroscopy (^{1}H MRS). J Comput Assist Tomogr 2011;35:406–10.

15. Rugg-Gunn FJ, Boulby PA, Symms MR, et al. Imaging the neocortex in epilepsy with double inversion recovery imaging. Neuroimage 2006;31:39–50.

16. Brewer JB, Magda S, Airriess C, et al. Fully-automated quantification of regional brain volumes for improved detection of focal atrophy in Alzheimer disease. AJNR Am J Neuroradiol 2009;30(3):578–80.

17. Sisodiya SM, Moran N, Free SL, et al. Correlation of widespread preoperative magnetic resonance imaging changes with unsuccessful surgery for hippocampal sclerosis. Ann Neurol 1997;41(4):490–6.

18. Farid N, Girard HM, Kemmotsu N, et al. Temporal lobe epilepsy: quantitative MR volumetry in detection of hippocampal atrophy. Radiology 2012; 264(2):542–50.

19. Ross DE, Ochs AL, Seabaugh JM, et al, Alzheimer's Disease Neuroimaging Initiative. Man versus machine: comparison of radiologists' interpretations and Neuro-Quant volumetric analyses of brain MRIs in patients with traumatic brain injury. J Neuropsychiatry Clin Neurosci 2013;25(1):32–9.

20. Haacke EM, Xu Y, Cheng YC, et al. Susceptibility weighted imaging (SWI). Magn Reson Med 2004; 52:612–8.

21. Tong KA, Ashwal S, Holshouser BA, et al. Hemorrhagic shearing lesions in children and adolescents with posttraumatic diffuse axonal injury: improved detection and initial results. Radiology 2003;227: 332–9.

22. Lee BC, Vo KD, Kido DK, et al. MR high-resolution blood oxygenation level dependent venography of occult (low-flow) vascular lesions. AJNR Am J Neuroradiol 1999;20:1239–42.

23. Essig M, Reichenbach JR, Schad LR, et al. High resolution MR venography of cerebral arteriovenous malformations. Magn Reson Imaging 1999;17: 1417–25.

24. Albayram S, Kilic F, Ozer H, et al. Gadolinium-enhanced MR cisternography to evaluate dural leaks in intracranial hypotension syndrome. AJNR Am J Neuroradiol 2008;29:116–21.

25. Aydin K, Terzibasioglu E, Sencer S, et al. Localization of cerebrospinal fluid leaks by gadolinium-enhanced magnetic resonance cisternography: a 5-year single-center experience. Neurosurgery 2008;62:584–9.

26. Algin O, Turkbey B. Intrathecal gadolinium-enhanced MR cisternography: a comprehensive review. AJNR Am J Neuroradiol 2013;34(1):14–22.

27. Algin O, Taskapilioglu O, Zan E, et al. Detection of CSF leaks with magnetic resonance imaging in intracranial hypotension syndrome. J Neuroradiol 2011; 38:175–7.

28. Lim RP, Shapiro M, Wang EY, et al. 3D time-resolved MR angiography (MRA) of the carotid arteries with time-resolved imaging with stochastic trajectories: comparison with 3D contrast-enhanced Bolus-Chase MRA and 3D time-of-flight MRA. AJNR Am J Neuroradiol 2008;29:1847–54.

29. Dehkharghani S, Kang J, Saindane AM. Improved quality and diagnostic confidence achieved by use of dose-reduced gadolinium blood-pool agents for time-resolved intracranial MR angiography. AJNR Am J Neuroradiol 2014;35(3):450–6.

30. Petkova M, Gauvrit JY, Trystram D, et al. Three-dimensional dynamic time-resolved contrast-enhanced MRA using parallel imaging and a variable rate k-space sampling strategy in intracranial arteriovenous malformations. J Magn Reson Imaging 2009;29:7–12.

31. Saindane AM, Boddu SR, Tong FC, et al. Contrast-enhanced time-resolved MRA for pre-angiographic evaluation of suspected spinal dural arterial venous fistulas. J Neurointervent Surg 2015;7:135–40.

32. Boddu SR, Tong FC, Dehkharghani S, et al. Contrast-enhanced time-resolved MRA for follow-up of intracranial aneurysms treated with the pipeline embolization device. AJNR Am J Neuroradiol 2014;35(11):2112–8.

33. Bradley WG, Daroff RB, Fenichel GM, et al, editors. Neurology in clinical practice: principles of diagnosis and management. 4th edition. Philadelphia: Elsevier; 2006. p. 306–9.

34. McGirt MJ, Nimjee SM, Fuchs HE, et al. Relationship of cine phase-contrast magnetic resonance imaging with outcome after decompression for Chiari I malformations. Neurosurgery 2006;59: 140–6.

35. Battal B, Kocaoglu M, Bulakbasi N, et al. Cerebrospinal fluid flow imaging by using phase-contrast MR technique. Br J Radiol 2011;84(1004):758–65.

36. Law M, Yang S, Wang H, et al. Glioma grading: sensitivity, specificity, and predictive values of perfusion MR imaging and proton MR spectroscopic imaging compared with conventional MR imaging. AJNR Am J Neuroradiol 2003;24:1989–98.

37. Cha S, Knopp EA, Johnson G, et al. Intracranial mass lesions: dynamic contrast-enhanced susceptibility-weighted echo-planar perfusion MR imaging. Radiology 2002;223:11–29.

38. Sugahara T, Korogi Y, Tomiguchi S, et al. Posttherapeutic intraaxial brain tumor: the value of perfusion-sensitive contrast-enhanced MR imaging for differentiating tumor recurrence from nonneoplastic contrast-enhancing tissue. AJNR Am J Neuroradiol 2000;21:901–9.

39. Gahramanov S, Raslan AM, Muldoon LL, et al. Potential for differentiation of pseudoprogression from true tumor progression with dynamic susceptibility-weighted contrast-enhanced magnetic resonance imaging using ferumoxytol vs gadoteridol: a pilot study. Int J Radiat Oncol Biol Phys 2011;79:514–23.

40. Detre JA, Rao H, Wang DJ, et al. Applications of arterial spin labeled MRI in the brain. J Magn Reson Imaging 2012;35(5):1026–37.

41. Oguz KK, Golay X, Pizzini FB, et al. Sickle cell disease: continuous arterial spin-labeling perfusion MR imaging in children. Radiology 2003;227(2): 567–74.

42. Ances BM, McGarvey ML, Abrahams JM, et al. Continuous arterial spin labeled perfusion magnetic resonance imaging in patients before and after carotid endarterectomy. J Neuroimaging 2004;14(2): 133–8.

43. Detre JA, Samuels OB, Alsop DC, et al. Noninvasive MRI evaluation of CBF with acetazolamide challenge in patients with cerebrovascular stenosis. J Magn Reson Imaging 1999;10:870–5.

44. Oz G, Alger JR, Barker PB, et al, the MRS Consensus Group. Clinical proton MR spectroscopy in central nervous system disorders. Radiology 2014;270(3):658–79.

45. van der Knaap MS, Pouwels PJ. Magnetic resonance spectroscopy: basic principles and application in white matter disorders. In: van der Knaap MS, Valk J, editors. Magnetic resonance of myelination and myelin disorders. 3rd edition. Berlin: Springer; 2005. p. 859–80.

46. Juli-Sap M, Coronel I, Majos C, et al. Prospective diagnostic performance evaluation of single-voxel 1H MRS for typing and grading of brain tumours. NMR Biomed 2012;25(4):661–73.

47. Poptani H, Gupta RK, Roy R, et al. Characterization of intracranial mass lesions with in vivo proton MR spectroscopy. AJNR Am J Neuroradiol 1995;16(8): 1593–603.

48. Matsusue E, Fink JR, Rockhill JK, et al. Distinction between gliomas progression and post-radiation change by combined physiologic MR imaging. Neuroradiology 2010;52(4):297–306.

49. de Carvalho Rangel C, Hygino Cruz LC Jr, Takayassu TC, et al. Diffusion MR imaging in central nervous system. Magn Reson Imaging Clin N Am 2011;19(1):23–53.

50. Gonzalez RG, Schaefer PW, Buonanno FS, et al. Diffusion-weighted MR imaging: diagnostic accuracy in patients imaged within 6 hours of stroke symptom onset. Radiology 1999;210:155–62.

51. Schlaug G, Siewert B, Benfield A, et al. Time course of the apparent diffusion coefficient (ADC) abnormality in human stroke. Neurology 1997;49:113–9.

52. Tsuruda J, Chew W, Moseley M, et al. Diffusion-weighted MR imaging of the brain: value of differentiating between extra-axial cysts and epidermoid tumors. AJNR Am J Neuroradiol 1990;11:925–31.

53. Ebisu T, Tanaka C, Umeda M, et al. Discrimination of brain abscess from necrotic or cystic tumors by diffusion-weighted echo planar imaging. Magn Reson Imaging 1996;14:1113–6.

54. Finkenstaedt M, Szudra A, Zerr I, et al. MR imaging of Creutzfeldt-Jakob disease. Radiology 1996;199: 793–8.

55. Tanenbaum LN. Clinical applications of diffusion imaging in the spine. Magn Reson Imaging Clin N Am 2013;21(2):299–320.

56. Conturo TE, Lori NF, Cull TS, et al. Tracking neuronal fiber pathways in the living human brain. Proc Natl Acad Sci U S A 1999;96:10422–7.

57. Wu JS, Zhou LF, Tang WJ, et al. Clinical evaluation and follow-up outcome of diffusion tensor imaging-based functional neuronavigation: a prospective, controlled study in patients with gliomas involving pyramidal tracts. Neurosurgery 2007;61:935–49.

58. Sunaert S. Presurgical planning for tumour resectioning. J Magn Reson Imaging 2006;23:887–905.

59. Majos A, Tybor K, Stefanczyk L, et al. Cortical mapping by functional magnetic resonance imaging in patients with brain tumors. Eur J Radiol 2005;15: 1148–58.

60. Spena G, Nava A, Cassini F, et al. Preoperative and intraoperative brain mapping for the resection of eloquent-area tumours. A prospective analysis of methodology, correlation, and usefulness based on clinical outcomes. Acta Neurochir 2010;152: 1835–46.

61. Chen CM, Hou BL, Holodny AI. Effect of age and tumor grade on BOLD functional MR imaging in preoperative assessment of patients with glioma. Radiology 2008;3:971–8.

62. Binder JR. Functional MRI is a valid noninvasive alternative to Wada testing. Epilepsy Behav 2011; 20(2):214–22.

Perfusion Imaging in Neuro-Oncology
Basic Techniques and Clinical Applications

Brent Griffith, MD[a],*, Rajan Jain, MD[b]

KEYWORDS

- MR perfusion • CT perfusion • DCE-T1 • DSC-T2* • ASL • Cerebral blood volume

KEY POINTS

- Perfusion imaging allows for assessment of changes occurring at the tumor microvasculature level.
- Perfusion-based parameters have the potential to serve as important quantitative imaging biomarkers, providing information not routinely available with standard morphologic imaging.
- Perfusion imaging is increasingly used for neuro-oncologic applications, including brain tumor grading, directing biopsies or targeted therapy, and evaluation of treatment response and disease progression.
- Perfusion-based quantitative biomarkers, when used in conjunction with standard morphologic imaging, have the potential to provide early indication of treatment failure or treatment response.
- Increased use of perfusion MR in the routine surveillance imaging of brain tumors allows for evaluation of relative cerebral blood volume (rCBV) trends, which may bolster its effectiveness as an imaging biomarker.

WHAT IS PERFUSION IMAGING?

Perfusion imaging is a method for assessing the flow of blood occurring at the tissue level.[1] Depending on the modality (eg, MR, CT) and method (eg, dynamic contrast enhanced [DCE], arterial spin labeled) used, several perfusion parameters can be evaluated, both qualitatively and quantitatively. These parameters include those related to the volume of blood within a given region of tissue, as well as those describing the movement of blood through that region over time. In addition to assessing blood volume and flow, these techniques also allow for the quantitative assessment of vessel leakiness through the measurement of vascular permeability.

WHAT IS MEASURED AND HOW IS IT USED?
Blood Volume and Blood Flow

Blood volume (BV), mean transit time (MTT), and blood flow (BF) are all parameters used to describe the flow of blood within a particular region of tissue.

- BV refers to the total volume of blood flowing within a given area of tissue and is measured in milliliters of blood per 100 g of tissue (mL/100 g).
- BF refers to the volume of blood flowing within a given area of tissue per unit time and is measured in milliliters of blood per 100 g of tissue per minute (mL/100 g/min).
- MTT refers to the average time blood takes to traverse through a given area of tissue and is measured in seconds (s).

Measuring the volume and flow of blood in a particular region of brain can have important clinical implications. In the setting of acute ischemia, measurement of CBV, MTT, and CBF helps in differentiating the "core" of irreversibly infarcted brain tissue from the ischemic, but potentially salvageable, brain tissue (ie, penumbra).[1] Similarly, CBV

[a] Department of Radiology, Henry Ford Health System, Detroit, MI, USA; [b] NYU School of Medicine, NYU Langone Medical Center, New York, NY, USA
* Corresponding author.
E-mail address: brentg@rad.hfh.edu

Radiol Clin N Am 53 (2015) 497–511
http://dx.doi.org/10.1016/j.rcl.2015.01.004
0033-8389/15/$ – see front matter © 2015 Elsevier Inc. All rights reserved.

has also been used successfully to identify patients with hemodynamic impairment in the setting of major arterial occlusive disease,[2] as well as in evaluating cerebrovascular reserve in patients with Moya-Moya.[3] In addition, assessment of CBV has been used extensively in neuro-oncologic applications, including for brain tumor grading and directing biopsies or targeted therapy, as well as for the evaluation of treatment response and disease progression.[4,5] These neuro-oncologic applications of perfusion imaging are the focus of this article.

Vessel Permeability

In addition to parameters describing the volume and flow of blood within a particular region of brain, perfusion imaging also allows for assessment of vessel permeability. This is particularly important for applications involving the brain, given the role of the blood–brain barrier (BBB), which serves as a physical barrier to the entry of lipophobic substances into the brain and can be disrupted by a number of disease processes, including brain tumors. This breakdown of the BBB, which accounts for the contrast enhancement seen on standard imaging, also provides a potential surrogate imaging marker. Various methods have been developed to quantify this vessel "leakiness," most notably by measurement of the permeability surface-area product (PS), which characterizes the diffusion of contrast agent from the blood vessels into the interstitial space, or by the transfer constant (K_{trans}).[6]

METHODS
CT Perfusion

CT perfusion (CTP) allows for the assessment of CBV and permeability with a single acquisition. The greatest advantage of CT perfusion is the linear relationship between iodine concentration and attenuation on CT. This easy conversion allows for a direct measurement of vascular parameters.

CTP protocols vary depending on the manufacturer and scanner model used, as well as depending on the reason for the examination (eg, tumor volume protocol vs acute stroke imaging). However, as a general concept, CTP is based on the principle of sequential acquisition of CT images during the washin and washout of iodinated contrast material from brain parenchyma (Fig. 1)[7] with the goal being to observe the distribution of contrast agent within tissues over time.

How Is It Done?

- Before obtaining the perfusion scan, a low radiation dose noncontrast CT head study can be performed.

- For the perfusion scan at our institution, 50 mL of nonionic contrast is injected at a rate of 4 to 5 mL/s through an intravenous line using an automatic power injector.
- A cine scan is then initiated at 5 seconds into the injection, using the following parameters: 80 kV (peak), 100 to 120 mÅ, and 1 second per rotation for a duration of 50 seconds. After the initial 50-s cine scan, 8 additional axial images are acquired, 1 image every 15 seconds for an additional 2 minutes, resulting in a total acquisition time of 170 seconds to assess delayed permeability.[8]
- Perfusion maps can then be obtained through the use of a number of commercially available software applications with the superior sagittal sinus generally used as the venous output function and the artery with the greatest peak and slope on the time–attenuation curves as the arterial input function.[8]

MR Perfusion

The measurement of vascular parameters with MR perfusion can be accomplished with both contrast-enhanced and non–contrast-enhanced (arterial spin labeling [ASL]) techniques. Dynamic contrast-enhanced MRI utilizes 2 techniques—a T1-weighted acquisition (DCE MR) and a T2*-based acquisition (DSC MR). Although the methods used by these techniques in quantifying cerebral perfusion differ, both rely on a trace of contrast agent concentration over time to estimate blood volume and permeability.[9] In contrast to these contrast-enhanced methods, evaluation of perfusion with ASL is accomplished through the use of magnetically labeled arterial blood water as a freely diffusible tracer.

In contrast with CT perfusion, which directly images the iodinated contrast agent, contrast agents utilized in MR perfusion are not imaged directly and instead rely on signal intensity to provide an estimate of CBV. However, regardless of the technique used, MR perfusion offers 2 major advantages over CT perfusion. First, MR perfusion requires no radiation, which is very important in oncologic imaging, because patients often require frequent imaging for tumor surveillance. Second, particularly in neuro-oncologic imaging, MR is the standard of care for assessing treatment response or progression of disease. Therefore, the acquisition of perfusion parameters with MR perfusion requires only additional sequences to be obtained rather than an entirely separate examination as in the case of CT perfusion.

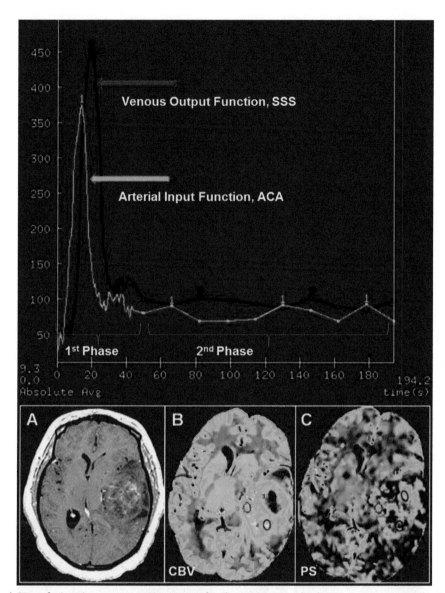

Fig. 1. (*Top*) CT perfusion time concentration curves for the anterior cerebral artery, representing the input artery (*green arrow*) and the superior sagittal sinus, representing the output vein (*red arrow*). (*Bottom row*) Postcontrast axial T1-weighted image shows a heterogeneously enhancing WHO grade III glioma centered in the left temporal region (*A*). CT perfusion maps show regions of interest placed in various regions of the tumor on both the cerebral blood volume map (*B*) and permeability surface area product map (*C*) showing heterogeneous areas of both increased CBV and permeability surface-area product (PS), suggesting a high-grade neoplasm.

Dynamic Contrast Enhanced-T1 Imaging

DCE-T1 imaging is based on the fact that an increase in the concentration of contrast agent results in a proportional increase in the rate of T1 relaxation from which a time–concentration curve can be generated and is tracked over a longer time period (5–10 minutes; **Fig. 2**).

DCE-T1 MR allows characterization of the vascular microenvironment through the measurement of a number of different parameters, including K_{trans} (influx transfer constant), K_b (reverse transfer constant), V_e (volume of the extravascular extracellular space), and V_P (blood plasma volume). The clinical application of these parameters, however, is often limited by the complicated, multicompartment physiologic models required to obtain the quantitative metrics. To improve the clinical utility, model-free "semiquantitative" indices have been developed to assess tissue perfusion.[10] These methods have been used to both assess the shape of the uptake and washout of contrast (ie, curveology), as well as to provide objective indices for

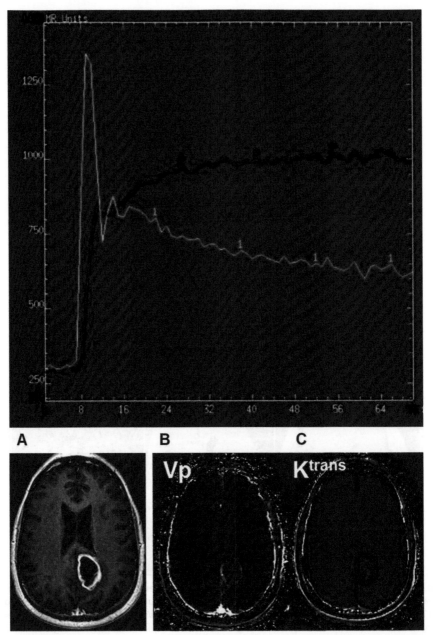

Fig. 2. (*Top*) DCE T1 time concentration curves from the arterial input function (*green*) and the tumor tissue (*red*). (*Bottom Row*) Post-contrast axial T1-weighted image shows a heterogeneously ring enhancing WHO grade IV glioma centered in the left medial occipital lobe (*A*). Plasma volume map (*B*) and K_{trans} map (*C*) showing markedly increased Vp and K_{trans} in the peripheral component of the tumor suggesting a high-grade neoplasm.

evaluation. These indices include maximum slope of enhancement in the initial vascular phase (MSIVP), which assesses change of signal intensity per second; normalized slope of the delayed equilibrium phase (nSDEP), which is the slope of the fitted linear curve to final 25% samples; as well as the initial area under the time–intensity curve (IAUC) at 60 and 120 seconds ($IAUC_{60}$ and $IAUC_{120}$).[10]

How Is It Done?

- At our institution DCE-MRI studies are performed on a 3T MR system using a standard 8-channel phased array radiofrequency (RF) coil and receiver with the following sequence parameters: TE/TR ~ 0.84/5.8 ms; flip angles, θi, of 2, 5, 10, 15, 20, and 25°; asset number = 2; matrix of 256 × 128; field of view, 240 mm; 16 slices of 5 mm; no gap.

- The precontrast T1 maps are used to establish baseline T1 values before the administration of contrast.

Dynamic Susceptibility Contrast T2* Imaging

DSC-T2* MRI is based on rapid imaging of the first pass of gadolinium-based contrast material through the tumor vasculature and utilizes susceptibility weighted imaging to generate a time–concentration curve after contrast administration. The contrast agent results in an initial drop in signal intensity owing to the T2* shortening effects, which in turn leads to loss and then recovery of signal in the tumor bed as the agent is redistributed or diluted (Fig. 3). This drop in signal intensity, also known as "negative enhancement," is proportional to the concentration of the contrast agent. As such, the area under the time concentration curve can be calculated and used to derive the rCBV map, which is the most widely used quantitative variable derived from DSC imaging.[11]

Because the bolus transit time for DSC-T2* imaging is so short, a fast acquisition technique, such as echo planar imaging (EPI) is typically performed, which provides the necessary temporal resolution to adequately characterize the transient drop in signal intensity.[12] Although both spin echo (SE) and gradient echo (GRE) techniques are used, GRE is most commonly used because it has been shown to be more sensitive to broader ranges of vessel size, an important feature when evaluating the morphologically abnormal vessels commonly seen in tumors undergoing neovascularization.[12] This finding is in contrast with the SE technique, which is more sensitive to capillary-sized vessels. The downside, of course, to the use of GRE DSC-MRI technique is its susceptibility to artifacts related to adjacent bony structures, air, or blood products, which is commonly encountered in the setting of brain tumors, particularly in the postoperative follow-up period.

In addition to these limitations related to susceptibility artifacts, DSC-T2* methods are also prone to errors related to contrast leakage, a common problem in high-grade gliomas owing to the leakiness of the BBB owing to significant neovascularization. The leakiness of the vessels, coupled with the use of low-molecular-weight extravascular contrast agents (eg, gadolinium-DTPA), results in rapid extravasation of contrast from the vascular compartment into the interstitium. This leakage results in both enhanced T1 relaxation effects, as well as increased or decreased T2* effects.[12] These effects can either result in overestimation or underestimation of rCBV, depending on the relative magnitude of the T2* or T1 effects, respectively.[12]

How Is It Done?

- At our institution, studies are performed on either a 1.5-T or 3-T MR system. Routine unenhanced MRIs are performed before the perfusion portion of the study.
- Perfusion images are performed during the injection of contrast agent, which is infused via a power injector at a constant rate of 5 mL/s.
- Perfusion images include the acquisition of a series of 95 phases of T2*-weighted GRE-EPI (repetition time ms/echo time ms, 1900/40; flip angle, 90°) with an acquisition matrix of 128 × 128 with a 26-cm field of view and 5-mm section thickness. The temporal resolution is 2.0 s. The number of sections obtained varies according to tumor size with the goal of including the entire tumor in the acquisition.
- T1-weighted contrast-enhanced images are then acquired after the perfusion study.

Arterial Spin Labeling

MR perfusion with ASL utilizes the magnetic labeling of arterial blood water through the use of an RF pulse.[13] After this proton labeling, a period of time referred to as the postlabeling delay is necessary to give the labeled blood time to reach the brain parenchyma.[14] In addition to the labeled images, all ASL techniques require the acquisition of control, or unlabeled, images. The signal remaining after subtraction of the labeled and control images can then be used to provide information regarding the CBF. Owing to the low signal-to-noise ratio between the labeled and control images, multiple control and label image pairs must be obtained.[14]

Different methods are used for labeling arterial water, including continuous ASL (CASL), pseudo-continuous ASL (PCASL), pulsed ASL (PASL), and velocity-selective ASL methods.[15] In CASL, a prolonged RF pulse continuously labels arterial blood water below the imaging slab.[13,14,16] The major advantage of CASL compared with the other labeling methods is its higher perfusion sensitivity.[14,15] The downside, however, to the prolonged RF pulse is 2-fold. First, the prolonged pulse lead to magnetization transfer effects that, if not appropriately balanced in the control acquisition, can lead to overestimation of perfusion.[13,16] In addition, these prolonged RF pulses result in greater energy deposition to the patient, which can exceed US Food and Drug Administration guidelines.[14,15] Finally, continuous RF transmit hardware is not available commonly on commercial MR scanners, which limits its widespread application in clinical practice.[14] In contrast with CASL, PASL utilizes a short RF pulse to label a thick slab of arterial blood at a single point in

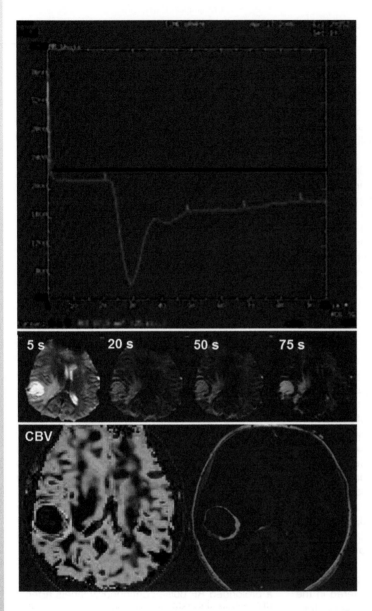

Fig. 3. (*Top*) Time concentration curve for a dynamic susceptibility contrast (DSC) T2* MR demonstrating the initial drop in signal intensity owing to the T2* shortening effects, which leads to signal loss and then recovery of signal as the contrast agent is redistributed (*green curve*). (*Second row*) Serial axial gradient echo images showing progressive signal drop through the brain as well as peripheral part of a necrotic tumor in right cerebral hemisphere, which was proven to be a GBM. (*Third row*) Cerebral blood volume map shows increased blood volume (*left*) corresponding with the enhancing rim of the tumor shown on the axial post-contrast T1-weighted image (*right*), suggesting a high-grade neoplasm.

time.[14,16] There are various methods of PASL differing in the labeling plane location and magnetic state of the labeled blood; however, this is beyond the scope of this article.[14] Whereas PASL offers a high labeling efficiency with lesser RF power deposition, its perfusion sensitivity is less when compared with CASL.[14] The third technique to discuss briefly is PCASL, which mimics CASL through the use of a train of RF pulses in addition to a synchronous gradient field.[14] PCASL offers high inversion efficiency, but with reduced magnetization transfer effects and RF power deposition when compared with CASL. Despite these advantages, however, PCASL is susceptible to both B0 inhomogeneity and eddy currents.[14,17]

Finally, once the blood has been labeled appropriately, ASL imaging is performed typically using an EPI technique, allowing for a fast acquisition speed. Unfortunately, as with DSC-T2* perfusion images, EPI is also sensitive to susceptibility artifacts caused by adjacent bony structures, air, or blood products, which are frequently encountered, particularly in neuro-oncologic applications.

Aside from the advantages of the various labeling methods described, in general there are several advantages to using ASL versus other perfusion imaging methods. First, as with contrast-enhanced MR perfusion techniques, ASL requires no radiation and requires only an additional sequence to the standard of care surveillance MRI, which provides important advantages over CT perfusion. Second, contrary to the other perfusion methods described, ASL does not rely on the use of an exogenous tracer, such as iodinated contrast material or gadolinium-based contrast material as is required for CT perfusion and contrast-enhanced MR perfusion techniques, respectively.[15] This is particularly advantageous in patients with chronic renal failure, given concerns regarding nephrogenic systemic fibrosis.[14,16]

CLINICAL UTILITY IN NEURO-ONCOLOGIC IMAGING

Although the regular use of perfusion imaging in oncologic imaging has been a more recent trend, its importance, particularly in the arena of tumor physiology, has been well-recognized for many years. In 1992, Folkman[18] discussed the role of angiogenesis in tumor growth, describing the neovascularization of a tumor as it moves from a prevascular to vascular phase, a phase that has the potential for rapid cell population expansion and a propensity for metastasis. This correlation between neovascularization and increasing aggressiveness of tumors has been well-documented in the brain tumor perfusion literature with both CT and MR perfusion methods, demonstrating a correlation between higher CBVs and permeability in higher grade tumors.[4,19–21]

Tumor Grading

The standard for grading of brain tumors is histopathologic assessment of tissue, for which a variety of classification systems are available, the most common being the World Health Organization (WHO) grading system. However, grading systems based on histopathology are plagued by a number of limitations, particularly sampling error and interobserver variation.[8] This is especially true in the case of gliomas, particularly high-grade gliomas, owing to their significant heterogeneity, which can lead to inaccurate grading and classification.[8]

Both MR and CT perfusion have been successfully used to grade gliomas on the basis of perfusion parameters. Previous studies by Shin and colleagues[21] and Jackson and colleagues[19] found that higher grade tumors demonstrated statistically significant higher mean values than lower grade tumors. By using an rCBV threshold value of 1.75, Law and colleagues[5] were able to differentiate low- and high-grade tumors with a sensitivity of 95% and specificity of 57.5%. In addition, Provenzale and colleagues[20] in 2002 found that permeability values for high-grade tumors obtained using a T2*-weighted method were significantly greater than those for low-grade tumors.

Similar to MR perfusion, CT perfusion has also demonstrated the ability to differentiate low grade and high grade tumors. A 2006 study by Ellika and colleagues[4] found that CT perfusion with a CBV normalized relative to a normal-appearing contralateral white matter threshold of 1.92 was able to differentiate low- and high-grade gliomas with a sensitivity of 85.7% and specificity of 100% (**Fig. 4**). Furthermore, Jain and colleagues[22] showed that in addition to differentiating low- and high-grade gliomas, PS measurements also enabled the differentiation of high-grade tumors into grades III and IV on the basis of PS measurements.

Differentiating Primary Gliomas from Tumefactive Demyelinating Lesions

In addition to tumor grading, perfusion imaging has also shown the ability to differentiate brain tumors from other masslike enhancing lesions, most notably from tumefactive demyelinating lesions (TDLs). TDLs have been described on imaging to demonstrate larger sizes with associated mass effect and edema, as well as atypical enhancement patterns, including ring enhancement.[23] This imaging appearance can make differentiation from primary gliomas, in particular glioblastoma multiforme (GBM), difficult, oftentimes requiring surgical biopsy for definitive diagnosis. However, not only can TDLs mimic an intracranial neoplasm on morphologic imaging, but these lesions can also simulate gliomas on histopathologic examination.[24] Given these similarities, preoperative suspicion of a demyelinating process can be helpful to ensure appropriate management.

One important difference that can be exploited by MR perfusion in differentiating these entities relates to differences in vascularity.[25] Whereas high-grade gliomas demonstrate neoangiogenesis and vascular endothelial proliferation, TDLs are characterized by inflamed vessels with mild inflammatory angiogenesis.[25,26] Given the lack of significant neoangiogenesis seen within TDLs, these lesions have been shown to demonstrate lower PS and CBV when compared with high-grade gliomas on CT perfusion, offering a potential in vivo means of differentiating the 2 entities (**Fig. 5**).[25] Similarly, rCBV measurements on MR perfusion have also

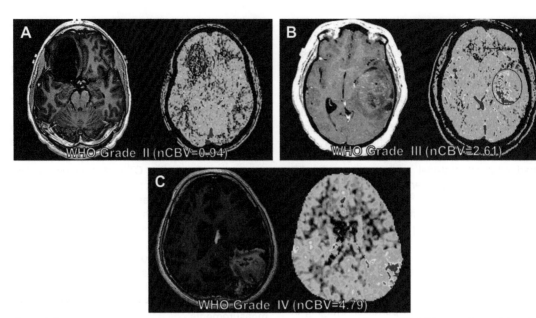

Fig. 4. (A) Postcontrast T1-weighted axial image (*left*) and CT perfusion CBV map (*right*) in a patient with a WHO grade II glioma showing a nonenhancing mass in the right frontal lobe with low CBV (nCBV = 0.94). (B) Postcontrast T1-weighted axial image (*left*) and CT perfusion CBV map (*right*) in a patient with a WHO grade III glioma showing a large, heterogeneously enhancing left temporal mass with significant mass effect and a nCBV of 2.61. (C) Postcontrast T1-weighted axial image (*left*) and CT perfusion CBV map (*right*) in a patient with a WHO grade IV glioma showing an enhancing mass in the left parietal region with very high CBV (nCBV = 4.79). (*From* Ellika S, Jain R, Patel SC, et al. Role of perfusion CT in glioma grading and comparison with conventional MRI features. AJNR Am J Neuroradiol 2007;28(10):1984; with permission.)

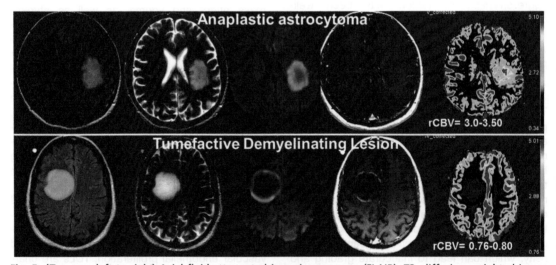

Fig. 5. (*Top row, left to right*) Axial fluid-attenuated inversion recovery (FLAIR), T2, diffusion-weighted image (DWI), T1 postcontrast, and rCBV map demonstrates a T2 FLAIR hyperintense lesion within the left hemispheric white matter, which demonstrates patchy enhancement and bright signal on DWI at its periphery. The lesion demonstrates an rCBV of 3.0 to 3.5, suggestive of a neoplastic process, proven to be a WHO grade III glioma with surgery and histopathology. (*Bottom row, left to right*) Axial FLAIR, T2, DWI, T1 postcontrast, and rCBV map demonstrates a T2 FLAIR hyperintense lesion within the right hemispheric white matter, which also demonstrates peripheral enhancement and bright signal on DWI, almost similar to the neoplasm from upper row. However, DSC T2* perfusion CBV map showing a very low rCBV of 0.76 to 0.80. At biopsy, this neoplasm was found to be a tumefactive demyelinating lesion. (*Courtesy of* Eytan Raz, MD, NYU.)

been shown to successfully discriminate between high-grade gliomas and TDLs,[27] although this differentiation does not extend to grade II/III gliomas, because these both can demonstrate similar level increases in rCBV.[28]

Differentiating Recurrent Tumor Versus Treatment Effects

One of the predominant roles of perfusion imaging in neuro-oncologic imaging is the accurate differentiation of treatment effects and disease progression, which has important implications for patient care, because correct differentiation can result in changes to a patient's treatment regimen.

Identifying disease progression or response by imaging has relied traditionally on measurement of the contrast-enhancing lesion, using either the RECIST or Macdonald criteria. However, brain tumor enhancement depends on the presence and integrity of the BBB, which can be affected by a number of factors other than disease response or progression, including effects related to particular treatments. Examples of this include both processes that can disrupt the BBB, such as postictal changes, postoperative infarcts, or treatment-related inflammatory processes, as well as those that stabilize the BBB, such as steroids or antiangiogenic therapies. The former, which results in disruption of the BBB, leads to increased enhancement, which mimics disease progression and has been termed 'pseudoprogression.' The latter, which improves the integrity of the BBB resulting in decreased enhancement in the absence of any true treatment response, thereby mimicking disease response, has been termed pseudoresponse (Fig. 6).[29,30]

Pseudoprogression

"Pseudoprogression" is the term applied to a treatment-related increase in enhancing lesion size and/or edema without a true increase in tumor burden, which shows either improvement or lack of progression on follow-up imaging. Pseudoprogression generally occurs in the 2- to 6-month period after chemoradiation therapy[31,32] and is believed to result from increased inflammation, edema, and abnormal vessel permeability in the local tissues, which leads to the movement of fluid into the interstitial space and subsequent brain edema.

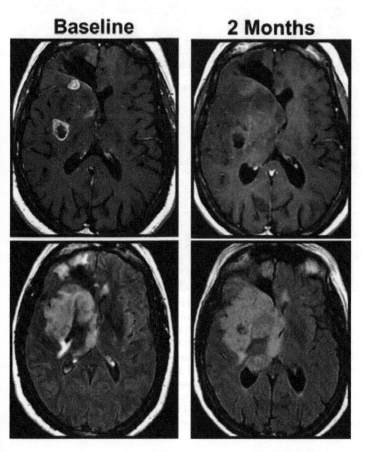

Baseline **2 Months**

Fig. 6. (*Left column*) Baseline axial postcontrast T1-weighted (*top row*) and axial fluid-attenuated inversion recovery (FLAIR) images demonstrate multiple enhancing lesions with surrounding FLAIR hyperintensity in the region of the right basal ganglia. (*Right column*) After treatment with bevacizumab, the 2-month follow-up demonstrates almost complete resolution of the previously seen enhancing lesions, but the degree of FLAIR hyperintensity has increased. This is consistent with a pseudoresponse owing to the addition of the antiangiogenic agent bevacizumab to the treatment regimen.

Differentiation of pseudoprogression from true tumor progression on MRI alone is not possible because both can demonstrate increased enhancement and edema. However, by evaluating changes occurring on the microvasculature level, perfusion imaging provides a potential tool for differentiating these entities.

Compared with recurrent tumor, enhancing lesions caused by treatment effects (eg, pseudoprogression) lack significant neoangiogenesis, which is the hallmark of recurrent tumor. This lack results in a lower microvascular density and lower vessel leakiness, which manifests as lower blood volume and permeability on perfusion imaging.[33,34]

A study by Mangla and associates[34] found that rCBV at 1 month was able to distinguish pseudoprogression from recurrent progressive disease with a sensitivity of 77% and specificity of 86%. A similar study by Young and colleagues[33] found that pseudoprogression demonstrated a lower median rCBV and permeability. In addition, model-free semiquantitative indices have also been used to differentiate recurrent tumor from treatment effects. By assessing the shape of the uptake and washout of the contrast agent, these semiquantitative methods, provide a more objective means of assessment with Jain and colleagues,[35] showing that pseudoprogression

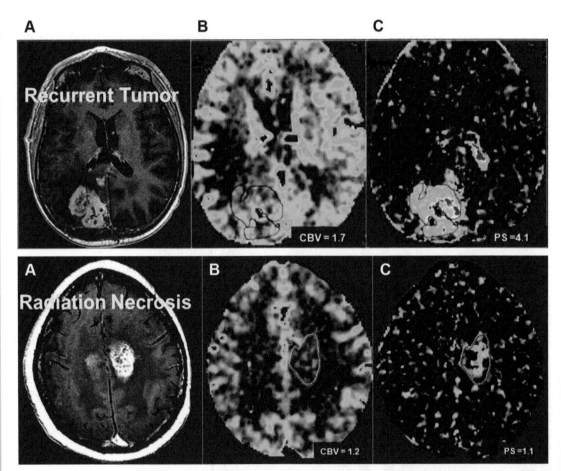

Fig. 7. (*Top row*) A 77-year-old man with initial diagnosis of GBM who underwent gross tumor resection, chemotherapy, and RT (external beam RT, 60 Gy). (*A*) Follow-up MRI shows a recurrent enhancing lesion 26 months after RT in the right parieto-occipital region within the radiation field. (*B, C*) CBV; (*B*) and PS; (*C*) maps show high rCBV and PS, suggesting recurrent progressive tumor, which was confirmed with histopathology. (*Bottom row*) A 41-year-old man with an initial diagnosis of WHO grade II astrocytoma who underwent chemotherapy and RT (intensity modulated RT, 63 Gy). (*A*) Follow-up MRI at 33 months after RT shows development of a recurrent enhancing lesion in the bilateral frontal regions. (*B, C*) CBV (*B*) and PS (*C*) maps show low rCBV and PS, suggesting treatment effects with treatment-induced necrosis suggested by biopsy. (*From* Jain R, Narang J, Schultz L, et al. Permeability estimates in histopathology-proved treatment-induced necrosis using perfusion CT: can these add to other perfusion parameters in differentiating from recurrent/progressive tumors? AJNR Am J Neuroradiol 2011;32:661; with permission.)

demonstrated a lower mean MSIVP, lower nlAUC[60], and higher nSDEP compared with early tumor progression.

Radiation Necrosis

Radiation necrosis is a delayed effect of radiation injury and is reported to occur in approximately 3% to 24% of patients undergoing standard radiation therapy.[36] Generally occurring between 3 and 12 months after radiation therapy, radiation necrosis most commonly occurs at the site of maximum radiation dose, which is usually in the vicinity of the original tumor and surrounding the surgical cavity.[29]

The clinical manifestations of radiation necrosis, including focal neurologic deficits, seizures, and cognitive dysfunction, as well as symptoms related to increased intracranial pressure and mass effect, are difficult to distinguish from tumor progression, which complicates patient management.[31,37] Similarly, the differentiation of radiation necrosis and recurrent tumor on standard morphologic imaging is also difficult, because both occur in close proximity to the original tumor site, enhance on postcontrast imaging, and demonstrate growth over time, surrounding edema, and mass effect.

As with pseudoprogression, both MR and CT perfusion techniques have shown promise in differentiating delayed radiation necrosis from tumor progression. The most commonly used parameter in this differentiation is relative cerebral blood volume (rCBV), which has been shown to be

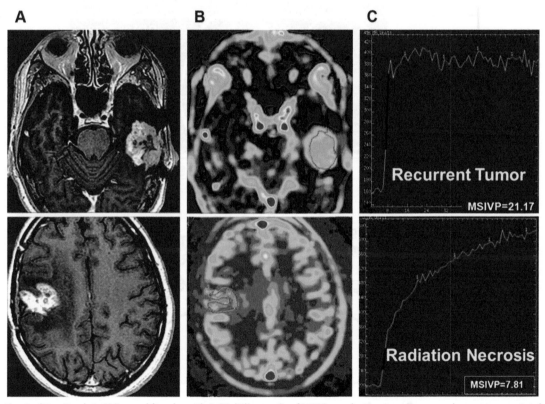

A   **B**   **C**

Recurrent Tumor

MSIVP=21.17

Radiation Necrosis

MSIVP=7.81

Fig. 8. (*Top Row*) A 40-year-old male with initial diagnosis of WHO grade III astrocytoma underwent gross total resection and received chemotherapy and external-beam radiotherapy (54 Gy). (*A*) Follow-up MRI showed appearance of a recurrent enhancing lesion 19 months postradiotherapy in the right temporal region within the radiation field. (*B*) Maximum slope of enhancement in initial vascular phase (MSIVP) parametric map and (*C*) graph of MSIVP showed high MSIVP, suggesting recurrent/progressive tumor (RPT), which was confirmed by histopathology. (*Bottom Row*) A 19-year-old female with initial diagnosis of GBM underwent chemotherapy and external beam radiotherapy (60 Gy). (*A*) Twelve months after radiotherapy, follow-up MRI showed development of a recurrent enhancing lesion in left parietal region. (*B*) Maximum slope of enhancement in the initial vascular phase (MSIVP) parametric map and (*C*) graph of MSIVP showed low MSIVP, suggesting treatment-induced necrosis, which was confirmed by histopathology. (*From* Narang J, Jain R, Arbab AS, et al. Differentiating treatment-induced necrosis from recurrent/progressive brain tumor using non–model-based semiquantitative indices derived from dynamic contrast-enhanced T1-weighted MR perfusion. Neuro Oncol 2011;13(9):1043; with permission.)

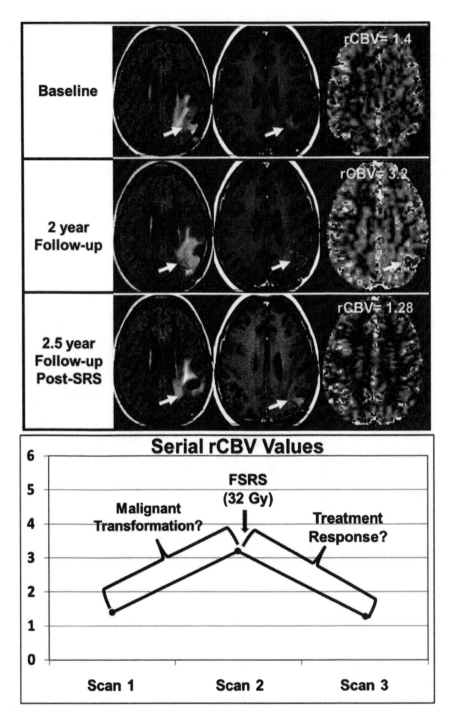

Fig. 9. A 35-year-old female with WHO grade III glioma, previously treated with radiation and temozolomide. Axial T2 FLAIR (*left*), axial T1 postcontrast (*middle*), and rCBV maps (*right*) show interval development of a T2 hyperintense, but predominantly nonenhancing lesion (*arrow*) at the posterior aspect of the surgical resection cavity on the 2-year follow-up study (*middle row*) with mean rCBV of 3.2 compared with 1.4 on the initial follow-up scan (*top row*). Based on an increase in CBV in the follow-up study compared with baseline, the patient underwent additional fractionated stereotactic radiosurgery (FSRS); 32 Gy) to the hot spot using perfusion maps for FSRS planning. At 6 months after FSRS, follow-up imaging (*bottom row*) shows slight improvement in the FLAIR signal, but more importantly marked reduction in rCBV (rCBV = 1.28), suggesting treatment response. A line graph demonstrates nicely this initial increase in rCBV suspicious for recurrent disease followed by a decrease after additional FSRS suggesting treatment response.

increased in the setting of recurrent tumor, whereas it is reduced in the setting of radiation necrosis.[38–40] Estimation of vascular leakiness (K_{trans} with MR perfusion or PS with CT perfusion) has also been used to differentiate tumor progression from treatment effects (eg, radiation necrosis; Fig. 7), because blood vessels within previously irradiated tissues tend to maintain an intact BBB versus the leaky BBB seen in recurrent tumor with neoangiogenesis, therefore demonstrating a lower K_{trans}.[41] Similarly, as is the case with pseudoprogression, radiation necrosis and recurrent tumor can also be differentiated using semiquantitative indices with recurrent tumor showing higher MSIVP (Fig. 8), nMSIVP, nIAUC$_{60}$, and nIAUC$_{120}$.

Tumor Surveillance

In an attempt to improve accurate tumor surveillance, the Response Assessment in Neuro-Oncology (RANO) working group recently developed new standardized response criteria for clinical trials in brain tumors. In addition to taking into account clinical factors such as patient clinical status and use of steroid, the updated criteria also added assessment of the nonenhancing portion of the tumor based on FLAIR/T2 imaging to assist in the differentiation of pseudoresponse from true treatment response after treatment with antiangiogenic agents.[42] However, although standard imaging provides insight into the gross morphologic changes occurring within and surrounding the tumor, it fails to provide an accurate assessment of the tumor physiology, vascularity, and metabolism.

Perfusion-based quantitative biomarkers, on the other hand, have the potential, when used in conjunction with standard morphologic imaging, to provide early indication of treatment failure or treatment response, which may allow clinicians to either switch a treatment that is not working, or to continue a treatment that may be effective. However, although perfusion imaging has become an important adjunct technique for tumor surveillance in many neuro-oncologic practices, its use at a single time-point limits its effectiveness as an imaging biomarker. One issue in particular has been the difficulty in establishing a definitive cutoff value for effectively distinguishing treatment effects from tumor progression when a new enhancing lesion in identified on follow-up imaging. A potential means to work around this limitation is through the rCBV trends, with a progressively increasing rCBV suggesting tumor progression (Fig. 9) and decreasing rCBV, suggesting treatment effects (Fig. 10). Evaluating rCBV trends has become possible recently with the increased use of perfusion MR in the routine follow-up imaging of brain tumors.

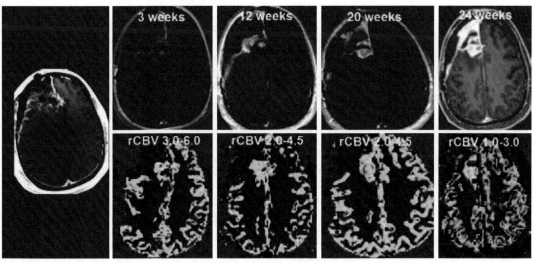

Fig. 10. (*Far left column*) Immediate postoperative axial T1-weighted postcontrast image shows a right frontal resection cavity with residual enhancing resection margins for a GBM. (*Columns 2–4*) Axial T1-weighted postcontrast images redemonstrate the right frontal resection cavity with a progressively increasing focus of nodular enhancement along the posterior aspect of the cavity from the 3 week follow-up scan to the 24 week follow-up scan. However, concurrent rCBV values progressively decreased from a mean of 4.5 at 3 weeks to a mean of 2.0 at 24 weeks. The patient underwent a second surgery and histopathology showed predominantly treatment induced necrosis with no viable tumor.

REFERENCES

1. Konstas AA, Goldmakher GV, Lee TY, et al. Theoretic basis and technical implementations of CT perfusion in acute ischemic stroke, part 1: theoretic basis. AJNR Am J Neuroradiol 2009;30(4):662–8.

2. Endo H, Inoue T, Ogasawara K, et al. Quantitative assessment of cerebral hemodynamics using perfusion-weighted MRI in patients with major cerebral artery occlusive disease: comparison with positron emission tomography. Stroke 2006;37(2):388–92.

3. Rim NJ, Kim HS, Shin YS, et al. Which CT perfusion parameter best reflects cerebrovascular reserve? Correlation of acetazolamide-challenged CT perfusion with single-photon emission CT in Moyamoya patients. AJNR Am J Neuroradiol 2008;29(9):1658–63.

4. Ellika SK, Jain R, Patel SC, et al. Role of perfusion CT in glioma grading and comparison with conventional MR imaging features. AJNR Am J Neuroradiol 2007;28(10):1981–7.

5. Law M, Yang S, Wang H, et al. Glioma grading: sensitivity, specificity, and predictive values of perfusion MR imaging and proton MR spectroscopic imaging compared with conventional MR imaging. AJNR Am J Neuroradiol 2003;24(10):1989–98.

6. Jain R, Griffith B, Narang J, et al. Blood-brain-barrier imaging in brain tumors: concepts and methods. Neurographics 2012;2(2):48–59.

7. Huang AP, Tsai JC, Kuo LT, et al. Clinical application of perfusion computed tomography in neurosurgery. J Neurosurg 2014;120(2):473–88.

8. Jain R. Perfusion CT imaging of brain tumors: an overview. AJNR Am J Neuroradiol 2011;32(9):1570–7.

9. Jain R. Measurements of tumor vascular leakiness using DCE in brain tumors: clinical applications. NMR Biomed 2013;26(8):1042–9.

10. Narang J, Jain R, Scarpace L, et al. Tumor vascular leakiness and blood volume estimates in oligodendrogliomas using perfusion CT: an analysis of perfusion parameters helping further characterize genetic subtypes as well as differentiate from astroglial tumors. J Neurooncol 2011;102(2):287–93.

11. Shiroishi MS, S Lacerda, Tang X, et al. Physical principles of MR perfusion and permeability imaging: gadolinium bolus technique, in functional neuroradiology: principles and clinical applications. In: Faro S, Mohamed FB, Yannes M, et al, editors. 2011.

12. Shiroishi MS, Castellazzi G, Boxerman JL, et al. Principles of T2*-weighted dynamic susceptibility contrast MRI technique in brain tumor imaging. J Magn Reson Imaging 2015;41:296–313.

13. Wolf RL, Detre JA. Clinical neuroimaging using arterial spin-labeled perfusion magnetic resonance imaging. Neurotherapeutics 2007;4(3):346–59.

14. Pollock JM, Tan H, Kraft RA, et al. Arterial spin-labeled MR perfusion imaging: clinical applications. Magn Reson Imaging Clin N Am 2009;17(2):315–38.

15. Watts JM, Whitlow CT, Maldjian JA. Clinical applications of arterial spin labeling. NMR Biomed 2013;26(8):892–900.

16. Essig M, Shiroishi MS, Nguyen TB, et al. Perfusion MRI: the five most frequently asked technical questions. AJR Am J Roentgenol 2013;200(1):24–34.

17. Wu WC, Fernández-Seara M, Detre JA, et al. A theoretical and experimental investigation of the tagging efficiency of pseudocontinuous arterial spin labeling. Magn Reson Med 2007;58(5):1020–7.

18. Folkman J. The role of angiogenesis in tumor growth. Semin Cancer Biol 1992;3(2):65–71.

19. Jackson A, Kassner A, Annesley-Williams D, et al. Abnormalities in the recirculation phase of contrast agent bolus passage in cerebral gliomas: comparison with relative blood volume and tumor grade. AJNR Am J Neuroradiol 2002;23(1):7–14.

20. Provenzale J, Wang GR, Brenner T, et al. Comparison of permeability in high-grade and low-grade brain tumors using dynamic susceptibility contrast MR imaging. AJR Am J Roentgenol 2002;178(3):711–6.

21. Shin JH, Lee HK, Kwun BD, et al. Using relative cerebral blood flow and volume to evaluate the histopathologic grade of cerebral gliomas: preliminary results. AJR Am J Roentgenol 2002;179(3):783–9.

22. Jain R, Ellika SK, Scarpace L, et al. Quantitative estimation of permeability surface-area product in astroglial brain tumors using perfusion CT and correlation with histopathologic grade. AJNR Am J Neuroradiol 2008;29(4):694–700.

23. Lucchinetti CF, Gavrilova RH, Metz I, et al. Clinical and radiographic spectrum of pathologically confirmed tumefactive multiple sclerosis. Brain 2008;131(Pt 7):1759–75.

24. Sugita Y, Terasaki M, Shigemori M, et al. Acute focal demyelinating disease simulating brain tumors: histopathologic guidelines for an accurate diagnosis. Neuropathology 2001;21(1):25–31.

25. Jain R, Ellika S, Lehman NL, et al. Can permeability measurements add to blood volume measurements in differentiating tumefactive demyelinating lesions from high grade gliomas using perfusion CT? J Neurooncol 2010;97(3):383–8.

26. Essig M, Nguyen TB, Shiroishi MS, et al. Perfusion MRI: the five most frequently asked clinical questions. AJR Am J Roentgenol 2013;201(3):W495–510.

27. Hourani R, Brant LJ, Rizk T, et al. Can proton MR spectroscopic and perfusion imaging differentiate between neoplastic and nonneoplastic brain lesions in adults? AJNR Am J Neuroradiol 2008;29(2):366–72.

28. Blasel S, Pfeilschifter W, Jansen V, et al. Metabolism and regional cerebral blood volume in autoimmune

inflammatory demyelinating lesions mimicking malignant gliomas. J Neurol 2011;258(1):113–22.

29. Clarke JL, Chang S. Pseudoprogression and pseudoresponse: challenges in brain tumor imaging. Curr Neurol Neurosci Rep 2009;9(3):241–6.

30. Vogelbaum MA, Jost S, Aghi MK, et al. Application of novel response/progression measures for surgically delivered therapies for gliomas: Response Assessment in Neuro-Oncology (RANO) Working Group. Neurosurgery 2012;70(1):234–43 [discussion: 243–4].

31. Sundgren PC, Cao Y. Brain irradiation: effects on normal brain parenchyma and radiation injury. Neuroimaging Clin N Am 2009;19(4):657–68.

32. Rabin BM, Meyer JR, Berlin JW. Radiation-induced changes in the central nervous system and head and neck. Radiographics 1996;16:1055–72.

33. Young RJ, Gupta A, Shah AD, et al. MRI perfusion in determining pseudoprogression in patients with glioblastoma. Clin Imaging 2013;37(1):41–9.

34. Mangla R, Singh G, Ziegelitz D, et al. Changes in relative cerebral blood volume 1 month after radiation-temozolomide therapy can help predict overall survival in patients with glioblastoma. Radiology 2010;256(2):575–84.

35. Jain R, Narang J, Arbab AS, et al. Role of non-model-based semi-quantitative indices obtained from DCE T1 MR Perfusion in differentiating pseudo-progression from true-progression [meeting abstract]. Neuro Oncol 2011;13:140.

36. Kim JH, Brown SL, Jenrow KA, et al. Mechanisms of radiation-induced brain toxicity and implications for future clinical trials. J Neurooncol 2008;87(3):279–86.

37. Giglio P, Gilbert MR. Cerebral radiation necrosis. Neurologist 2003;9(4):180–8.

38. Hu LS, Baxter LC, Smith KA, et al. Relative cerebral blood volume values to differentiate high-grade glioma recurrence from posttreatment radiation effect: direct correlation between image-guided tissue histopathology and localized dynamic susceptibility-weighted contrast-enhanced perfusion MR imaging measurements. AJNR Am J Neuroradiol 2009;30(3):552–8.

39. Cha S, Lupo JM, Chen MH, et al. Differentiation of glioblastoma multiforme and single brain metastasis by peak height and percentage of signal intensity recovery derived from dynamic susceptibility-weighted contrast-enhanced perfusion MR imaging. AJNR Am J Neuroradiol 2007;28(6):1078–84.

40. Barajas RF, Chang JS, Sneed PK, et al. Distinguishing recurrent intra-axial metastatic tumor from radiation necrosis following gamma knife radiosurgery using dynamic susceptibility-weighted contrast-enhanced perfusion MR imaging. AJNR Am J Neuroradiol 2009;30(2):367–72.

41. Cao Y, Tsien CI, Shen Z, et al. Use of magnetic resonance imaging to assess blood-brain/blood-glioma barrier opening during conformal radiotherapy. J Clin Oncol 2005;23(18):4127–36.

42. Wen PY, Macdonald DR, Reardon DA, et al. Updated response assessment criteria for high-grade gliomas: response assessment in neuro-oncology working group. J Clin Oncol 2010;28(11):1963–72.

Focus on Advanced Magnetic Resonance Techniques in Clinical Practice

Magnetic Resonance Neurography

Elizabeth L. Carpenter, MD*, Jenny T. Bencardino, MD

KEYWORDS

• MR imaging • Neurography • Upper extremity • Lower extremity

KEY POINTS

- Magnetic resonance neurography (MRN) provides the greatest degree of soft tissue contrast in the evaluation of peripheral nerves.
- Utilization of MRN relies on (1) peripheral nerve anatomy, (2) the spectrum of pathology, and (3) familiarity with dedicated MR imaging techniques.
- Although there remain several pitfalls in MRN imaging, awareness of these pitfalls improves imaging quality and limits misinterpretation.

INTRODUCTION

There has been significant development in the field of MRN imaging techniques since its initial description in rabbit forelimbs.[1] Expansion of this technique for human use occurred in 1993, and, to date, its utility is ever expanding.[2]

The strength of MRN rests on that in comparison with any other imaging technique, it provides the greatest degree of soft tissue contrast in the evaluation of peripheral nerves. As such, it allows for optimal evaluation of peripheral nerve morphology and alterations in nerve caliber and signal as well as location-specific detection of nerve compression due to anatomic variations or space-occupying lesions. Additionally, MRN provides exceptional assessment of regional muscle and nerve anatomy, which allows for elucidation of systemic versus local pathology. Furthermore, MRN provides radiologists with the ability to generate high-resolution, 3-D images, which have proved useful for preoperative assessment and planning.

Utilization of MRN in the evaluation of the peripheral nervous system relies on 3 facets of knowledge: (1) peripheral nerve anatomy, (2) the spectrum of pathology, and (3) familiarity with dedicated MR imaging techniques.[3]

PERIPHERAL NERVE ANATOMY

Evaluation of the peripheral nervous system through MRN allows for visualization of sub–5-mm peripheral nerves.[4] The nerves are typically symmetric in size bilaterally, gradually decrease in caliber from proximal to distal, and are similar in size relative to their adjacent arteries. In addition, delineation of peripheral nerves from adjacent vessels is essential for accurate image interpretation. Peripheral nerves generally follow a straight course, do not branch, and should not exhibit flow voids. Familiarity with the basic structure of the nerve unit is also essential for image interpretation, where an individual nerve is often likened to an insulated cable: nerves are comprised of multiple axons, which are grouped together into fascicles. At the deepest level, each axon is surrounded by endoneurium, whereas individual

The authors have nothing to disclose.

Department of Radiology, New York University Hospital for Joint Diseases, 301 East 17th Street, 6th Floor, New York, NY 10003, USA

* Corresponding author.

E-mail address: elizabeth.carpenter@alumni.med.nyu.edu

Radiol Clin N Am 53 (2015) 513–529

http://dx.doi.org/10.1016/j.rcl.2014.12.002

fascicles are surrounded by perineurium and groups of fascicles are surrounded by epineurium.

Understanding this compartmentalization of the nerve unit is important for imaging because it allows for detection of nerve pathology. Similar to the brain, fluid bathing each axon and fascicle allows for optimal transmission of electrical impulses and accounts for approximately 70% of peripheral nerve water content.[5,6] The flow of this fluid is regulated by the endoneurium and perineurium, which act together to form a functional, relatively impermeable barrier known as the blood-nerve interface (BNI).

Similar to the blood-brain barrier, the ability of the BNI to regulate the endoneurial microenvironment protects the peripheral nervous system. Like the brain, the endoneurial space lacks a lymphatic system and is regulated according to hydrostatic pressure mechanisms. In this way, how hydrostatic pressure within the endoneurial fluid increases after trauma can be understood, and, therefore, these changes in the microenvironment through MR imaging can be identified.

NERVE INJURY: PATHOPHYSIOLOGY AND CLASSIFICATION
Technical Considerations

The magnet
Performing MRN at 3T is preferable compared with 1.5T due to the improved signal-to-noise ratio (SNR), which allows for thinner slices, greater contrast, and overall better spatial resolution. Furthermore, there is also less magnetic field inhomogeneity at 3T, which provides for better, more uniform fat suppression and thus greater conspicuity of fluid signal. Additionally, utilization of specialized phased-array surface coils in conjunction with parallel imaging techniques allows for faster acquisition time. An exception to this general rule includes the performance of MRN in patients with metallic implants and hardware located in the field of view (FOV), where imaging at 1.5T is preferable.

Although SNR is optimized through the use of high-field, 3T imaging, the use of a 3-D acquisition is preferable to a 2-D acquisition. This is in part due to generation of a data set, which is derived from isotropic voxels, thereby allowing for high-resolution 3-D reconstructions in any desired plane. Furthermore, compared with a 2-D acquisition, a 3-D acquisition lacks interslice gaps and limits cross-talk between slices, which can further decrease SNR.[7]

Magnetic resonance protocol
Field of view Determination of the FOV relies on the physician request and the nerve being evaluated. Ideally, the FOV should be kept as small as possible to maintain high-resolution images (Fig. 1). Ideally, patients should also receive correlative electrodiagnostic testing prior to MRN to further narrow the anatomic location of interest.

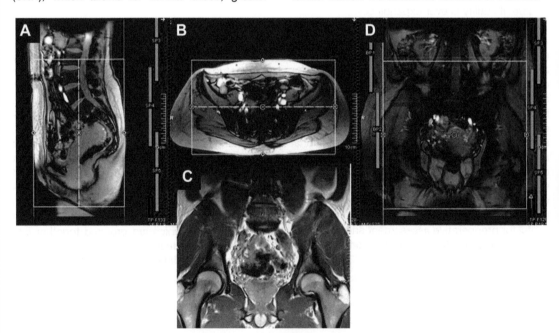

Fig. 1. FOV. Imaging planes for the lumbosacral plexus. (A) Sagittal STIR. (B) Transaxial fast spin-echo proton density. (C) Coronal T1, thin section (4 mm). Superior arrow points to right L3 nerve root. (D) Thin coronal fast spin-echo proton density.

T1-weighted imaging Evaluation of peripheral nerve anatomy is best assessed through use of high-resolution, thin-section (4-mm), T1-weighted (T1W) images. Peripheral nerves can be identified as linear T1-hypointense structures in the expected anatomic location and after an expected course. Delineation of peripheral nerves from their adjacent blood vessels is often possible through analysis of the T1W transaxial images, where adjacent arteries exhibit flow voids and adjacent veins produce T1-hyperintense venous signal due to inflow phenomenon. Furthermore, detection of T1-hyperintense perineural fat surrounding larger peripheral nerves creates a reverse tram-track appearance, a characteristic finding specific to the nerve unit.

T2-weighted imaging Evaluation of edematous changes involving the peripheral nervous system is best assessed through T2-weighted (T2W) sequences, which are sensitive to fluctuations of fluid content in the endoneurial environment. To maximize T2 signal abnormalities, long TEs of approximately 90 to 130 milliseconds are utilized, which also function to minimize the effects of magic angle. Furthermore, radiofrequency saturation pulses are necessary to dull the T2 signal from adjacent vessels. Use of frequency selective or adiabatic inversion recovery fat suppression (SPAIR) allows for assessment of nerve signal

and nerve size as well as fascicle configuration and epineurial thickness. For assessment of peripheral nerves in the upper and lower extremities, SPAIR is generally favored because it provides uniform fat suppression with a better SNR than short tau inversion recovery (STIR).[8]

3-D imaging As discussed previously, the generation of isotropic 3-D images is essential for peripheral nerve evaluation, especially in regard to elucidation of pathologic change for preoperative planning and discussion with referring clinicians. Because peripheral nerves are longitudinally oriented structures, which often follow an oblique course, 3-D images allow for overall assessment of nerve orientation as well as signal changes, which may otherwise be overlooked through analysis of transaxial images alone. For these reasons, the advent of the 3-D–sampling perfection with application-optimized contrasts using different flip angle evolutions (SPACE) sequence (Siemens, Erlangen, Germany) has significantly advanced the value of MRN. This is because the 3-D–SPACE sequence allows for multiplanar reconstructions, consistent projection reconstructions, and maximum intensity projection (MIP) reconstructions through an isotropic single-slab acquisition, whereas retaining optimal SNR and contrast-to-noise ratio (Fig. 2) has significantly advanced the value of MRN. Coapplication of fat-suppression

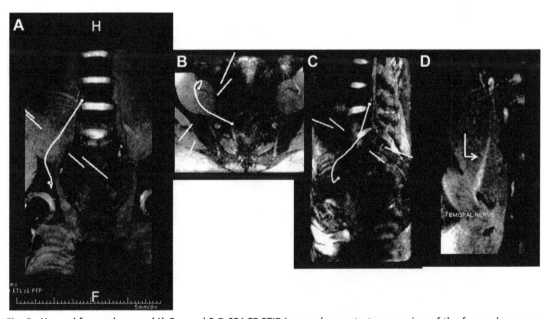

Fig. 2. Normal femoral nerve. (*A*) Coronal 3-D SPACE STIR image demonstrates mapping of the femoral nerve on consecutive overlapped images. (*B*) Transaxial 3-D SPACE STIR image demonstrates mapping of the femoral nerve on consecutive overlapped images. (*C*) Sagittal 3-D SPACE STIR image demonstrates mapping of the femoral nerve on consecutive overlapped images. (*D*) MIP 3-D SPACE STIR demonstrates the normal course of the right femoral nerve (*arrow*).

techniques (SPAIR and STIR) to the SPACE sequence further highlights any T2 signal abnormalities, where SPAIR is preferred for evaluation of the extremities and STIR is preferred for evaluation of the lumbosacral plexus given its more homogeneous performance at large FOV imaging.

Despite the utility of 3-D–SPACE sequences with fat-suppression, frequent contamination from adjacent vessels may confound image interpretation (Fig. 3). This is especially true for smaller peripheral nerves, where the size and signal intensity of the nerve are similar to adjacent vessels. For this reason, the utility of a 3-D sequence, which can suppress signal from blood flow in adjacent vessels, becomes evident. This is the role of the 3-D diffusion-weighted reversed fast imaging with steady state precession sequence (3-D DW-PSIF), which is flow sensitive and allows for generation of nerve-specific images (Fig. 4). The continued investigation into the quantification of water proton diffusion within the nerve itself through diffusion tensor imaging also holds great promise in the functional evaluation of peripheral nerves.[9]

Contrast Gadolinium administration is of limited value in MRN, because normal nerves do not enhance due to the BNI, as described previously. The use of gadolinium contrast, however, may prove advantageous in the identification of soft tissues abnormalities within the nerve, as in diffuse polyneuropathy, or adjacent to the nerve, as in cases of suspected infection or neoplasm.

Pitfalls and technical limitations Although T2 signal changes are predominantly relied on to indicate pathology, there are many nonspecific causes of T2 signal abnormality in MRN. These include nonspecific, spurious T2 hyperintensity along the course of a given nerve, commonly seen in the ulnar nerve in the cubital tunnel. Additional causes include heterogeneous fat suppression as well as magic angle effect. The magic angle effect is due to the orientation of the nerve to the main magnetic field (B_0), and may result in spurious increases in intraneural signal intensity on T1 and proton density sequences. One way to minimize the effects of the magic angle effect is to increase the echo time (TE) to greater than 60 milliseconds.

Although implementation of nerve selective imaging through diffusion weighting is advantageous in that it suppresses the signal from adjacent vessels, it may also result in degraded image quality secondary to inherently reduced SNR. For this reason, a b-value in the range of 80 to 120 mm^2 is most often utilized (Fig. 5).[10] Because 3-D DW-PSIF also provides T2-type contrast, it is useful to avoid confounding artifacts from the bowel and bladder by scheduling the study during fasting (early morning hours) and emptying the bladder prior to the examination (Fig. 6). Patients should also be reminded to remain as still as possible before this sequence, because it is particularly sensitive to motion, which results in ghosting artifact.

Imaging Findings

A systematic approach to peripheral nerve evaluation through MRN is recommended, beginning with evaluation of the large FOV images first to assess regional abnormalities.[3] This is followed

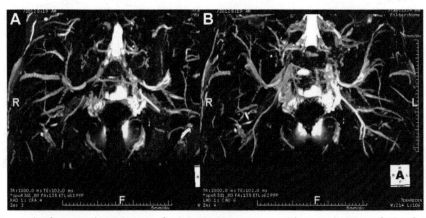

Fig. 3. (A) Coronal reformatted MIP image of a 3-D SPACE sequence with coapplication of T2W fat suppression utilizing SPAIR demonstrates normal appearance of the lumbar sacral plexus and associated vessels. (B) Coronal reformatted MIP image of a 3-D SPACE sequence with coapplication of T2W fat suppression utilizing SPAIR, just ventral to image in (A), demonstrates normal appearance of the lumbar sacral plexus and associated vessels. Note that the vessels are also projected in the reformatted MIP images.

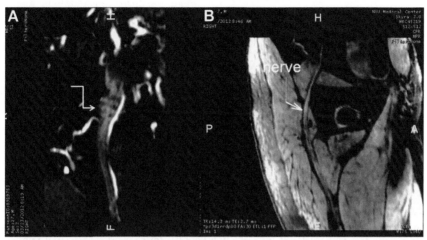

Fig. 4. (A) Curved reformatted MIP 3-D SPAIR sequence demonstrates the normal sciatic nerve (arrow) and associated vessels. (B) Curved reformatted MIP 3-D PSIF demonstrates the normal sciatic nerve with suppression of vascular flow signal.

by evaluation of the transaxial T1W and T2W sequences to distinguish peripheral nerves from the adjacent blood vessels while also assessing nerve signal, caliber, fascicle configuration, and epineurial thickness.[11] Finally, the 3-D images are evaluated and additional regional changes noted, such as the presence or absence of denervation edema in muscle.

MRN allows for evaluation of both direct and indirect signs of peripheral nerve compromise. Direct evidence of peripheral nerve injury includes an alteration in the size of the nerve, altered signal intensity within or surrounding the nerve, loss of the fascicular pattern, nerve displacement, and increased enhancement (Table 1). Peripheral nerves are similar in size to the adjacent artery and taper distally. In pathologic disease states, the nerve demonstrates either focal or diffuse enlargement, such that it becomes larger than the adjacent artery. Furthermore, in the absence of magic angle artifact, abnormal peripheral nerves demonstrate T2-hyperintense signal similar to adjacent veins, which is in direct contrast to the signal intensity of normal peripheral nerves, which are isointense to skeletal muscle on both T1W and T2W images with preservation of the characteristic

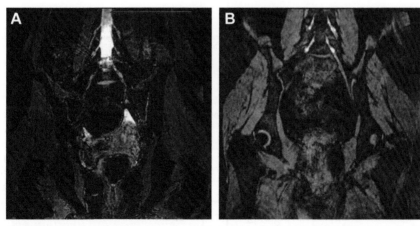

Fig. 5. Role of b-value selection. (A) Coronal reformatted MIP image of a 3-D SPACE sequence with fat suppression performed with a b-value of 0 mm² demonstrates high signal intensity of the cerebrospinal fluid (red arrow), which reduces conspicuity of the exiting lumbar nerve roots. (B) Coronal reformatted MIP image of a 3-D SPACE sequence with fat suppression performed with a b-value of 80 mm² demonstrates suppression of cerebrospinal fluid signal, with increased conspicuity of the exiting lumbar nerve roots. The application of a b-value ranging from 80 to 120 mm² allows for nerve selective imaging through suppression of adjacent fluid and vascular signal, whereby focally increased nerve signal can be detected.

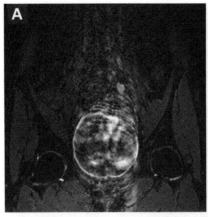 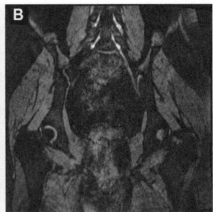

Fig. 6. Patient preparation. (*A*) Coronal reformatted MIP image of a 3-D DW-PSIF sequence demonstrates ghosting artifact secondary to bowel activity and a full bladder. (*B*) Coronal reformatted MIP image of a 3-D DW-PSIF sequence demonstrates improved anatomic resolution of the exiting L4 and L5 lumbar nerve roots in a patient who fasted and emptied the bladder prior to the examination.

tram-track appearance of the nerve fascicles, in conjunction with delineation of the perineural fat planes.

Indirect signs of peripheral nerve injury relate to loss of the normal perineural fat planes, perineural edema, and stages of muscle denervation (see Table 1). The earliest evidence of muscle denervation manifests as denervation-like edema, with diffuse, homogenously increased T2 signal intensity throughout a given muscle belly. In contrast to myositis, these signal changes demonstrate sharp demarcation from the adjacent musculature and surrounding soft tissues and lack of intermuscular and perifascial fluid (Table 2).

For peripheral nerves, which have a purely sensory function, there are no indirect signs of nerve damage (ie, saphenous nerve).

MAGNETIC RESONANCE IMAGING OF COMMON NERVE DISORDERS
Upper Extremity

Brachial plexopathy: thoracic outlet syndrome and Parsonage-Turner syndrome
The brachial plexus is formed by the ventral rami of C5 through T1. The nerve roots descend through the supraclavicular fossa along the course of the subclavian neurovascular bundle. In general, the nerve roots converge to form 3 trunks: the superior

Table 1
Direct and indirect signs of magnetic resonance neuropathy

Direct	Indirect
Increased size	Infiltration of surrounding soft tissue planes
Increased signal	Perineural edema
Irregular shape, loss of normal fascicular morphology	Muscle denervation "edema" • Diffuse • Homogeneous • Sharp margins/demarcation • Spares surrounding fascia and soft tissues (compared with myositis)
Abnormal course	Muscle atrophy
Increased enhancement	

Table 2
Differential diagnosis of abnormal muscle signal on magnetic resonance

Focal/Patchy	Diffuse
Infectious myositis	Denervation
Inflammatory myositis	Polymyositis
Delayed-onset muscle soreness	Postinfectious/inflammatory (Parsonage-turner syndrome)
Trauma (contusion)	Diabetes mellitus
Muscular/tendon strain	Disuse/atrophy
Polymyositis	Geographic margins Homogeneous
Tumor	No associated fluid/fascial abnormality Corresponds to nerve distribution

trunk (C5-C6), the middle trunk (C7), and the inferior trunk (C8, T1). Each of these trunks then splits into anterior and posterior divisions, for a total of 6 divisions, which then reconverge to form 3 cords. The 3 cords are named in reference to the axillary artery: medial, lateral, and posterior. Several important branches then arise from these 3 cords, some of which are reviewed later.

The thoracic outlet refers to the space bounded by the clavicle and the first rib, through which the brachial plexus and subclavian vessels traverse. Thoracic outlet syndrome (TOS) refers to compression of the neurovascular bundle within this space, often secondary to arm elevation. Typical causes of TOS include the presence of cervical ribs and posttraumatic soft tissue and osseous deformities as well as muscular hypertrophy and fibrous band formation. Clinical manifestations may be attributable to vessel ischemia and/or nerve compression, although neurologic symptoms are more common. The site of compression is thought to occur within 1 or more anatomic compartments: the costoclavicular space, the interscalene triangle, and the retropectoralis minor space. Imaging manifestations include asymmetric enlargement and increased T2W signal intensity on the affected side (Fig. 7).

Treatment of neurogenic TOS (NTOS) is initially managed nonsurgically and consists of lifestyle modification along with physical therapy. Although a majority of patients respond well to such conservative measures, if symptoms persist, chemodenervation of the anterior scalene muscle can be performed through image-guided injection of botulinum toxin type A or local anesthetic agents (bupivacaine and lidocaine).[12]

In patients with symptoms refractory to conservative management, surgical release can be pursued, most commonly through supraclavicular thoracic outlet decompression. Surgical management of NTOS, however, is controversial owing to variability in diagnosis, surgical technique, and defined outcome measures.[13]

Parsonage-Turner syndrome refers to idiopathic brachial plexopathy, which may present after surgery, infection, or vaccination. Patients typically present with an insidious onset of unilateral shoulder pain followed by progressive upper extremity motor and sensory deficits. The proposed pathophysiology is related to denervation along the peripheral branch(es) of the brachial plexus, where it is not uncommon for more than 1 nerve to be involved, and the suprascapular and axillary nerves are most frequently affected.[14]

Diagnosis of parsonage-turner syndrome is a combination of clinical history and physical examination findings, along with electromyography results and characteristic diffuse denervation-like edema on T2W images within the muscles innervated by the brachial plexus. Depending on the time course of disease, T1W images may also demonstrate muscular atrophy. Absent in this patient cohort is a history of excessive overhead activity, such as in certain athletic populations, as well as an identifiable morphologic cause of nerve compression on MR imaging. Parsonage-turner syndrome is a self-limited disease, and treatment consists of conservative and supportive measures, including analgesia and physical therapy.

Suprascapular neuropathy

The suprascapular nerve arises from the superior branch of the brachial plexus trunk, which is generally comprised of the C5 and C6 nerve roots. Patients with suprascapular neuropathy (SSN) manifest clinically with shoulder girdle pain and paresthesia, which may initially overshadow associated muscle weakness. Differential diagnosis

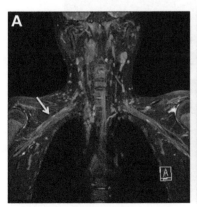
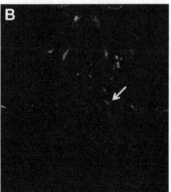
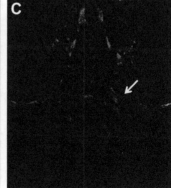

Fig. 7. (A) Coronal 3-D SPACE SPAIR image demonstrates right brachial plexus enlargement and increased signal intensity (*yellow arrow*). (B) Coronal 3-D SPACE SPAIR image in a different patient demonstrating thickening of the left brachial plexus (*yellow arrow*). (C) Coronal 3-D SPACE SPAIR image in the same patient as in (B), demonstrating thickening of the left brachial plexus (*yellow arrow*).

includes, but is not limited to, cervical radiculopathy, paralabral cyst formation, and quadrilateral space syndrome. Imaging findings include denervation-like edema and/or fatty infiltration/atrophy involving the supraspinatus and/or infraspinatus muscles.

In contrast to parsonage-turner syndrome, SSN is related to physical entrapment of the suprascapular nerve, and the site of compression determines whether there is isolated infraspinatus denervation (spinoglenoid notch) or combined supraspinatus and infraspinatus denervation findings (suprascapular notch) (Fig. 8). Causes of entrapment include extrinsic compression secondary to a labral cyst or soft tissue tumor; repetitive stretch injury, such as can be found in overhead athletes; and thickened transverse scapular or spinoglenoid ligaments. Management of acute SSN includes rest and corticosteroid therapy, whereas management of chronic SSN may include image-guided percutaneous needle aspiration followed by therapeutic corticosteroid injection. If medical therapy fails to relieve symptoms, then surgical decompression can be pursued.

Cubital tunnel syndrome

The ulnar nerve arises from the medial cord of the brachial plexus, which is comprised of the C8 and T1 nerve roots. It descends through the medial aspect of the upper arm, and, at the elbow, it travels along the posterior margin of the medial epicondyle prior to entering the forearm. It is here that the ulnar nerve travels through the cubital tunnel, which extends from the medial epicondyle to the olecranon. The cubital tunnel is an important anatomic landmark because it functions as the primary constraint for the ulnar nerve as it descends into the anterior compartment of the forearm.

Cubital tunnel syndrome most commonly refers to compressive neuropathy of the ulnar nerve as a result of increased pressure within the cubital tunnel. Considering the effects of dynamic motion at the elbow joint on the cubital tunnel, which is

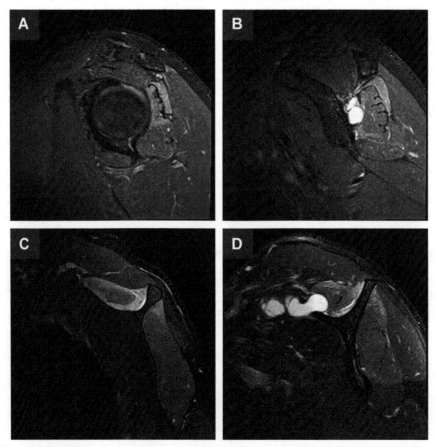

Fig. 8. (*A, B*) Sagittal T2 FS images demonstrate denervation-like edema of the infraspinatus muscle secondary to compression of the suprascapular nerve within the spinoglenoid notch by a ganglion cyst. (*C, D*) Sagittal T2 FS images in a different patient demonstrate denervation-like edema of the supraspinatus and infraspinatus muscle secondary to compression of the suprascapular nerve within the suprascapular notch by a large ganglion cyst.

taut on flexion and lax on extension, how anything that compromises this space renders the ulnar nerve susceptible to impingement can be understood. Some of these causes include medial condylar osteophyte formation, soft tissue tumor, ganglion cyst, accessory anconeus epitrochlearis muscle, low-lying medial head of triceps, and posttraumatic deformity.[15]

Imaging manifestations include thickening and signal hyperintensity of the ulnar nerve proximal to the cubital tunnel, flattening of the nerve within the tunnel, and denervation-like edema of the flexor carpi ulnaris muscle (Fig. 9). Treatment options include initial conservative management with rest, physical therapy, and splinting, with progression to surgical management in patients whose symptoms do not regress. Operative intervention depends on the cause of ulnar nerve impingement and most commonly includes surgical release via neurolysis and/or anterior submuscular or subcutaneous ulnar nerve transposition.

Posterior interosseous nerve syndrome

The radial nerve arises from the posterior cord of the brachial plexus, which is comprised of the C5 through T1 nerve roots. It descends through the posterior compartment of the upper arm and at the level of distal humerus passes into the anterior compartment of the forearm through the radial tunnel. The radial tunnel extends from the lateral epicondyle to the distal margin of the supinator muscle.[16] At the level of the radiohumeral joint, just proximal to the supinator muscle, the radial nerve divides into a superficial sensory branch and a deep motor branch. The deep branch of the radial nerve (DBRN) innervates all of the forearm extensors, except for extensor carpi radialis longus, which is innervated by the radial nerve

proper. As the deep motor branch courses posteriorly through the supinator muscle, it becomes known as the posterior interosseous nerve (PIN). The PIN innervates the common and deep forearm extensors. The superficial sensory branch travels alongside the radial artery, and, as it courses distally, it supplies sensory innervation to the dorsolateral forearm, wrist, and hand.

The most common site of entrapment along the course of the radial nerve and its branches involves the PIN at the arcade of Fröhse, which corresponds to the proximal border of the superficial portion of the supinator muscle. Additional sites of entrapment include recurrent radial vessels at the level of the radial neck (leash of Henry), thickened extensor carpi radialis brevis fascia, space-occupying lesions (ganglion), and posttraumatic deformity of the radial head.

Entrapment of the DBRN or PIN within the radial tunnel results in 2 clinically distinct syndromes: radial tunnel syndrome (RTS) and PIN syndrome (PINS).[17] In PINS, patients present with metacarpal and wrist weakness on extension, associated with radial wrist deviation. This is due to preserved innervation of extensor carpi radialis longus and weakness of extensor carpi ulnaris. Patients with PINS lack sensory deficits, whereas patients with RTS present with pain along the proximal aspect of the lateral forearm and no associated motor deficit.

Imaging manifestations of PINS include denervation-like muscle edema involving the common extensors (extensor digitorum communis, extensor digiti minimi, extensor carpi ulnaris, and variably extensor carpi radialis brevis) and deep extensors (abductor pollicis longus, extensor pollicis longus and brevis, extensor indicis proprius, and variably supinator) (Fig. 10). These findings

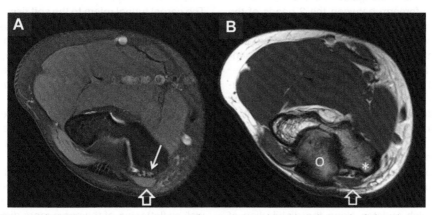

Fig. 9. (A) Transaxial T2 FS image demonstrates enlargement and increased signal of the ulnar nerve (arrow) within the cubital tunnel secondary to external compression by an accessory epitrochlearis muscle (open arrow). (B) Transaxial proton density image of the accessory epitrochlearis muscle (open arrow) inserting into the olecranon (O) and the medial humeral epicondyle (asterisk).

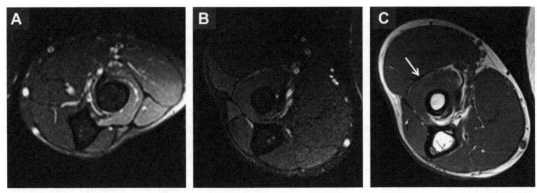

Fig. 10. (*A*) Transaxial T2 FS image of the pattern of T2 denervation-like edema affecting the forearm extensor muscles, including the supinator, extensor carpi ulnaris, extensor digitorum communis, and extensor carpi radialis brevis. This patient was diagnosed with PINS secondary to recurrent radial vessels at the level of the radial neck (leash of Henry). (*B*) Transaxial T2 FS image in a different patient demonstrating subtle T2 denervation-like edema affecting the supinator, extensor carpi ulnaris, and extensor digitorum communis muscles, secondary to entrapment of the PIN in the proximal radial tunnel by a prominent proximal fascial edge of the extensor carpi radialis brevis muscle. (*C*) Same patient as in (*B*), demonstrating the prominent fascial edge of the extensor carpi radialis brevis muscle (*arrow*).

are not present in RTS, which is a clinical diagnosis.

In the absence of a space-occupying lesion, treatment of RTS and PINS is initially managed conservatively with activity modification and antiinflammatories. In the setting of focal nerve compression, radial tunnel decompression is performed surgically. Additionally, in patients with paralysis secondary to PINS, surgery is typically indicated by 3 months time.[18]

Pronator syndrome

The median nerve arises from the medial and lateral cords of the brachial plexus, receiving contributions from the C5 through T1 nerve roots. It descends along the anteromedial compartment of the upper arm alongside the brachial artery, entering the forearm between the 2 heads of the pronator teres muscle and biceps tendon. At this level, the median nerve provides motor innervation to most of the forearm and hand flexors, with sensory innervation to the palm and several fingers.

Although there are several potential sites of median nerve entrapment, pronator syndrome was originally described in relation to entrapment of the median nerve between the 2 heads of the pronator teres muscle and is thus also known as pronator teres syndrome (PTS).[19] Causes include muscle hypertrophy and posttraumatic soft tissue and osseous abnormalities. Patients typically present with pain and numbness in the proximal volar forearm, which radiates along the distribution of the median nerve, involving the thumb and index and middle fingers as well as the radial half of the ring finger.

Imaging findings of PTS include muscle denervation-like edema, which may progress to subsequent atrophy, involving the pronator teres, flexor carpi radialis, palmaris longus, and flexor digitorum superficialis muscles. In this way, MR imaging can be especially helpful in elucidating a diagnosis of PTS, because there is significant overlap between the clinical presentation of PTS and carpal tunnel syndrome (CTS).

Clinical management of PTS is similar to other forms of compressive neuropathy, where initial conservative treatment is recommended through activity modulation and antiinflammatory therapy. Failure to improve with conservative management may be followed by surgical decompression.

Carpal tunnel syndrome

The carpal tunnel refers to the soft tissue compartment along the palmar aspect of the wrist, containing 9 flexor tendons and the median nerve. CTS is the most common cause of neuropathy, often secondary to repetitive motion and/or vibration. Additional causes include synovial inflammation, soft tissue tumor, hormonal changes, and an anomalous muscle. Patients typically present with nocturnal pain as well as numbness and tingling corresponding to median nerve distribution (as detailed previously).

Interrogation of transaxial MR images in the setting of CTS reveals median nerve enlargement within the proximal aspect of the carpal tunnel as well as flattening of the nerve more distally, which may be associated with bowing of the flexor retinaculum (**Fig. 11**). It is also not uncommon to observe increased fluid-sensitive signal within the

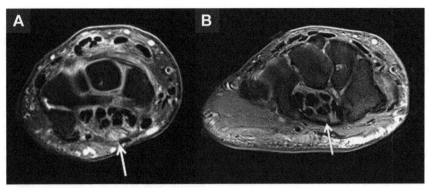

Fig. 11. (*A*) Transaxial T2 FS image in a patient with CTS demonstrates thickening and increased T2W signal of the median nerve in the proximal carpal tunnel (*arrow*). (*B*) Transaxial T2 FS image in the same patient depicts marked flattening of the median nerve (*arrow*) under the carpal ligament proper.

nerve itself as it courses through the carpal tunnel. In patients with severe CTS, denervation-like edema of the thenar muscles may be observed.

Clinical management often begins with conservative treatment, which often consists of wrist splinting. Depending on the severity of CTS, however, local steroid injection may be performed in mild cases, and surgical release of the carpal tunnel may be performed in more severe cases.

Guyon canal syndrome

Ulnar nerve compression may also occur at Guyon canal, which refers to the soft tissue compartment extending from the proximal carpal ligament to the origin of the hypothenar muscles. Both the ulnar nerve and artery travel through Guyon canal, which measures approximately 4 cm in length.

Ulnar nerve impingement may be secondary to external compression, as can be seen in cyclists with handlebar palsy, or after traumatic dislocation of the pisiform or fracture of the hook of the hamate. Sources of internal compression include space-occupying lesions, such as ganglion cyst or lipoma, ulnar artery enlargement secondary to thrombosis/aneurysm, and an accessory muscle.

Clinical presentation of Guyon canal syndrome is dependent on the site of ulnar nerve entrapment, because 3 zones have been described, which correspond to motor and sensory divisions of the nerve.[20] Thus, the presence of isolated motor, isolated sensory, or combined motor and sensory deficits provides clues as to the site of ulnar nerve compression. Furthermore, as discussed previously, denervation-like muscle edema only occurs in those muscles where motor innervation is disrupted. In this way, entrapment of the deep motor branch of the ulnar nerve may result in increased T2W signal within the hypothenar muscles, deep head of flexor pollicis brevis, adductor pollicis, dorsal and palmar interosseous, and third and

fourth lumbrical muscles.[21] Clinical management predominantly relies on conservative treatment, especially in cases related to repetitive trauma. Operative release of the volar carpal ligament may be performed, however, in those patients with compressive causes, such as ganglion cyst formation.

Lower Extremity

Lumbosacral plexopathy

The lumbar plexus is formed by the ventral rami of L1 through L4, with a small contribution from the T12 nerve. The nerve roots descend through the psoas muscle or dorsal to it, emerging along its medial and lateral margins. The obturator nerve and lumbosacral trunk arise medially, whereas the iliohypogastric, ilioinguinal, genitofemoral, lateral femoral cutaneous, and femoral nerves arise laterally.

The sacral plexus is formed by the lumbosacral trunk and the ventral rami of the S1 through S3 nerve roots. The nerve roots converge along the inferior margin of the greater sciatic notch, interposed between the piriformis muscle and the pelvic fascia. The major branches that arise from the sacral plexus include the sciatic, pudendal, and inferior and superior gluteal nerves.

Multiple peripheral branches from the lumbosacral plexus provide both motor and sensory innervation to the pelvis and lower limbs. For this reason, there is no specific syndrome or set of symptoms referable to lumbosacral plexopathy, and often, there is no specific imaging manifestation of disease. In patients with retroperitoneal pathology, however, such as a psoas abscess, hematoma, tumor, or aneurysm, branches of the lumbosacral plexus may be affected. Similarly, patients with disorders of the sacroiliac joints, such as arthropathy or tumor, may present with symptoms referable to sacral plexopathy. Additionally, in the setting of inherited neurologic disorders, such as Charcot-Marie-Tooth disease, imaging findings may include focal nerve enlargement and atrophy of the affected musculature.

Piriformis syndrome and deep gluteal syndrome

The sciatic nerve is formed by branches of the L4, L5, S1, S2, and S3 nerve roots and descends along the course of the piriformis muscle. It is the largest nerve in the body and gives rise to the tibial and peroneal nerves as it exits the greater sciatic foramen and descends in the thigh between the adductor magnus and gluteus maximus muscles. The sciatic nerve provides motor innervation to the hamstrings and all muscles below the knee. It provides sensory innervation to the entire lower limb with the exception of the medial leg (innervated by obturator and femoral nerves). The sciatic nerve is often prone to injury, given both its size and anatomic course (Fig. 12).

Piriformis syndrome is a result of sciatic nerve entrapment by the piriformis muscle at the level of the greater sciatic notch. It may be caused by an aberrant intramuscular course of the sciatic nerve through the piriformis muscle as well as any muscle pathology, such as hypertrophy, inflammation, and spasticity. In general, patients with piriformis syndrome present with nonspecific symptoms attributable to various forms of sciatica: radiating unilateral buttock or posterior thigh pain, aggravated by activity and relieved with rest. Additionally, given that there are many causes of sciatica, a diagnosis of piriformis syndrome is typically advised only after excluding more common causes, such as lumbar/lumbosacral discogenic degenerative disease and spinal stenosis. When evaluating the sciatic nerve, it is especially important to analyze for sciatic nerve symmetry with respect to anatomic course, contour, size, and signal intensity on T2W images. Careful investigation of the sciatic nerve in piriformis syndrome may reveal unilateral enlargement along with increased T2W signal of both the nerve and piriformis muscle itself (Fig. 13).

The subgluteal space is the fat-filled plane interposed between the deep fascia of the gluteus maximus muscle and the superfical border of the muscles that parallel it: gluteus medius and minimus, superior and inferior gemellus, obturator internus, and quadratus femoris. This is the space where it is often with greatest ease that the sciatic nerve is identified, because it is both large and surrounded by fat. Anything that impinges on the fat within the subgluteal space may result in deep gluteal syndrome, including trauma, inflammation/infection, and soft tissue masses. Additionally, entrapment of the sciatic nerve may occur as it travels underneath the piriformis muscle and over the superior gemellus/obturator internus muscles (see Fig. 13).[22]

Treatment of piriformis and deep gluteal syndromes begins with conservative treatment, which includes physical therapy, antiinflammatory medication, and image-guided corticosteroid injection into either the piriformis muscle itself or the deep gluteal space. Chronic forms of these syndromes in which the sciatic nerve is entrapped by the surrounding musculature may also be treated with botulinum toxin type A. In patients whose symptoms are refractory to the aforementioned treatments, surgical release through endoscopy has been described.[23]

Superior and inferior gluteal neuropathy

The superior and inferior gluteal nerves arise from the posterior roots of L4, L5, and S1. They emerge

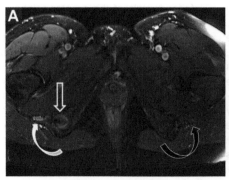 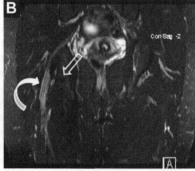

Fig. 12. (*A*) Transaxial T2 FS image through the lower pelvis demonstrates right sciatic neuropathy secondary to adhesions from hamstring suture anchor repair at the ischial tuberosity (*open arrow*). Compare the increased size and T2 signal of the right sciatic nerve (*curved white arrow*) with the normal, left sciatic nerve (*curved black arrow*). (*B*) Coronal T2 FS of the same patient demonstrating an enlarged, T2-hyperintense right sciatic nerve (*curved white arrow*) adjacent to hamstring suture anchor repair (*open arrow*).

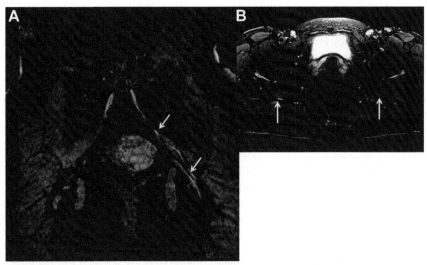

Fig. 13. (A) Coronal 3-D SPACE MIP demonstrating entrapment of the left sciatic nerve (*yellow arrows*) as it courses through a bifid left piriformis muscle. (B) Transaxial T2 FS image in a different patient demonstrating entrapment of the left sciatic nerve (*yellow arrow*) within the subgluteal space. Note the increased size and signal intensity of the left sciatic nerve compared with the right (*white arrow*).

from the pelvis underneath the roof of the greater sciatic foramen, above the piriformis muscle. Both branches travel between gluteus medius and minimus, with the superior branch terminating in the gluteus minimus and the inferior branch terminating in the tensor fascia lata. Motor innervation is provided to the gluteus medius, minimus, and tensor fascia lata muscles. There is no associated sensory component.

Patients with superior and inferior gluteal neuropathy present with weakness on abduction, limping gait, and positive Trendelenburg sign. The most common cause of these symptoms is iatrogenic in etiology and related to prior total hip replacement or fracture fixation. Imaging manifestations include denervation-like edema within the gluteus medius, gluteus minimus, and tensor fascia lata, which may progress to muscle atrophy. Treatment includes conservative management and continued physical therapy to strengthen the muscles on the affected side.

Obturator neuropathy
The obturator nerve is formed by the ventral divisions of the L2, L3, and L4 nerve roots and descends through the psoas muscle. The obturator nerve exits at the obturator foramen, which is located at the pelvic brim. It is here that the nerve divides into anterior and posterior branches. It is also in this location where the nerve can become injured or compressed secondary to osseous or soft tissue trauma, tumors, hernias, and fibrous band formation as a result of chronic adductor inflammation. As with superior and inferior gluteal neuropathy, the most common causes of obturator neuropathy are iatrogenic in etiology and occur after prolonged lithotomic positioning, such as during gynecologic or genitourinary surgery as well as total hip arthroplasty.

The anterior division provides motor innervation to gracilis, adductor longus, adductor brevis, and pectineus, with sensory innervation to the hip and medial thigh. The posterior division provides motor innervation to obturator externus, adductor magnus, and adductor brevis, with sensory innervation to the knee.

Patients with obturator neuropathy may manifest with groin or medial thigh pain as well as adductor muscle weakness. On imaging, these patients may demonstrate denervation-like edema of the adductor musculature, although adductor brevis may be spared due to dual innervation. Treatment includes image-guided selective blockade of the obturator nerve, with progression to surgical neurolysis in chronic cases.

Pudendal neuropathy
The pudendal nerve is formed by the S2 ventral rami and the S3 and S4 rami. It descends between the piriformis and coccygeus muscles, exiting the pelvis through the greater sciatic foramen. From here, it crosses the ischial spine, reenters the pelvis by way of the perineum through the lesser sciatic foramen, and travels through the pudendal canal. The pudendal canal is also known as Alcock canal and is a compartment within the obturator fascia along the lateral wall of the ischiorectal fossa, which contains the pudendal nerve and

vessels. As with other forms of nerve entrapment, Alcock canal is a common site of pudendal nerve entrapment (PNE), especially in cyclists and individuals who sit for prolonged periods of time. Additional causes of pudendal neuralgia include stretching of the nerve during gynecologic or obstetric procedures.

The major branches of the pudendal nerve include the inferior rectal nerve, perineal nerve, and dorsal nerve of the penis/clitoris. Motor innervation is provided to the bulbospongiosis and ischiocavernosis muscles as well as the external urethral and rectal sphincters. Sensory innervation is provided to the perineum, scrotum, and anus. Thus, patients with PNE may present clinically with perineal and genital numbness as well as urinary and fecal incontinence.

Imaging manifestations of PNE can often be overshadowed by the nerve's complex anatomy. Therefore, it is important to investigate 4 separate sites of possible entrapment: piriformis muscle/ greater sciatic foramen, ischial spine, Alcock canal/obturator internus muscle, and distal branches.[24] The spectrum of imaging findings includes asymmetry of the obturator internus and piriformis muscles as well as increased T2W signal within the muscle itself or along the course of the nerve. Treatment of PNE is most often performed via image-guided selective nerve blockade.[25]

Common peroneal neuropathy

The common peroneal nerve arises from the lateral branch of the sciatic nerve at the level of the upper popliteal fossa. It courses inferolaterally within the distal popliteal fossa, posteromedial to the biceps femoris muscle, and courses obliquely toward the proximal fibula. At the level of the fibular neck, it trifurcates into 3 terminal branches: the recurrent articular nerve, the superficial peroneal nerve, and the deep peroneal nerve.

The superficial and deep peroneal nerves supply motor innervation to the lower leg musculature. The superficial peroneal nerve courses anteriorly along the fibula in the lateral compartment, supplying the peroneus longus and brevis muscles. The deep peroneal nerve descends anteriorly along the interosseous membrane, supplying the anterior compartment muscles: anterior tibialis, extensor hallucis longus, extensor digitorum longus, extensor digitorum brevis, and peroneus tertius.

Common peroneal neuropathy (CPN) proximal to the level of trifurcation is most often related to knee joint pathology and proximal fibular fracture. Additional causes are often related to compartment syndrome, whether due to extrinsic compression as a result of space-occupying lesions or posttraumatic compartment syndrome.

Clinical manifestations of CPN include foot drop and slapping gait. On imaging, focal nerve compression can often be identified as well as denervation-like edema affecting the musculature innervated by the branches of the common peroneal nerve (Fig. 14). Treatment of CPN often depends on the duration and intensity of symptoms and ranges from conservative therapy to surgical neurolysis.

Tarsal tunnel syndrome

The tibial nerve arises from the medial branch of the sciatic nerve and is the largest branch of the sciatic nerve. It descends within the posterior compartment of the thigh and lower leg, and, at the level of the ankle, it passes posteroinferior to the medial malleolus, where it is referred to as the posterior tibial nerve. The posterior tibial nerve divides into the medial and lateral plantar nerves and provides motor and sensory innervation to the plantar foot.

Tarsal tunnel syndrome (TTS) refers to compression of the posterior tibial nerve or its branches along the course of the flexor retinaculum. The tunnel is divided into a proximal component at the level of the tibiotalar joint and a distal component at the level of the subtalar joint. Posterior tibial nerve entrapment may occur as a result of alterations in hindfoot alignment, as can be seen with congenital conditions, such as tarsal coalition, or acquired deformities as a result of trauma and degenerative change (Fig. 15). Additional causes of TTS include space-occupying lesions, such as nerve-sheath tumors and ganglia, as well as systemic diseases, such as diabetes and peripheral vascular disease.

Clinical manifestations of TTS most commonly include paresthesia and weakness along the plantar foot. MR imaging allows for assessment of pathologic change along the course of the tibial nerve within the tarsal tunnel. Nonoperative management includes antiinflammatory medication and corticosteroid injection, activity modification, and orthotics. Operative management is considered after failure of conservative therapy and when a definite point of entrapment is identified.[26]

Interventional procedures

Although MR imaging is essential in the evaluation of peripheral nerve pathology, treatment of peripheral neuropathy can often be achieved through ultrasound-guided locoregional anesthesia administration. With the advent of ultrasound–magnetic resonance fusion, which syncs real-time ultrasound images with previously acquired MR

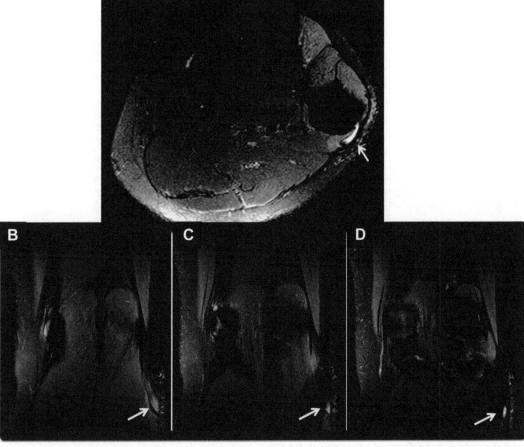

Fig. 14. (*A*) Transaxial T2 FS image demonstrating enlargement and hyperintensity of the peroneal nerve (*yellow arrow*) as it courses around the fibular neck. (*B–D*) Coronal T2 FS images in the same patient demonstrating enlargement and hyperintensity of the peroneal nerve (*yellow arrows*) as it courses around the fibular neck.

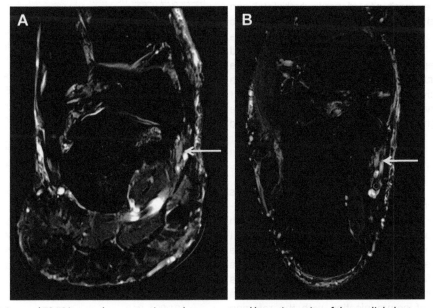

Fig. 15. (*A*) Coronal T2 FS image demonstrating enlargement and hyperintensity of the medial plantar nerve (*yellow arrow*) secondary to subtalar (talocalcaneal) coalition. (*B*) Transaxial T2 FS image in the same patient demonstrating enlargement and hyperintensity of the medial plantar nerve (*yellow arrow*) secondary to subtalar coalition.

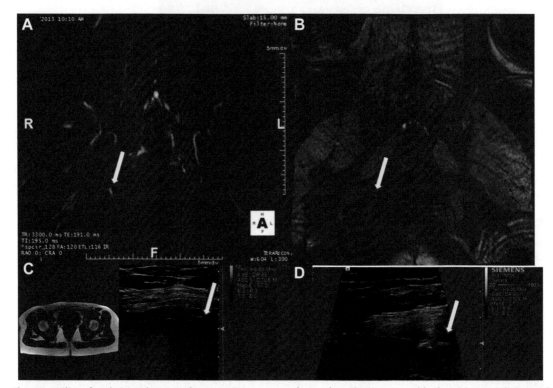

Fig. 16. Utility of real-time ultrasound–magnetic resonance fusion for selective nerve block guidance. (*A*) Coronal 3-D SPACE SPAIR image demonstrates asymmetric enlargement in T2-hyperintensity of the right pudendal nerve in Alcock canal (*yellow arrow*). (*B*) 3-D PSIF demonstrates focal signal hyperintensity of the right pudendal nerve in Alcock canal (*yellow arrow*). (*C*) Ultrasound–magnetic resonance fusion demonstrates real-time guidance to target the right pudendal nerve (*yellow arrow*). (*D*) Ultrasound image demonstrates the pathologic right pudendal nerve identified on the prior MR images (*yellow arrow*).

images, the exact site of nerve pathology can be targeted further (**Fig. 16**). Ultrasound–magnetic resonance fusion already has proved advantageous for guidance during both prostate and breast biopsies.[27,28] This technology will be most useful for targeting nerve pathology in anatomically complex locations, such as the pudendal nerve within the pelvis, with greater ease than magnetic resonance–guided therapeutic injections.

SUMMARY

The role of MRN in peripheral nerve pathology is becoming increasingly refined, both through advances in magnetic resonance technology and in the ability to accurately interpret direct and indirect signs of neuropathic change. Although there remain several pitfalls in MRN imaging, awareness of these pitfalls improves imaging quality and limits misinterpretation. Most importantly, maintaining a direct line of communication with the referring clinician allows for the greatest degree of diagnostic accuracy.

REFERENCES

1. Howe FA, Filler AG, Bell BA, et al. Magnetic resonance neurography. Magn Reson Med 1992;28: 328–38.
2. Filler AG, Howe GA, Hayes CE, et al. Magnetic resonance neurography. Lancet 1993;341:659–61.
3. Chabra A. Peripheral MR neurography: approach to interpretation. Neuroimaging Clin N Am 2014; 24:79–89.
4. Chabra A, Andreisek G. "Magnetic resoance neurography of tunnels – part ii: lower extremity nerves." Magnetic resonance neurography. 1st edition. New Dehli (India): Jaypee Brothers Medical Publishers; 2012. p. 109. Print.
5. Azuelos A, Coro L, Alexandre A. Femoral nerve entrapment. Acta Neurochir Suppl 2005;92:61–2.
6. Mizisin A, Weerasuriya A. Homeostatic regulation of the endoneurial microenvironment during development, aging and in response to trauma, disease and toxic insult. Acta Neuropathol 2011; 121:291–312.
7. Runge VM, Nitz WR, Schmeets SH. "3D imaging: basic principles." the physics of clinical MR taught

through images. 2nd edition. New York: Thieme Medical Publishers, Inc; 2009. p. 72. Print.

8. Delaney H, Bencardino J, Rosenberg ZS. Magnetic resonance neurography of the pelvis and lumbosacral plexus. Neuroimaging Clin N Am 2014;24:127–50.

9. Chhabra A, Andreisek G. "Magnetic resonance neurography technique." Magnetic resonance neurography. 1st edition. New Dehli (India): Jaypee Brothers Medical Publishers; 2012. p. 16. Print.

10. Chhabra A, Padua A, Flammang A, et al. Magnetic resonance neurography – techniques and interpretation. 2012. Available at: http://www.healthcare. siemens.com/siemens_hwem-hwem_ssxa_web-sites-context-root/wcm/idc/groups/public/@global/@imaging/@mri/documents/download/mdaw/mjq1/~edisp/mr_neurography_techniques_interpretation-00277343.pdf. Accessed May, 2014.

11. Chhabra A, Andreisek G. "Magnetic resonance neurography interpretation." Magnetic resonance neurography. 1st edition. New Dehli (India): Jaypee Brothers Medical Publishers; 2012. p. 23–36. Print.

12. Danielson K, Odderson IR. Botulinum toxin type a improves blood flow in vascular thoracic outlet syndrome. Am J Phys Med Rehabil 2008;87:956–9.

13. Caputo FJ, Wittenberg AM, Vemuri C, et al. Supraclavicular decompression for neurogenic thoracic outlet syndrome in adolescent and adult populations. J Vasc Surg 2013;57(1):149–57.

14. Gaskin CM, Helms CA. Parsonage-turner syndrome: MR imaging findings and clinical information of 27 patients. Radiology 2006;240(2):501–7.

15. Beltran LS, Lerman O, Sharma S, et al. Transient pain and parestheisas in the hand—ulnar neuropathy secondary to compression from a low-lying medial triceps muscle and tendon insertion. Skeletal Radiol 2014;43:63.

16. Konjengbam M, Elangbam J. Radial nerve in the radial tunnel: anatomic sites of entrapment neuropathy. Clin Anat 2004;17:21–5.

17. Dong Q, Jacobsen JA, Jamadar D, et al. Entrapment neuropathies in the upper and lower limbs: anatomy and MRI features. Radiol Res Pract 2012;2012:1–12. http://dx.doi.org/10.1155/2012/230679. Article ID: 230679.

18. Knutsen EJ, Calfee RP. Uncommon upper extremity compression neuropathies. Hand Clin 2013;29:443–53.

19. Seyffarth H. Primary myoses in the M. pronator teres as cause of lesion of the N. medianus (the pronator syndrome). Acta Psychiatr Neurol Scand Suppl 1951;74:251–4.

20. Chalian M, Behzadi AH, Williams EH, et al. High-resolution magnetic resonance neurography in upper extremity neuropathy. Neuroimaging Clin N Am 2014;24:109–25.

21. Kim SJ, Hong SH, Jun WS, et al. MR imaging mapping of skeletal muscle denervation in entrapment and compressive neuropathies. Radiographics 2011;31:319–32.

22. Fernandez Hernando M, Cerezal L, Perez Carro L. Deep gluteal syndrome: anatomy, imaging and management of the sciatic nerve entrapments in the subgluteal space. 2013. Available at: http://dx.doi.org/10.1594/ecr2013/C-2006. Accessed May, 2014.

23. Martin HD, Shears SA, Johnson JC, et al. The endoscopic treatment of sciatic nerve entrapment/deep gluteal syndrome. Arthroscopy 2011;27(2):172–81.

24. Filler AG. Diagnosis and treatment of pudendal nerve entrapment syndrome subtypes: imaging, injections, and minimal access surgery. Neurosurg Focus 2009;26(2):E9.

25. Fritz J, Chhabra A, Wang KC, et al. Magnetic resonance neurography-guided nerve blocks for the diagnosis and treatment of chronic pelvic pain syndrome. Neuroimaging Clin N Am 2014;24:211–34.

26. Ahmad M, Tsang K, Mackenney PJ, et al. Tarsal tunnel syndrome: a literature review. Foot Ankle Surg 2012;18(3):149–52.

27. Lawrence EM, Tang SY, Barrett T, et al. Prostate cancer: performance characteristics of combined T2W and SW-MRI scoring in the setting of template transperineal re-biopsy using MR-TRUS fusion. Eur Radiol 2014;24:1497–505.

28. Pons EP, Azcon FM, Casas MC, et al. Real-time NRI navigated US: role in diagnosis and guided biopsy of incidental breast lesions and axillary lymph nodes detected on breast MRI but not on second look US. Eur J Radiol 2014;83:942–50.

Metal Artifact Reduction

Standard and Advanced Magnetic Resonance and Computed Tomography Techniques

 CrossMark

Amit Gupta, MD[a], Naveen Subhas, MD[a],*, Andrew N. Primak, PhD[b], Mathias Nittka, PhD[c], Kecheng Liu, PhD, MBA[d]

KEYWORDS

- Metal artifact reduction • Techniques • MR • CT • Hardware

KEY POINTS

- MR imaging and computed tomography (CT) artifacts from metallic implants are related to various factors, such as the type, size, and shape of the metal and the imaging parameters that are used.
- MR imaging artifacts can be reduced using standard techniques, such as scanning on lower-field-strength systems and using fast spin echo and short tau inversion recovery sequences with high bandwidth parameters, as well as using advanced techniques, such as view angle tilting, slice encoding for metal artifact correction, and multi-acquisition variable-resonance image combination.
- CT artifacts can be reduced using standard techniques, such as using high kilovolts peak and milliampere second, narrow collimation, and thinner slices, as well as advanced techniques, such as monoenergetic dual-energy CT and sinogram inpainting methods.

INTRODUCTION

An increasing number of joint replacements are being performed in the United States[1,2] owing to several factors, including increased life expectancy of the population, increased demand by younger patients seeking a better quality of life,[3,4] and increased access, with more surgeons performing these procedures. Between 1990 and 2002, the annual number of primary and revision total hip replacements (THR) per 100,000 persons increased by 46% and 60%, respectively; the annual number of primary and revision total knee replacements (TKR) per 100,000 persons increased by 295% and 166%, respectively.[2] Similarly, the number of shoulder arthroplasties increased by 236% per annum in 2008 compared with 1993.[1] It is projected that this trend will continue and that by 2030 the number of primary and revision THR will increase by 174% and 137%, respectively, in comparison with 2005; for TKR, these numbers will increase by 673% and 605%, respectively.[5]

Patients undergoing these procedures can have various complications, including loosening of the implant (both infectious and aseptic), fracture, dislocation, component failure and wear of the

Financial Disclosures and Conflicts of Interest: None (A. Gupta); research support from Siemens Healthcare for computed tomography metal artifact reduction (N. Subhas); employee of Siemens Healthcare (A.N. Primak, M. Nittka, and K. Liu).
[a] Department of Diagnostic Radiology, Imaging Institute, Cleveland Clinic, 9500 Euclid Avenue, A21, Cleveland, OH 44195, USA; [b] Computed Tomography, Siemens Healthcare USA, 51 Valley Stream Parkway, Malvern, PA 19355, USA; [c] Magnetic Resonance Imaging, Siemens AG, Allee am Roethelheimpark 2, Erlangen 91052, Germany; [d] Magnetic Resonance Imaging, Siemens Healthcare USA, 51 Valley Stream Parkway, Malvern, PA 19355, USA
* Corresponding author.
E-mail address: subhasn@ccf.org

radiologic.theclinics.com

implant, synovitis, bursitis, and tendon tears. Imaging is usually one of the primary means of diagnosing these complications. Radiography has been and continues to be the first-line modality for the evaluation of patients with implants. However, radiographs may significantly underestimate the extent of any complication. Cross-sectional imaging techniques, such as computed tomography (CT) and MR imaging, are more sensitive than radiographs for the evaluation of complications (**Fig. 1**). In a study by Walde and colleagues,[6] the sensitivity of radiographs in detecting osteolysis was found to be only 52%; the sensitivities for CT and MR imaging were 75% and 95%, respectively. CT, MR imaging, and ultrasound are also superior to radiography for the evaluation of periprosthetic soft tissues.[7,8] However, the use of CT and MR imaging in patients with metallic implants is limited by the presence of artifacts, which can obscure pathologic findings and lower the reader's confidence. These artifacts can be reduced through the use of metal artifact reduction (MAR) techniques. This review discusses the causes of metal artifacts on MR imaging and CT, contributing factors, and both conventional and novel methods to reduce the effects of these artifacts on scans.

CAUSES OF METAL ARTIFACTS ON MR IMAGING

Metallic objects cause artifacts on MR imaging because of their magnetic susceptibility, which is the tendency of a substance to become magnetized when exposed to an external magnetic field. When an object becomes magnetized, it exerts its own magnetic field, thereby distorting the external magnetic field (B_0). This distortion results in a field inhomogeneity near the metal, which in turn alters the phase and frequency of the local spins. Alteration in phase results in loss of signal intensity by intravoxel dephasing (also known as the T2* effect). Alteration in frequency results in spatial misregistration, primarily in the frequency-encoding and the slice selection direction. This misregistration results in distortion of the image within the x-y plane of the image (in-plane distortion) and in the z-direction (through-plane distortion).

FACTORS THAT DETERMINE THE DEGREE OF METAL ARTIFACT ON MR IMAGING
Composition of the Implant

The degree of artifact caused by a metallic implant depends on its magnetic susceptibility, which in turn depends on the implant's composition. Metals with higher magnetic susceptibility demonstrate more artifacts than metals with lower magnetic susceptibility. Materials can be broadly divided into diamagnetic, paramagnetic, and ferromagnetic substances based on their magnetic susceptibility, with ferromagnetic substances having the highest susceptibility, followed by paramagnetic materials; diamagnetic materials have the lowest susceptibility.[9] Implants composed of ferromagnetic metals, such as iron, nickel, and cobalt, generate more artifacts than those composed of titanium, which is paramagnetic.[10,11] In clinical practice, orthopedic implants composed of stainless steel or cobalt-chromium (CoCr) alloys will result in greater artifact than implants composed of titanium (**Fig. 2**).

Size, Shape, and Orientation of the Implant

The size, shape, and orientation of the implant relative to the B_0 direction contribute to the degree of artifact. A larger implant will result in a greater

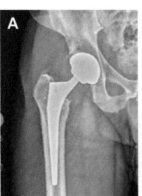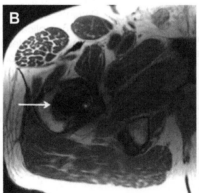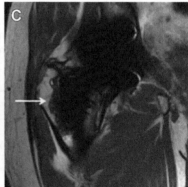

Fig. 1. Radiograph (*A*), axial (*B*), and coronal (*C*) non–fat-suppressed high-bandwidth proton density MR images in a patient with a metal-on-metal right hip arthroplasty. Several radiographs performed in the preceding 2 years had been interpreted as normal. However, because the patient reported chronic pain, MR imaging was performed; the images demonstrated osteolysis (*arrows*) adjacent to the femoral component.

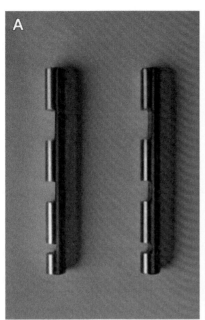 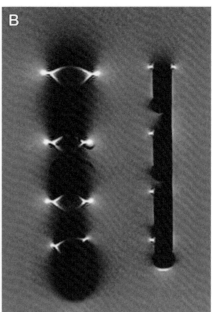

Fig. 2. Two metallic rods (*A*), one composed of stainless steel (*left*) and the other composed of titanium (*right*), were imaged in a water bath on a 1.5T magnetic resonance scanner. Coronal high-bandwidth images with view angle tilting (*B*), with the long axis of the rods oriented along the main magnetic field of the scanner, demonstrate significantly worse susceptibility artifact with the stainless steel rod than with the titanium rod.

area of distortion of the external magnetic field. As a result, the size of the artifact increases with an increase in the size of the implant.[10,11] The shape of the implant also affects the degree to which the B_0 is distorted. The distortion is greatest adjacent to spherical objects and lowest adjacent to cylindrical objects.[11,12] In the case of hip arthroplasty, for example, there are more artifacts adjacent to the femoral head than to the femoral stem. The relationship between the long axis of the implant and the direction of the B_0 also affects the degree of the artifact. The degree of artifact is lowest when the long axis of the implant is parallel to B_0, increases with an increased angle between the two, and is greatest when the long axis of the implant is perpendicular to B_0.[9–11]

Strength of the Main Magnetic Field

The effect of magnetic susceptibility of a metal increases with an increase in the strength of B_0. In other words, imaging with higher-field-strength MR imaging systems will result in greater artifacts than imaging on lower-field-strength systems.[13] In contrast to most musculoskeletal applications, in which the use of 3T scanners is preferred for the improved signal-to-noise ratio (SNR), when imaging metallic implants, a 1.5T scanner is preferred. Although there will be reduction in the artifact, the drawback is that SNR will also be reduced when moving to a lower-field-strength system.

Imaging Pulse Sequence

Susceptibility artifacts can vary depending on the pulse sequence used. Artifacts are less prominent on spin echo (SE) sequences than on gradient-recalled echo (GRE) sequences because of the loss of signal intensity from intravoxel dephasing that occurs around metallic components.[9] In SE sequences, the 180° refocusing reduces this dephasing and helps to recover the transverse signal loss. Because GRE sequences do not use a refocusing pulse, there is no correction for the increased intravoxel dephasing that occurs from implant-induced field inhomogeneity, resulting in signal loss. Fast SE (FSE) sequences are preferred over conventional SE sequences because of their higher efficiency with respect to SNR per scan time. This improved efficiency is particularly valuable to help compensate for the SNR loss that results from other MAR techniques that are discussed in later sections. The primary drawback of FSE techniques is the image blurring that occurs with long echo train lengths for tissues with short T2 signal components.

Signal loss and signal pileups from spatial misregistration related to alteration of the frequency of the spins near the metallic implant will not be corrected by the use of SE sequences.[9,12] Additional techniques are needed to correct for both in-plane and through-plane spatial misregistration.

Imaging Parameters

Frequency-encoding gradient strength

The degree of artifact along the frequency-encoding direction is inversely proportional to the strength of the frequency-encoding gradient or readout gradient.[14,15] This in-plane distortion (ie, distortion occurring along the frequency-encoding direction) can, therefore, be partially offset by using a high-frequency–encoding gradient (ie, high receiver bandwidth) during readout. In practical terms, this equates to increasing the receiver bandwidth. The drawback of this technique is that it results in decreased SNR.

Frequency-encoding gradient direction

In contrast to frequency encoding, the phase-encoding process is not affected by field distortions.[11] With this in mind, the frequency-encoding and phase-encoding directions can be chosen in a way to minimize artifact in the area of interest. This approach must be balanced with the fact that the artifact is increased when the long axis of the implant is perpendicular to the direction of the frequency-encoding gradient, irrespective of the direction on B_0, as discussed earlier.[10] Additionally, swapping phase- and frequency-encoding directions can result in longer imaging times.

Slice thickness and voxel size

A smaller voxel size results in less susceptibility artifact.[11,14] The voxel size is determined by the image matrix, the size of the field of view (FOV), and the slice thickness of the image. The use of a larger matrix, a smaller FOV, and thin section images will minimize susceptibility artifacts. The primary drawback of a smaller voxel size is decreased SNR (fewer protons in each voxel from which to acquire a signal). One way to compensate for the loss of SNR is to increase the number of excitations (NEX), which will lead to increased imaging time.

Fat-suppression imaging

In musculoskeletal imaging, fat suppression is usually achieved using the frequency-selective fat-saturation technique, also known as spectral fat suppression. Frequency-selective fat suppression is the preferred technique because it achieves good fat suppression in a time-efficient manner while minimizing the loss in SNR. Frequency-selective fat saturation takes advantage of the fact that water protons are resonating at a slightly different frequency than fat protons (which also accounts for chemical shift artifact). Application of a narrow-bandwidth radiofrequency (RF) pulse centered on the resonance frequency of fat before the main excitation pulse selectively destroys the longitudinal magnetization of the fat protons such that they do not contribute to the signal during readout. In the presence of a metallic implant, the resultant magnetic field inhomogeneity causes the water and fat protons adjacent to the implant to spin at different frequencies. As a result, application of an RF pulse centered on the resonance frequency of fat will not have the intended effect of nulling the signal from all of the fat protons. Instead, it may result in incomplete suppression of the fat signal or, even worse, it may (locally) null signal from water protons instead of fat protons, resulting in water suppression. Alternative fat-suppression techniques such as inversion recovery sequences (eg, short tau inversion recovery [STIR]) provide improved fat suppression in patients with implants.[9,16] With inversion recovery sequences, tissues are isolated by their inherent T1 characteristics rather than by their resonance frequencies and, therefore, are not affected by frequency shifts caused by the presence of metallic implants. In environments with strong off-resonance conditions, such as the presence of metallic implants, the STIR sequence can be optimized such that the bandwidth of the inversion pulse is matched to that of the excitation pulse to properly invert the signal close to metal.[17] The Dixon technique is another imaging method that has a certain degree of insensitivity to magnetic field heterogeneity and can be used for fat suppression in patients with implants; however, if the static field gradient close to the metal is too strong, the ability to separate fat and water may be hampered and fat suppression may fail.

TECHNIQUES TO REDUCE METAL ARTIFACTS ON MR IMAGING

As discussed earlier, the severity of the artifacts from metal implants depends on several factors. Some of these factors cannot be controlled or modified by radiologists, such as composition, size, and shape of the implant. Other factors can be modified to help decrease susceptibility artifacts. These factors include the type of magnetic resonance (MR) scanner, orientation of the hardware in the scanner, type of sequences used, and imaging parameters. In this section, MAR techniques are broadly divided into 2 categories: (1) standard artifact reduction methods (using optimized acquisition parameters) and (2) advanced artifact reduction (artifact correction) methods (using dedicated acquisition and postprocessing methods).

Standard Metal Artifact Reduction Techniques on MR Imaging

Scanning on a low-field-strength magnetic resonance system

Scanning on a lower-field-strength magnet reduces the degree of susceptibility artifact by decreasing the magnetization of the implant, as illustrated in **Fig. 3**. The tradeoff with this technique is lower SNR. When the choice is between a 3T or 1.5T system, the SNR with a 1.5T system is sufficient to justify this tradeoff for most musculoskeletal applications, especially when the distortions are severe such as for large structures or high-susceptibility metal (stainless steel, CoCr alloys). On the other hand, artifacts related to smaller implants made of titanium (eg, screws) may be controlled even at 3T, especially if the main region of interest is not too close to the implant.

Orientating the long axis of the hardware parallel to external magnetic field

When possible, the orientation of the hardware should be aligned parallel to the B_0 direction, as this reduces the artifact (**Fig. 4**). For example, when scanning the wrist of a patient with a scaphoid screw, orienting the wrist in the scanner such that the long axis of the screw is parallel to the direction of B_0 will minimize the susceptibility artifact. In most cases, however, this is not possible because of the geometry or location of the hardware.

Orienting the frequency-encoding gradient parallel to external magnetic field

Because metal artifacts are most pronounced in the direction of the frequency-encoding gradient, the gradient should be applied in a way such that artifacts are directed away from the area of interest, keeping in mind that artifacts are minimized if the long axis of the implant is parallel to the frequency-encoding gradient. For example, in a scan of a metallic rod in the tibia, the frequency-encoding direction should be directed along the craniocaudal length of the rod (z-direction), not in the mediolateral (x) or anteroposterior (y) directions (**Fig. 5**).

Increasing the receiver bandwidth

Increasing the strength of the frequency-encoding gradient decreases the metal susceptibility artifact.[14,15] This increase can be achieved by increasing the receiver bandwidth while keeping the FOV constant (**Fig. 6**). A wider receiver bandwidth, however, decreases the SNR. In most cases, this tradeoff is acceptable. If the SNR is not sufficient, other compensatory changes will need to be made, such as increasing the NEX, which will lead to a longer scan time.

Using fast spin echo sequences with short echo spacing

FSE sequences minimize the loss of signal related to intravoxel dephasing and result in less artifact compared with GRE sequences (**Fig. 7**). FSE sequences can be optimized in the presence of metal with the use of high bandwidth, with short readout times and short RF pulses. Increasing the echo train length will allow faster scan times to minimize SNR loss related to high readout bandwidth, and shortening the echo spacing (ie, the time between the echoes) will reduce image blurring from the T2 signal decay.

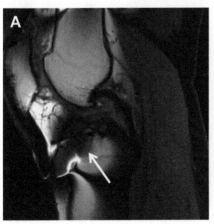 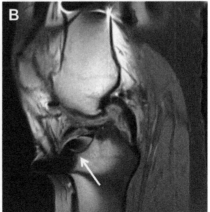

Fig. 3. MR imaging of the knee in a patient with anterior cruciate ligament reconstruction. Sagittal non–fat-saturated FSE proton density–weighted MR images of the knee obtained at 3T (*A*) and at 1.5T (*B*) at the same location. The image obtained at the higher magnetic field strength of 3T shows more metallic artifact than the image obtained at 1.5T (*arrows*).

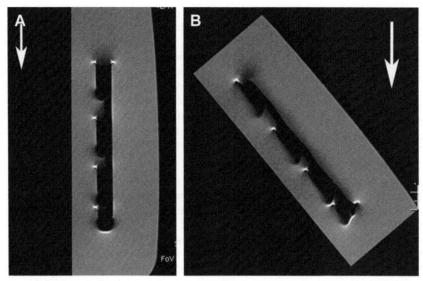

Fig. 4. Titanium rod in a water bath imaged on a 1.5T MR scanner, first with the long axis of the rod oriented parallel to the main magnetic field (B_0) of the scanner (A) and subsequently after rotating the rod approximately 45° with respect to B_0 (B). The frequency-encoding gradient (*arrows*) was parallel to B_0 during both acquisitions. The distortions are reduced when the long axis of the rod is oriented parallel to B_0 (A), and the distortions are increased when the angle between the long axis of the rod and B_0 is increased (B).

Using short tau inversion recovery for fat suppression

Techniques that are relatively insensitive to magnetic field heterogeneity (eg, STIR and Dixon techniques) produce less artifact compared with frequency-selective fat-suppression techniques (Fig. 8). The drawbacks of these techniques include decreased SNR and increased imaging time; these drawbacks are acceptable in most cases. The Dixon technique provides better SNR than

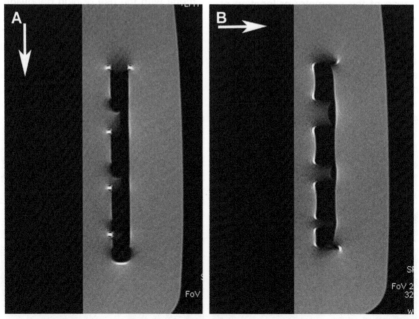

Fig. 5. Titanium rod in a water bath imaged on a 1.5T MR scanner with the long axis of the rod parallel to the main magnetic field (B_0). The images were then obtained with the frequency-encoding direction parallel (A) and perpendicular (B) to the long axis of the rod (*arrows* indicate the direction of the frequency-encoding gradient). The distortions are reduced when the long axis of the rod and frequency-encoding gradient direction are parallel (A) compared with when they are perpendicular (B).

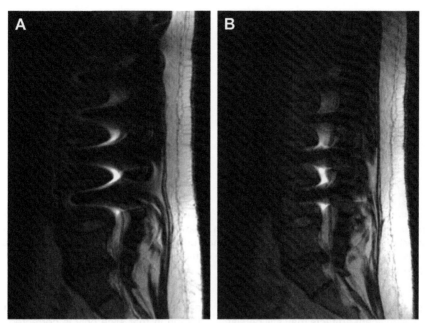

Fig. 6. Sagittal FSE T2-weighted images from MR imaging of lumbar spine. Image obtained with a receiver bandwidth of 130 Hz per pixel (*A*) shows worse artifact than image obtained with a receiver bandwidth of 400 Hz per pixel (*B*). Both images were obtained after a single excitation.

inversion recovery sequences,[16] whereas STIR provides more homogeneous fat suppression. As discussed earlier, fat suppression with the Dixon technique may fail in regions very close to metal.

Modifying voxel size, field of view, imaging matrix, and slice thickness

A smaller voxel size is associated with lesser artifact, as discussed previously. The voxel size can be decreased by using a high-resolution matrix and a small FOV and by obtaining thin slice images. This approach must be balanced with the

resulting loss in SNR and increase in imaging time. In clinical practice, the most effective method for achieving a smaller voxel is increasing the matrix in the frequency-encoding direction, which does not add to the imaging time.

Advanced Metal Artifact Reduction Techniques on MR Imaging

The aforementioned conventional methods of MAR can be performed on most MR systems without special software or hardware modifications.

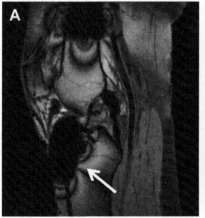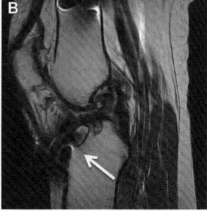

Fig. 7. Sagittal images from MR imaging of the knee in a patient with anterior cruciate ligament repair. (*A*) Image obtained with GRE sequence. (*B*) Image obtained with FSE sequence. There is blooming of the susceptibility artifact on the GRE sequence, which obscures anatomic details (*arrow*); on the FSE sequence, the distortions are significantly reduced and anatomic details are better visualized (*arrow*).

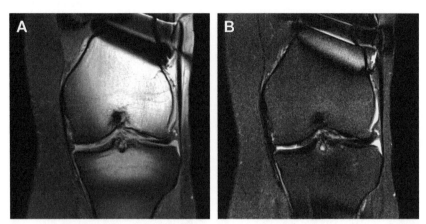

Fig. 8. Coronal images from MR imaging of the knee in a patient with hardware from an anterior cruciate ligament reconstruction. (*A*) Fat-suppression image obtained using a frequency-selective technique demonstrates inhomogeneous suppression. (*B*) Fat-suppression image obtained using STIR demonstrates much more homogeneous fat suppression.

Depending on the composition, size, and shape of the hardware, significant artifacts may still persist, which may limit the evaluation of bone and soft tissues adjacent to the implant. The magnetic field inhomogeneity results in both in-plane and through-plane artifacts. In-plane artifact is caused by improper frequency encoding at the time of readout and occurs in the readout direction. Through-plane distortions are caused by improper spatial encoding at the time of slice selection and occur in the z-direction. Newer MAR techniques are now available for clinical use from different vendors; these techniques address both in-plane and through-plane distortions to reduce susceptibility artifact. Three of these techniques that are discussed in greater detail are view angle tilting (VAT), slice encoding for metal artifact correction (SEMAC), and multi-acquisition variable-resonance image combination (MAVRIC).

View angle tilting
VAT, although first described by Cho and colleagues[18] in 1988, has only recently been used clinically. A modification to a conventional 2-dimentionsal (2D) SE sequence, this technique is now available commercially to reduce metal artifact. VAT corrects the in-plane distortion caused by metal hardware by applying a gradient along the z-direction with the same amplitude as the slice select gradient during readout (ie, at the same time as the frequency-encoding gradient). The application of this additional gradient results in viewing the slice at an angle that is a function of the strength of the two gradients. Viewing the slice at this angle helps to correct the linear malposition of spins along the readout direction caused by the metal artifact. Because this gradient is applied to a particular slice, the spatial misregistration in that slice only is corrected (ie, in-plane distortion). Distortions resulting in spatial misregistration above or below the selected slice (ie, through-plane distortion) are not corrected by this technique. As a result, although susceptibility artifact is reduced further with the use of VAT than with conventional MAR techniques,[18–20] a significant amount of artifact remains (**Fig. 9**). Therefore, VAT is usually used in combination with SEMAC, a technique that corrects through-plane distortion.

The main drawback of VAT is that it results in blurring of the entire image (not just the area adjacent to the implant). This blurring has been proposed to be the result of slice profile modulation and tilting of the view angle, with the former being the primary factor.[21] Several techniques have been described to reduce this blurring, including increasing the bandwidth of the RF pulse, increasing the readout bandwidth, using a quadratic phase RF pulse, and using a multiple readout method in which each readout is shorter in duration than the main lobe of the RF pulse.[21] Other techniques, such as increasing the readout-encoding gradient, can also compensate for the blurring; but these methods result in a decrease in SNR. This decrease in SNR, however, does not compromise the interpretability of the image.[19,22]

Slice encoding for metal artifact correction
SEMAC is a newer MAR technique that corrects through-plane distortions caused by metal. This method uses a 2D excitation pulse combined with a 3-dimensional (3D) FSE acquisition to capture signal from the slice that has been distorted

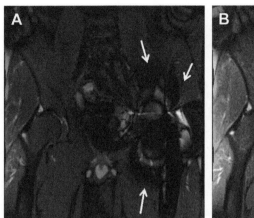
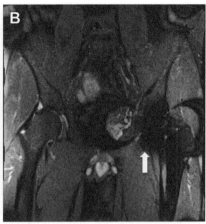

Fig. 9. Coronal MR images obtained with a conventional STIR technique with high bandwidth (*A*) and STIR technique with addition of VAT (*B*) in a patient with left hip replacement. A significant decrease in the susceptibility artifact (*arrows*) is seen on the STIR image with VAT (*B*) compared with the conventional STIR image (*A*). A significant amount of susceptibility artifact (*arrows*) is still present with VAT (*B*) because of a lack of correction of the through-plane distortions.

above or below the slice. SEMAC works in tandem with the previously described MAR techniques (ie, FSE imaging technique to reduce the intravoxel dephasing and VAT technique to correct the in-plane distortion).

In the presence of magnetic susceptibility, the application of a slice-selective RF pulse may excite not only the protons in the slice of interest but also protons in other slices above and below the slice of interest that happen to be spinning at the excited frequency. As a consequence, signal seen in an image section may actually belong to a very different slice position. SEMAC is able to resolve the true location of all excited signal by acquiring signal not only from the excited slice but also from the slices above and below the excited slice with an additional phase-encoding

gradient applied along the z-axis. Postprocessing techniques are then used to combine the signal from all of the individual slices from the volume to generate a corrected 2D image for each particular slice.[23] The use of SEMAC corrects through-plane distortion but not in-plane distortion that occurs with susceptibility artifact along the frequency-encoding direction. Therefore, this technique is used in combination with VAT. SEMAC has been shown to provide better artifact reduction than conventional MAR techniques.[24] **Figs. 10** and **11** show the drastic reduction in artifact when images are obtained with SEMAC and VAT in comparison with standard imaging.

The main limitation with SEMAC is that the imaging time with this technique is significantly longer than for a standard 2D FSE technique because

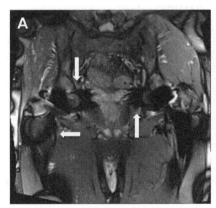
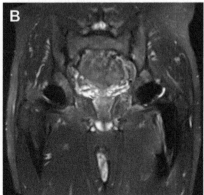

Fig. 10. Coronal STIR MR images of the pelvis in a patient with bilateral hip replacements. (*A*) Conventional STIR image with high bandwidth (imaging time, 2 minutes) demonstrates distortion and signal voids near the implants, obscuring areas of bone and soft tissue (*arrows*). (*B*) Distortion and signal voids are significantly reduced on an STIR image with SEMAC/VAT (imaging time, 6 minutes).

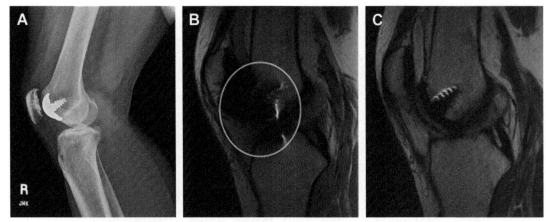

Fig. 11. Lateral radiograph of the knee (*A*), sagittal image of the knee with conventional FSE proton density (PD)–weighted high-bandwidth technique (*B*), and sagittal image of the knee with FSE PD-weighted image with SEMAC and VAT technique (*C*) in a patient with metallic screw in femoral trochlea. On conventional FSE PD-weighted image (*B*), there is extensive artifact with obscuration of the anatomy in the area adjacent to the screw (*circle*); this artifact is significantly reduced with the use of SEMAC and VAT (*C*).

to generate each 2D slice with SEMAC, a volume of data must be acquired. Because the additional SEMAC encoding increases the SNR, methods to reduce the scan time, such as partial Fourier imaging and parallel imaging, can be applied efficiently.[25]

Multi-acquisition variable-resonance image combination

MAVRIC is a new imaging technique that reduces both through-plane and in-plane susceptibility artifact by combining the signal from a volume of data excited with RF pulses over a range of frequencies centered around the resonance frequency. As previously described, the magnetic susceptibility of a metallic implant changes the resonance frequency of the protons spinning adjacent to it. If the altered resonance frequency is different from but close to the resonance frequency of the tissue, the protons can be excited by using a wider bandwidth RF pulse and a signal can be recorded. However, if the frequencies of the spins are vastly different from the resonance frequency, as is the case near metallic hardware, even the widest bandwidth RF pulse cannot excite all of these protons. As a result, signal voids will occur adjacent to the implant. With MAVRIC, these spins are excited through the use of multiple narrow bandwidth RF pulses with a range of frequencies at, above, and below the resonance frequency. A 3D FSE technique is used to acquire volumetric data for each frequency range, and the final image is then generated by combining the data for all of these volumes. Because the 3D excitation is performed without any slice selection gradient, all of the acquired signal is restricted to the rather narrow

excitation bandwidth, which also means that MAVRIC does not suffer from the severe in-plane distortions that occur with 2D FSE techniques. MAVRIC has been shown to provide superior artifact reduction when compared with standard MAR techniques (**Fig. 12**).[26,27]

The main drawback of MAVRIC, similar to SEMAC, is a long scan time, as multiple volume sets must be acquired for a single imaging volume.[26] Because of the increased SNR gained from multiple volume acquisitions, the scan time can be reduced by using techniques such as parallel imaging and a compressed sensing algorithm.[27] Another limitation with MAVRIC is its non-slice-selective excitation, which can result in significant wrap artifact (aliasing) in the z-direction that can degrade the images. A recently described SEMAC-MAVRIC hybrid technique MAVRIC-SL (MAVRIC selective) combines the application of a slice-encoding gradient during acquisition with the MAVRIC technique. This hybrid approach takes advantage of both techniques to provide the spectral selectivity of MAVRIC and the slice selectivity of SEMAC to obtain images with good SNR and minimal aliasing.[28]

Other Metal Artifact Reduction Techniques on MR Imaging

In addition to the aforementioned MAR techniques, several other techniques have been proposed to reduce susceptibility artifacts, such as single-point imaging,[29] prepolarized MR imaging,[30] and dual reversed-gradient acquisitions.[31] These techniques suffer from various technical limitations, such as low spatial resolution, lengthy

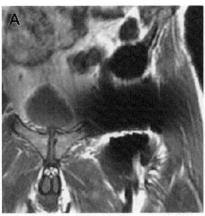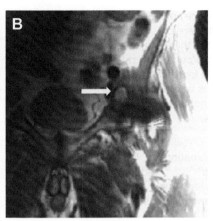

Fig. 12. Coronal proton density–weighted MR images of the pelvis obtained with standard FSE technique (*A*) and MAVRIC technique (*B*) in a patient with a left total hip arthroplasty. Susceptibility artifact with the MAVRIC technique (*B*) is significantly reduced compared with artifact on the standard technique (*A*), allowing visualization of cystic changes in the acetabulum (*arrow*) with the MAVRIC technique that are not visible with the standard technique. (*Courtesy of* Richard Kijowski, MD, University of Wisconsin.)

imaging times, and need for dedicated hardware; so these methods are not available for clinical use.[26]

METAL ARTIFACT ON COMPUTED TOMOGRAPHY IMAGING

Patients with metal implants may undergo CT imaging for complaints related to the implant itself or for other unrelated complaints. In such cases, the artifacts caused by the metal degrade image quality by obscuring the anatomy, making it difficult or sometimes even impossible to evaluate the implant-bone interface and the adjacent soft tissues. The primary causes of metal artifact on CT imaging are from photon starvation, beam hardening, scatter, and partial volume averaging.[32] The degree of artifact is also affected by the composition of the metal and the size and orientation of the implant. Similar to MR imaging, implants containing titanium alloys cause less artifact than implants composed of CoCr or stainless steel alloys[33]; implants oriented with their long axis along the z-direction of the scanner cause less artifact. Therefore, when possible, the patient positioning during scanning should be adjusted so that the x-ray beam traverses the smallest possible cross-sectional area of the implant.[34,35]

TECHNIQUES TO REDUCE METAL ARTIFACTS ON COMPUTED TOMOGRAPHY IMAGING

As with MR imaging, the severity of artifacts from metal implants depends on several factors. Some of these factors cannot be controlled or modified by radiologists, such as composition,

size, and shape of the implant. Other factors can be modified to help decrease the artifacts. In this section, MAR techniques are broadly divided into 2 categories[1]: standard artifact reduction methods (using optimized acquisition parameters) and[2] advanced artifact reduction (artifact correction) methods (using dedicated acquisition and postprocessing methods).

Standard Metal Artifact Reduction Techniques on Computed Tomography Imaging

Several measures can be taken to reduce metal artifact on CT on most CT scanners without the need for special hardware or software.

Increasing tube potential (kilovolts peak)
Increasing the kilovolts peak increases the mean energy of the x-ray photons, which results in reducing photon starvation and beam hardening.[9,32,36]

Increasing tube current (milliampere second)
Increasing the milliampere second reduces photon starvation by increasing the total number of photons in the x-ray beam.[32,35]

The benefits in artifact reduction with increases in kilovolts peak and milliampere second, especially with respect to increased radiation risk, have not been fully investigated; there are no established values for kilovolts peak or milliampere second when imaging metallic implants.[33]

Reducing beam width
Most scanners (except those with ultrawide detectors) use one-dimensional scatter grids that only block the photons in the x-y plane, the photons

in z-direction are not blocked. A decrease in beam width would, therefore, result in reduced scatter.[37] However, very thin beams reduce the dose efficiency (umbra/penumbra ratio) and can result in unacceptably long scan times; therefore, detector configurations with beam widths less than 10 mm are typically not used in clinical protocols on modern scanners.

Using narrow collimation and thin slices
A narrow collimation (eg, 0.6 mm vs 1.2 mm) and thinner slices[9,32,36,38] reduce partial volume averaging. However, thinner slices have increased image noise and decreased SNR (at a matched dose).

Reconstructing thicker slices and using a smooth reconstruction algorithm
Many of the MAR techniques discussed earlier can lead to decreased SNR. For interpretation of 2D images, thicker slices can be reconstructed to reduce noise.[9,35] Additionally, a smoother reconstruction kernel can be beneficial both for 2D interpretation as well as for 3D volume rendering applications.[34] At the authors' institution, a 2-mm slice thickness for 2D interpretation is used along with a smooth soft tissue reconstruction kernel.

Using an extended computed tomography scale
The standard CT scale uses the 12-bit range that extends from −1024 to +3071 Hounsfield units (HU). Some scanners have the ability to scale the raw data using a higher bit range that can increases the range of attenuation values by 10-fold or greater.[39] With the extended CT scale, the attenuation values can be displayed over a much wider range to help separate these attenuation differences. The extended scale, however, does not restore accurate HU values, and its benefits are limited.[40]

Advanced Metal Artifact Reduction Techniques on Computed Tomography Imaging

Monoenergetic dual-energy computed tomography
One of the primary causes of metal artifact is beam hardening. This occurs because x-ray tubes generate a polyenergetic beam. If all of the photons were of the same energy (ie, monoenergetic or monochromatic), beam hardening would be eliminated, as the photon energy would remain the same before and after passing through the metal. Unfortunately, current-generation x-ray tubes cannot generate a monochromatic beam of sufficient intensity. However, with the use of

dual-energy CT (DECT) and special postprocessing techniques, pseudo or virtual monoenergetic images can be reconstructed.[41]

DECT refers to imaging the same volume of tissue with 2 different polychromatic energies.[42] Current-generation DECT scanners accomplish this by one of 3 methods depending on the vendor. The first method uses 2 x-ray tubes, one at a higher energy (typically 140 kVp) and the second at a lower energy (80 or 100 kVp).[43] The second method uses a single x-ray tube that rapidly alternates between generating a high-energy and a low-energy beam (fast kilovolts peak switching, also known as gemstone spectral imaging).[44] The third method uses a single x-ray tube with dual-layer detector, each capturing photons of different energies.[45]

Regardless of how the data sets from the two energies are obtained, this information can then be postprocessed to reconstruct images as if the data were acquired using a monochromatic energy. This postprocessing is based on a 2-material decomposition that represents the attenuation of the imaging object as a sum of attenuations from the two objects made of the basis materials (water and iodine). Because the attenuation behavior for the two basis materials is well known and tabulated for any given photon energy (kiloelectron volt), one can calculate the attenuations of the two objects for any given kiloelectron volt and then combine them to obtain the attenuation of the imaging object at this kiloelectron volt. Using this method, it is possible to obtain virtual monoenergetic images for kiloelectron volt values ranging from as low as 40 keV (right above the iodine K-edge value) to as high as 190 keV (more than 140 keV, which corresponds to the highest photon energy in the 140-kVp spectrum).[41]

Several recent studies have reported both qualitative and quantitative reductions in metal artifact with the monoenergetic DECT technique (**Fig. 13**).[46–55] In these studies, optimal monochromatic energies varied between 95 and 150 keV, depending on the composition and size of the metal implant.[46] Although most of these studies were performed using either dual-source[46,48–51,53] or fast kilovolts peak switching[47,52,54,55] technologies, a recent study demonstrated that the DECT MAR technique can also be applied to the dual-energy data obtained with 2 consecutive spiral scans.[56] Therefore, in principle, this technique can be used on any modern scanner (provided the necessary postprocessing is available). Although the dual-energy monoenergetic technique is effective for artifact reduction by reducing effects of beam hardening, when the metal artifact is dominated by photon starvation (eg, large size

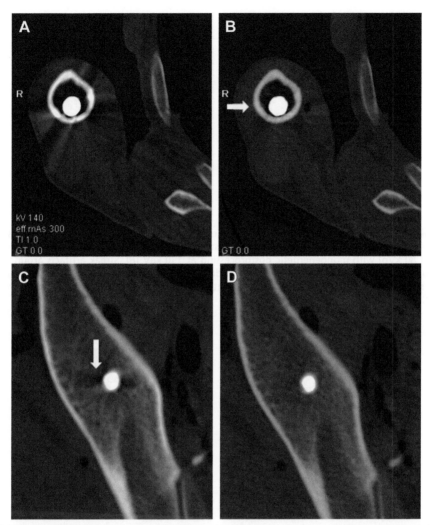

Fig. 13. Axial CT images (*A, B*) in a cadaver with a right shoulder arthroplasty; axial CT images in a cadaver with a metallic nail (*C, D*) in the right iliac bone. Images in (*A*) and (*C*) were acquired using a standard single-energy technique (140 kVp, 300 reference mAs) and FBP, and images in (*B*) and (*D*) were acquired using a dose-matched DECT technique (140 kVp and 80 kVp) with monoenergetic postprocessing at 130 keV. The images obtained with DECT have significantly reduced beam-hardening artifacts when compared with the images obtained with the standard technique (*arrows*).

or very dense metal), the performance of the DECT technique is limited (**Fig. 14**).

Replacing corrupted raw data (sinogram inpainting)

Several new techniques are emerging that reduce metal artifacts by replacing the corrupted data. Only some of these techniques are commercially available, with others still in various stages of prototyping. All of these techniques follow a similar approach (sometimes referred to as *sinogram inpainting*) in which the projection data corrupted by metal is identified in the raw data (sinogram) space and replaced with the approximated or interpolated data using various algorithms.[57] In principle, the inpainting-based approach can be realized exclusively in the image space by using the synthetic raw data obtained with the forward-projection operation. This solution seems attractive because it is generic and does not require access to the actual scanner-specific raw data; however, its performance has been limited in comparison with the solution implemented in the projection space.[58] To the best of the authors' knowledge, the only commercially available MAR product implemented in the image space is MARIS (metal artifact reduction in image space) (Siemens Healthcare, Forchheim, Germany).[59] All other

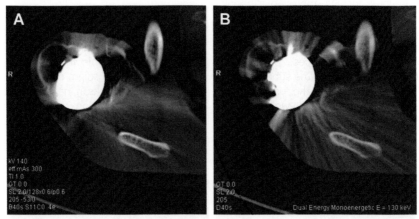

Fig. 14. Axial CT images in a cadaver with right shoulder arthroplasty acquired using a standard single-energy technique (140 kVp, 300 reference mAs) and FBP reconstruction (*A*) and using a dose-matched DECT technique (140 kVp and 80 kVp) with monoenergetic postprocessing at 130 keV (*B*). Streak artifacts around the implant with DECT (*B*) are more prominent than with the standard technique (*A*). This paradoxic result is likely related to the large size and composition (CoCr) of the implant, resulting in significant photon starvation that cannot be corrected.

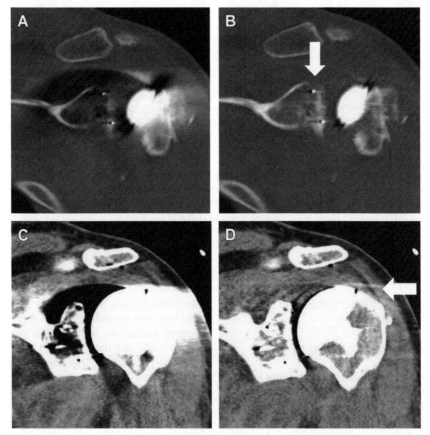

Fig. 15. Axial (*A*, *B*) and coronal (*C*, *D*) CT images in 2 different patients with left shoulder arthroplasty obtained using a standard 140-kVp, 300 reference mAs technique. Images in (*A*) and (*C*) were reconstructed with standard FBP, and images in (*B*) and (*D*) were reconstructed with IMAR. The IMAR images (*B*, *D*) have significantly reduced streak artifacts, allowing better visualization of the glenoid (*arrow*) and supraspinatus tendon (*arrow*), compared with images reconstructed with FBP (*A*, *C*).

commercial MAR products, such as MARS (GE Medical Systems, Milwaukee, WI), O-MAR (metal artifact reduction for orthopedic implants) (Philips Healthcare System, Cleveland, OH), and SEMAR (single energy metal artifact reduction) (Toshiba Medical Systems, Otawara, Japan), use the projection space. The technical details of these solutions are beyond the scope of this article but can be found (to the extent they are revealed) in the provided references.[47,52,54,55,60,61]

The main advantage of sinogram inpainting-based techniques is that they can be applied to the data acquired on any CT scanner (provided the MAR software is available). However, they can also introduce new artifacts and suffer from data loss near the metal edge, which has limited their clinical utility in the past. To address these limitations, new prototype software from Siemens known as IMAR (iterative metal artifact reduction) implements additional steps, such as normalizing the sinogram before interpolation[62] and incorporating the high-frequency data from the original filtered back projection (FBP) reconstruction into the final MAR-corrected image.[63] In recent studies, the IMAR technique was demonstrated to produce more accurate attenuation values and improved image quality in patients with hip arthroplasties[64] and shoulder arthroplasties[53,65] when compared with FBP (Fig. 15).

The main drawback of these techniques is that their clinical availability as of yet is still limited (usually restricted to the latest-generation scanners or as prototypes for select academic centers); these techniques also require increased image reconstruction times compared with FBP. Although early studies have been promising in their ability to improve image quality, further studies are needed to determine whether these techniques are helpful in clinical practice.

SUMMARY

Standard and advanced MR and CT techniques can reduce artifacts related to metallic implants. Standard MR techniques to reduce metal artifact include scanning on lower-field-strength systems; optimal positioning of hardware; and using high-bandwidth parameters, smaller voxels, and appropriate sequences (eg, FSE and STIR) and frequency-encoding direction. Advanced MR techniques to further reduce metal artifact include the use of specialized sequences, such as VAT, SEMAC, and MAVRIC. Standard MAR CT techniques include optimal positioning of the implant, using a high kilovolts peak and milliampere second technique, using narrow collimation to acquire images and thicker sections to reconstruct the data, and using smooth reconstruction algorithms and extended CT scales. Further reduction in metal artifact can be achieved by using advanced techniques, such as monoenergetic DECT, and metal subtraction techniques, such as sinogram inpainting.

With the projected increase of patients with metallic implants, the need for MAR techniques will undoubtedly continue to grow in the future. Knowledge of and familiarity with these techniques will allow better visualization of anatomy and pathology and better evaluation of complications related to metal implants.

REFERENCES

1. Kim SH, Wise BL, Zhang Y, et al. Increasing incidence of shoulder arthroplasty in the United States. J Bone Joint Surg Am 2011;93(24):2249–54.
2. Kurtz S, Mowat F, Ong K, et al. Prevalence of primary and revision total hip and knee arthroplasty in the United States from 1990 through 2002. J Bone Joint Surg Am 2005;87(7):1487–97.
3. Losina E, Thornhill TS, Rome BN, et al. The dramatic increase in total knee replacement utilization rates in the United States cannot be fully explained by growth in population size and the obesity epidemic. J Bone Joint Surg Am 2012;94(3):201–7.
4. Ravi B, Croxford R, Reichmann WM, et al. The changing demographics of total joint arthroplasty recipients in the United States and Ontario from 2001 to 2007. Best Pract Res Clin Rheumatol 2012;26(5): 637–47.
5. Kurtz S, Ong K, Lau E, et al. Projections of primary and revision hip and knee arthroplasty in the United States from 2005 to 2030. J Bone Joint Surg Am 2007;89(4):780–5.
6. Walde TA, Weiland DE, Leung SB, et al. Comparison of CT, MRI, and radiographs in assessing pelvic osteolysis: a cadaveric study. Clin Orthop Relat Res 2005;437:138–44.
7. Weiland DE, Walde TA, Leung SB, et al. Magnetic resonance imaging in the evaluation of periprosthetic acetabular osteolysis: a cadaveric study. J Orthop Res 2005;23(4):713–9.
8. Potter HG, Nestor BJ, Sofka CM, et al. Magnetic resonance imaging after total hip arthroplasty: evaluation of periprosthetic soft tissue. J Bone Joint Surg Am 2004;86A:1947–54.
9. Lee MJ, Kim S, Lee SA, et al. Overcoming artifacts from metallic orthopedic implants at high-field-strength MR imaging and multi-detector CT. Radiographics 2007;27(3):791–803.
10. Ganapathi M, Joseph G, Savage R, et al. MRI susceptibility artefacts related to scaphoid screws: the effect of screw type, screw orientation and imaging parameters. J Hand Surg Br 2002;27(2):165–70.

11. Suh JS, Jeong EK, Shin KH, et al. Minimizing artifacts caused by metallic implants at MR imaging: experimental and clinical studies. AJR Am J Roentgenol 1998;171(5):1207–13.

12. Naraghi AM, White LM. Magnetic resonance imaging of joint replacements. Semin Musculoskelet Radiol 2006;10(1):98–106.

13. Guermazi A, Miaux Y, Zaim S, et al. Metallic artefacts in MR imaging: effects of main field orientation and strength. Clin Radiol 2003;58(4):322–8.

14. Petersilge CA, Lewin JS, Duerk JL, et al. Optimizing imaging parameters for MR evaluation of the spine with titanium pedicle screws. AJR Am J Roentgenol 1996;166(5):1213–8.

15. Ludeke KM, Roschmann P, Tischler R. Susceptibility artefacts in NMR imaging. Magn Reson Imaging 1985;3(4):329–43.

16. Del Grande F, Santini F, Herzka DA, et al. Fat-suppression techniques for 3-T MR imaging of the musculoskeletal system. Radiographics 2014;34(1):217–33.

17. Ulbrich EJ, Sutter R, Aguiar RF, et al. STIR sequence with increased receiver bandwidth of the inversion pulse for reduction of metallic artifacts. AJR Am J Roentgenol 2012;199(6):W735–42.

18. Cho ZH, Kim DJ, Kim YK. Total inhomogeneity correction including chemical shifts and susceptibility by view angle tilting. Med Phys 1988;15(1):7–11.

19. Chang SD, Lee MJ, Munk PL, et al. MRI of spinal hardware: comparison of conventional T1-weighted sequence with a new metal artifact reduction sequence. Skeletal Radiol 2001;30(4):213–8.

20. Lee MJ, Janzen DL, Munk PL, et al. Quantitative assessment of an MR technique for reducing metal artifact: application to spin-echo imaging in a phantom. Skeletal Radiol 2001;30(7):398–401.

21. Butts K, Pauly JM, Gold GE. Reduction of blurring in view angle tilting MRI. Magn Reson Med 2005;53(2): 418–24.

22. Olsen RV, Munk PL, Lee MJ, et al. Metal artifact reduction sequence: early clinical applications. Radiographics 2000;20(3):699–712.

23. Lu W, Pauly KB, Gold GE, et al. SEMAC: slice encoding for metal artifact correction in MRI. Magn Reson Med 2009;62(1):66–76.

24. Chen CA, Chen W, Goodman SB, et al. New MR imaging methods for metallic implants in the knee: artifact correction and clinical impact. J Magn Reson Imaging 2011;33(5):1121–7.

25. Hargreaves BA, Chen W, Lu W, et al. Accelerated slice encoding for metal artifact correction. J Magn Reson Imaging 2010;31(4):987–96.

26. Hayter CL, Koff MF, Shah P, et al. MRI after arthroplasty: comparison of MAVRIC and conventional fast spin-echo techniques. AJR Am J Roentgenol 2011;197(3):W405–11.

27. Koch KM, Lorbiecki JE, Hinks RS, et al. A multispectral three-dimensional acquisition technique for imaging near metal implants. Magn Reson Med 2009;61(2):381–90.

28. Koch KM, Brau AC, Chen W, et al. Imaging near metal with a MAVRIC-SEMAC hybrid. Magn Reson Med 2011;65(1):71–82.

29. Ramos-Cabrer P, van Duynhoven JP, Van der Toorn A, et al. MRI of hip prostheses using single-point methods: in vitro studies towards the artifact-free imaging of individuals with metal implants. Magn Reson Imaging 2004;22(8):1097–103.

30. Venook RD, Matter NI, Ramachandran M, et al. Prepolarized magnetic resonance imaging around metal orthopedic implants. Magn Reson Med 2006;56(1):177–86.

31. Skare S, Andersson JL. Correction of MR image distortions induced by metallic objects using a 3D cubic B-spline basis set: application to stereotactic surgical planning. Magn Reson Med 2005;54(1):169–81.

32. Barrett JF, Keat N. Artifacts in CT: recognition and avoidance. Radiographics 2004;24(6):1679–91.

33. Haramati N, Staron RB, Mazel-Sperling K, et al. CT scans through metal scanning technique versus hardware composition. Comput Med Imaging Graph 1994;18(6):429–34.

34. Douglas-Akinwande AC, Buckwalter KA, Rydberg J, et al. Multichannel CT: evaluating the spine in postoperative patients with orthopedic hardware. Radiographics 2006;26(Suppl 1):S97–110.

35. Stradiotti P, Curti A, Castellazzi G, et al. Metal-related artifacts in instrumented spine. Techniques for reducing artifacts in CT and MRI: state of the art. Eur Spine J 2009;18(Suppl 1):102–8.

36. Moon SG, Hong SH, Choi JY, et al. Metal artifact reduction by the alteration of technical factors in multidetector computed tomography: a 3-dimensional quantitative assessment. J Comput Assist Tomogr 2008;32(4):630–3.

37. Goldman LW. Principles of CT: radiation dose and image quality. J Nucl Med Technol 2007;35(4):213–25 [quiz: 226–8].

38. Glover GH, Pelc NJ. Nonlinear partial volume artifacts in x-ray computed tomography. Med Phys 1980;7(3):238–48.

39. Glide-Hurst C, Chen D, Zhong H, et al. Changes realized from extended bit-depth and metal artifact reduction in CT. Med Phys 2013;40(6):061711.

40. Gosheger G, Ludwig K, Hillmann A, et al. An extended CT scale technique for evaluating periprosthetic bone lesions - an in vitro study. Rofo 2001;173(12):1099–103.

41. Yu L, Leng S, McCollough CH. Dual-energy CT-based monochromatic imaging. AJR Am J Roentgenol 2012;199(Suppl 5):S9–15.

42. Johnson TR. Dual-energy CT: general principles. AJR Am J Roentgenol 2012;199(Suppl 5):S3–8.

43. Johnson TR, Krauss B, Sedlmair M, et al. Material differentiation by dual energy CT: initial experience. Eur Radiol 2007;17(6):1510–7.

44. Chandra N, Langan DA. Gemstone detector: dual energy imaging via fast kVp switching. In: Johnson TR, Fink C, Schönberg SO, et al, editors. Dual energy CT in clinical practice. Heidelberg, Germany: Springer-Verlag GmbH; 2011. p. 35–41.

45. Vlassenbroek A. Dual layer CT. In: Johnson TR, Fink C, Schönberg SO, et al, editors. Dual energy CT in clinical practice. Heidelberg, Germany: Springer-Verlag GmbH; 2011. p. 21–34.

46. Bamberg F, Dierks A, Nikolaou K, et al. Metal artifact reduction by dual energy computed tomography using monoenergetic extrapolation. Eur Radiol 2011; 21(7):1424–9.

47. Lee YH, Park KK, Song HT, et al. Metal artefact reduction in gemstone spectral imaging dual-energy CT with and without metal artefact reduction software. Eur Radiol 2012;22(6):1331–40.

48. Meinel FG, Bischoff B, Zhang Q, et al. Metal artifact reduction by dual-energy computed tomography using energetic extrapolation: a systematically optimized protocol. Invest Radiol 2012;47(7):406–14.

49. Zhou C, Zhao YE, Luo S, et al. Monoenergetic imaging of dual-energy CT reduces artifacts from implanted metal orthopedic devices in patients with factures. Acad Radiol 2011;18(10):1252–7.

50. Guggenberger R, Winklhofer S, Osterhoff G, et al. Metallic artefact reduction with monoenergetic dual-energy CT: systematic ex vivo evaluation of posterior spinal fusion implants from various vendors and different spine levels. Eur Radiol 2012; 22(11):2357–64.

51. Lewis M, Reid K, Toms AP. Reducing the effects of metal artefact using high keV monoenergetic reconstruction of dual energy CT (DECT) in hip replacements. Skeletal Radiol 2013;42(2):275–82.

52. Pessis E, Campagna R, Sverzut JM, et al. Virtual monochromatic spectral imaging with fast kilovoltage switching: reduction of metal artifacts at CT. Radiographics 2013;33(2):573–83.

53. Winklhofer S, Benninger E, Spross C, et al. CT metal artefact reduction for internal fixation of the proximal humerus: value of mono-energetic extrapolation from dual-energy and iterative reconstructions. Clin Radiol 2014;69(5):e199–206.

54. Wang F, Xue H, Yang X, et al. Reduction of metal artifacts from alloy hip prostheses in computer tomography. J Comput Assist Tomogr 2014;38:828–33.

55. Wang Y, Qian B, Li B, et al. Metal artifacts reduction using monochromatic images from spectral CT: evaluation of pedicle screws in patients with scoliosis. Eur J Radiol 2013;82(8):e360–6.

56. Mangold S, Gatidis S, Luz O, et al. Single-source dual-energy computed tomography: use of monoenergetic extrapolation for a reduction of metal artifacts. Invest Radiol 2014;49:788–93.

57. Kalender WA, Hebel R, Ebersberger J. Reduction of CT artifacts caused by metallic implants. Radiology 1987;164(2):576–7.

58. Joemai RM, de Bruin PW, Veldkamp WJ, et al. Metal artifact reduction for CT: development, implementation, and clinical comparison of a generic and a scanner-specific technique. Med Phys 2012;39(2): 1125–32.

59. Raupach R, Shukla H, Amies C, et al. MARIS – metal artifact reduction in image space – technical principles. Siemens white paper. 2013.

60. Li H, Noel C, Chen H, et al. Clinical evaluation of a commercial orthopedic metal artifact reduction tool for CT simulations in radiation therapy. Med Phys 2012;39(12):7507–17.

61. Gondim Teixeira PA, Meyer JB, Baumann C, et al. Total hip prosthesis CT with single-energy projection-based metallic artifact reduction: impact on the visualization of specific periprosthetic soft tissue structures. Skeletal Radiol 2014;43:1237–46.

62. Meyer E, Raupach R, Lell M, et al. Normalized metal artifact reduction (NMAR) in computed tomography. Med Phys 2010;37(10):5482–93.

63. Meyer E, Raupach R, Lell M, et al. Frequency split metal artifact reduction (FSMAR) in computed tomography. Med Phys 2012;39(4):1904–16.

64. Morsbach F, Bickelhaupt S, Wanner GA, et al. Reduction of metal artifacts from hip prostheses on CT images of the pelvis: value of iterative reconstructions. Radiology 2013;268(1):237–44.

65. Subhas N, Primak AN, Obuchowski NA, et al. Iterative metal artifact reduction: evaluation and optimization of technique. Skeletal Radiol 2014;43: 1729–35.

Advanced Noncontrast MR Imaging in Musculoskeletal Radiology

Sasan Partovi, MD[a],*, Hendrik von Tengg-Kobligk, MD[b],
Nicholas Bhojwani, MD[a], Christof Karmonik, PhD[c],
Martin Maurer, MD[b], Mark R. Robbin, MD[a]

KEYWORDS

- Skeletal muscle • Blood-oxygen-level-dependent MR imaging • Arterial spin labeling
- Diffusion-weighted imaging • Diffusion-tensor imaging • Peripheral arterial occlusive disease
- Soft-tissue and bone tumors

KEY POINTS

- The blood-oxygen-level-dependent (BOLD) MR imaging signal in the skeletal muscle provides information about the muscle microcirculation. The most common paradigm applied in clinical settings is the cuff-compression paradigm, leading to ischemia followed by hyperemia. Impaired muscle microcirculation has been demonstrated with BOLD MR imaging in patients with peripheral arterial occlusive disease (PAOD) and systemic sclerosis.
- Arterial spin labeling (ASL) is an MR imaging method without the need of exogenous contrast to measure skeletal muscle tissue perfusion. ASL is valuable in assessing PAOD but has several limitations.
- DWI of the musculoskeletal system is a relatively fast and robust technique that can be implemented for evaluation of soft-tissue and bone tumors. DTI and related techniques, originally developed for visualizing white matter fibers in the brain, have been translated to musculoskeletal imaging for visualizing muscle fiber groups. DTI has been applied to study various diseases, such as ischemia of the skeletal muscle, cervical spine disorders, and recurrent carpal tunnel syndrome.

MUSCLE BLOOD-OXYGEN-LEVEL-DEPENDENT MR IMAGING

Introduction

The technique of skeletal muscle blood-oxygen-level-dependent (BOLD) MR imaging has been derived from functional MR imaging of the brain. In neuroimaging, the BOLD technique is used to localize areas in the brain that are responsible for execution of specific tasks, such as the motor, sensory, or language function.[1] These areas are activated by performing a variety of paradigms, such as the word or sentence generation paradigm.[2]

Skeletal muscle BOLD MR imaging, similarly, uses blood as an endogenous contrast agent.[3] The technique detects changes in the intravascular ratio of oxyhemoglobin, which is diamagnetic to deoxyhemoglobin, which is paramagnetic. The magnetic properties of both forms of hemoglobin have an impact on the magnetic susceptibility of adjacent water protons.[4] An increase in the ratio of oxyhemoglobin to deoxyhemoglobin is leading

[a] Department of Radiology, University Hospitals Case Medical Center, Case Western Reserve University, 11100 Euclid Avenue, Cleveland, OH 44106, USA; [b] Institute of Diagnostic, Interventional and Pediatric Radiology, Inselspital University Hospitals Bern, Freiburgstrasse 4, Bern 3010, Switzerland; [c] MRI Core, Houston Methodist Research Institute, 6565 Fannin ST944, Houston, TX 77030, USA
* Corresponding author.
E-mail address: sasan.partovi@uhhospitals.org

Radiol Clin N Am 53 (2015) 549–567
http://dx.doi.org/10.1016/j.rcl.2015.01.005
0033-8389/15/$ – see front matter © 2015 Elsevier Inc. All rights reserved.

radiologic.theclinics.com

to a decrease in the transverse relaxation time and to an increase in the measured T2* signal. BOLD MR imaging is measured with a T2*-weighted MR imaging sequence. The BOLD signal is multifactorial, but it reflects primarily skeletal muscle microcirculation. As discussed earlier, paradigms are essential for clinical functional MR imaging of the brain. Similarly, to transfer the technique to the skeletal muscle, it was essential to develop suitable paradigms. Exercise, drugs, and oxygen ventilation paradigms have been suggested for usage in skeletal muscle BOLD MR imaging.[5–7] An approach that has been successfully applied in clinical practice for calf muscle BOLD MR imaging is the ischemia-hyperemia paradigm. For this paradigm, cuff compression is performed at the mid thigh level. With patients in the supine position, initially a resting phase imaging of approximately 5 minutes is performed; in the last 60 seconds of this resting phase, magnetic resonance (MR) signal detection can be started. That means that there is no acquisition performed in the initial 4 minutes. Then the occlusion pressure is applied with 30 to 50 mm Hg more than the individual systolic blood pressure by cuff inflation, and the MR signal is detected for 240 seconds (ischemia phase) followed by rapid deflation of the cuff to prevent extensive filling of the venous system. Once the cuff is rapidly deflated, the hyperemia phase starts and the MR signal is detected for another 600 seconds. The experimental setup is demonstrated in **Fig. 1**.

MR Imaging Protocol

Patients are imaged in the supine position. Muscle BOLD MR imaging is based on the echo-planar imaging (EPI) principle. A fat-saturated multi-shot multi-echo gradient-echo EPI sequence is acquired without administration of exogenous contrast material. The temporal resolution of the sequence can be one acquisition every 2 seconds, and the slice thickness is 5 mm with a gap of 5 mm at the maximum calf diameter. In previous studies, the following imaging parameters have been used: field of view (FOV) 384×192 mm^2, matrix size 192×96 leading to a voxel size of $2 \times 2 \times 5$ mm^3, repetition time (TR) of 2000 milliseconds, and flip angle of 25°.[4] The multi-echo component of the sequence is important to reduce inflow artifacts and separate the oxygenation-dependent T2* signal. Nearly identical increasing echo times (TE) are used, and they are usually between 7 and 80 milliseconds. For example, on a 1.5-T scanner TEs can be 8.1, 19.1, 30.1, 41.0, 52.0, and 63.0 milliseconds; and for a 3-T scanner, TEs can be 8.1, 18.9, 29.7, 40.5, 51.3, and 62.1 milliseconds. The gradient-echo component is of value because of its high oxygen sensitivity and its superior temporal resolution.[8] T1-weighted images of the corresponding muscle regions are performed for anatomic reference.

Previous studies in functional MR imaging of the brain have shown that using higher field strengths of MR magnets leads to a superior signal-to-noise ratio (SNR) and higher differences in BOLD signal changes.[9–11] In the calf muscle, it was demonstrated that a higher relative T2* signal change can be achieved when using a 3.0-T in comparison with a 1.5-T MR scanner. In one study, the ratio of activation-induced changes in the transverse relaxation rate of 3.0 T to 1.5 T ranged between 1.6 and 2.2.[4] These results indicate that skeletal

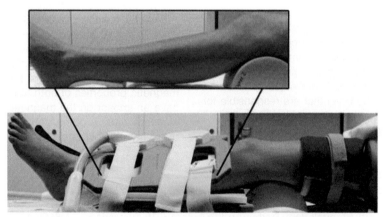

Fig. 1. The experimental setup of the ischemia-hyperemia paradigm for muscle BOLD MR imaging is depicted. The vascular array coils are appreciated. The standard leg sphygmomanometer is fixed at mid thigh level and will be inflated for the ischemia phase and then rapidly deflated for the hyperemia phase. (*From* Jacobi B, Bongartz G, Partovi S, et al. Skeletal muscle BOLD MRI: from underlying physiological concepts to its usefulness in clinical conditions. J Magn Reson Imaging 2012;35(6):1256; with permission.)

muscle BOLD MR imaging studies in patients should be ideally conducted on a standard 3.0-T MR scanner.

Postprocessing

Initial signal intensity (I0) is influenced by the T1 signal, proton density, and inflow alterations. T2* and I0 are separated, from multi-echo datasets using a pixel-by-pixel least-square fit of the mono-exponential decay to the signal intensities of the TEs to create T2* maps. Once the T2* parametric maps are created, motion correction is applied and the region of interest (ROI) needs to be determined. The ROI is usually rectangular and is set into the calf muscle, most commonly the gastrocnemius and/or soleus muscle. These ROIs have to be set careful to exclude larger vascular structures. The T2* time courses are then normalized to baseline, which is defined as the initial 30 to 45 seconds during the resting phase (equals 1 or 100% on the T2* time course graph). For motion correction and setting of the ROIs, a variety of software solutions are available. The T2* time course is then analyzed quantitatively using MatLab (MathWorks, Natick, MA). BOLD key parameters, as described in the following section, are extracted from the T2* time course of the study population.

Blood-Oxygen-Level-Dependent Key Parameters and Normal Blood-Oxygen-Level-Dependent Time Course

A thorough understanding of the normal T2* time course with its BOLD key parameters is of importance in order to recognize abnormal T2* time courses, which may reflect impaired microcirculation. In a healthy volunteer in the ischemia period during cuff inflation, the signal decreases until it reaches a minimum value. This minimum value is often described as *T2* minimum* or *minimum ischemic value*. The time from cuff inflation until reaching half of the minimum value can be used as a BOLD key parameter (time to half ischemic minimum) to further describe the ischemia phase. Once the cuff is rapidly deflated, the curve peaks within a short time frame, reaching its maximum; the T2* signal thereafter decreases until it reaches a steady value, the end value. The maximum value is termed *T2* maximum* or *hyperemia peak value*. The time from cuff deflation until reaching T2* maximum is named the *time to peak* (TTP). The time from cuff deflation until reaching half of the maximum value can be used as a BOLD key parameter (time to half peak value) to further describe the hyperemia phase. The declining slope after the T2* maximum value when decreasing towards the end value can also been used as a BOLD key parameter

during hyperemia. A typical BOLD time course with key parameters is depicted in **Fig. 2**.

Correlation with Other Techniques

The BOLD signal itself has been correlated with several other imaging techniques. One of the early skeletal muscle BOLD imaging studies performed a comparison with myoglobin proton spectroscopy. This study showed that the BOLD signal decrease during ischemia is related to hemoglobin deoxygenation rather than myoglobin desaturation.[12] During reactive hyperemia, the increase in muscle perfusion measured by arterial spin labeling (ASL) is correlated with the BOLD signal time course. However, this correlation was influenced in the study by the filling state of the blood vessels in the legs.[13] Skeletal muscle BOLD MR imaging has been correlated with laser Doppler flowmetry (LDF) and transcutaneous oxygen pressure (TcPO2) measurements in several studies. LDF and TcPO2 are frequently used in the clinical arena, for instance in patients with peripheral arterial occlusive disease. LDF is regarded as a representative measurement method for tissue perfusion.[14,15] TcPO2 is regarded as a representative measurement method for tissue oxygenation at the skin level underneath the sensor.[16] One study demonstrated in 15 healthy volunteers moderate

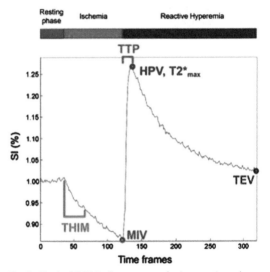

Fig. 2. Typical BOLD time course during resting phase, ischemia, and reactive hyperemia with key parameters marked in the curve. HPV, hyperemia peak value; MIV, minimum ischemic value; TEV, T2* end value; THIM, time to half ischemic minimum; T2* max, T2* maximum. (*From* Jacobi B, Bongartz G, Partovi S, et al. Skeletal muscle BOLD MRI: from underlying physiological concepts to its usefulness in clinical conditions. J Magn Reson Imaging 2012;35(6):1257; with permission.)

to good correlation between calf muscle BOLD MR imaging using the ischemia-hyperemia paradigm and LDF measurements as well as TcPO2 measurements.[17] Two other studies assessed the relationship of LDF and TcPO2 with muscle BOLD MR imaging in both patients with systemic sclerosis and healthy volunteers. One of the 2 studies demonstrated a very good correlation between BOLD MR imaging and TcPO2, suggesting that T2* alterations are reflecting reoxygenation deficits in the muscle tissue of the systemic sclerosis patient population.[18] The other study demonstrated a close correlation between muscle BOLD MR imaging and LDF in patients with systemic sclerosis reflecting tissue microperfusion.[19] These correlative studies allow the interpretation of the BOLD signal as perfusion-induced changes of oxygenation on the muscle tissue level.

Multifactorial Blood-Oxygen-Level-Dependent Signal

A variety of factors have an impact on the BOLD signal.

1. The age of the individual impacts the skeletal muscle BOLD signal. There are statistically significant age-dependent differences in the BOLD signal when comparing an elderly healthy population (mean age older than 60 years) as opposed to a younger healthy population (mean age around 30 years) during the reactive hyperemia phase.[20] In a further study, the previous results were confirmed for the reactive hyperemia phase and expanded to the ischemic phase when imaging the calf and foot muscles simultaneously with BOLD MR imaging.[21] Thus, it is imperative to compare age- and sex-matched study populations.
2. The physical activity/exercise level is of importance as it may influence the BOLD signal. More physically active people demonstrate higher BOLD signal increases after muscle contractions.[22]
3. Furthermore, the muscle with its predominant fiber type needs to be considered. The soleus is a slow-twitch oxidative muscle with a higher capillary density in comparison with the gastrocnemius muscle, which is a fast-twitch glycolytic muscle.[23–25] Therefore, it is not only important to compare the same calf muscle with regard to the BOLD time course but also ideally always include in the analysis at least one slow-twitch oxidative and one fast-twitch glycolytic muscle.

Given the multiple influencing factors, before enrolling patients for a study, the inclusion and exclusion criteria need to be defined strictly; a pre-enrollment screening with regard to past medical history and current medications is highly recommended. Drugs can impair the muscle BOLD signal. For example, antihistamines are known to be strong intramuscular vasoconstrictors during exercise. Therefore, in patients on antihistamines, the BOLD signal increases less strongly when performing the exercise paradigm.[26]

Clinical Applications

Peripheral arterial occlusive disease

Muscle BOLD MR imaging has been used to assess the microcirculation in different patient populations. Early studies were conducted in patients with peripheral arterial occlusive disease (PAOD), a disease in which the macrocirculation is affected by progressively stenotic and occluded lower extremity arteries.[27] The disease becomes symptomatic with intermittent claudication due to lack of perfusion of the functional end organs of interest including the skeletal muscle.[28] The calf musculature has been studied with BOLD applying the ischemia and hyperemia paradigm. Significantly altered BOLD time courses and key BOLD parameters were appreciated during reactive hyperemia and ischemia in comparison to healthy volunteers.[29] During hyperemia patients with PAOD had decreased T2* maximum values and delayed TTP as opposed to healthy volunteers.[30] During ischemia the T2* minimum value was higher in comparison to an age-matched control group.[31] The BOLD time courses of a healthy volunteer and a patient with PAOD are demonstrated in **Fig. 3**. Another study in patients with PAOD was focusing on treatment assessment after percutaneous transluminal angioplasty (PTA) of the superficial femoral artery using muscle BOLD MR imaging. Muscle BOLD MR imaging was done with the hyperemia paradigm in 10 patients at the calf musculature 1 day prior and 6 weeks after intervention. Even though nonsignificant, it was shown that the T2* maximum value increased and the time-to-peak value decreased between the preintervention and postintervention measurements.[32] These changes reflect a trend towards normalization of the BOLD time course after intervention. Regarding the reproducibility, a study was performed evaluating a variety of morphologic and functional MR imaging techniques in patients with PAOD, including BOLD imaging. The investigators found poor reproducibility of the functional sequences including BOLD and dynamic contrast-enhanced MR imaging.[33] Therefore, to improve reproducibility standardization and optimization of the muscle BOLD MR imaging technique,

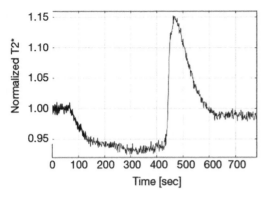

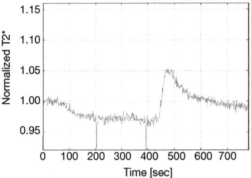

Fig. 3. Muscle BOLD MR imaging in a healthy individual and a patient with PAOD performing the ischemia-hyperemia paradigm. The upper part is demonstrating the T2* time course in a healthy volunteer, whereas the lower part shows the altered T2* time course in a patient with PAOD. (*From* Aschwanden M, Partovi S, Jacobi B, et al. Assessing the end-organ in peripheral arterial occlusive disease-from contrast-enhanced ultrasound to blood-oxygen-level-dependent MR imaging. Cardiovasc Diagn Ther 2014;4(2):169; with permission.)

including the use of applied paradigms, is warranted.

Systemic sclerosis

Skeletal muscle BOLD MR imaging has also been performed for evaluation of the microcirculation in patients with autoimmune diseases. Systemic sclerosis is a systemic disease associated with vascular alterations and endothelial damage, essentially leading to microangiopathy and associated organ dysfunction.[34] Muscle weakness and atrophy as well as elevated creatinine kinase are potential hallmarks of systemic sclerosis.[35] Comparing patients with systemic sclerosis with healthy volunteers, the T2* time courses in the soleus and gastrocnemius muscle demonstrated significant differences. Furthermore BOLD key parameters T2* minimum and T2* maximum were both lower in the patient population compared

with healthy volunteers, and the TTP was significantly delayed in the patient population.[36] These findings indicate pronounced impairment of the muscle microcirculation in patients with systemic sclerosis caused by small vessel disease. Muscle BOLD MR imaging, thus, might be a valuable aid in the evaluation of patients with systemic sclerosis.

Granulomatosis with polyangiitis

A published case report of severe myalgia in a patient with granulomatosis with polyangiitis also illustrates the usefulness of calf muscle BOLD MR imaging performed with the ischemia-hyperemia paradigm. In this reported case morphologic imaging including MR imaging was unremarkable, and there were no signs of inflammation in the lower extremities musculature. However, muscle BOLD MR imaging revealed a significantly altered microcirculatory network with a markedly reduced minimum ischemia value (T2* minimum) and a decreased hyperemia peak value (T2* maximum) in comparison with a matched healthy volunteer. These findings of marked impairment of the microcirculatory network at the calf muscle level in this patient may explain her underlying symptoms.[37]

Clinical Perspectives

The muscle BOLD signal is primarily reflecting skeletal muscle microcirculation, which is considered an end organ in a variety of disease processes. The skeletal muscle as the end organ of interest is eventually responsible for symptoms, such as claudication in PAOD or myalgia in rheumatic diseases. In PAOD muscle BOLD imaging enables quantitative and objective evaluation of the end organ at risk and may be helpful for assessment of therapeutic approaches, including novel devices, medications, and stem cell therapy. In rheumatic diseases imaging the skeletal muscle as one of the functional end organs helps in narrowing the differential diagnosis of muscle weakness, muscle pain, and fatigue, which are frequently encountered symptoms in patients with systemic sclerosis. Also studies imply that skeletal muscle involvement is an early sign of microangiopathy in the systemic sclerosis population and, therefore, could be an interesting tool for noninvasive risk stratification.

ARTERIAL SPIN LABELING
Introduction

The ASL technique allows characterization and quantification of tissue perfusion without the need of gadolinium contrast agent. This ability is of great importance in patients with renal impairment. In this technique, water hydrogen within arterial blood that is flowing into a region of tissue is magnetically labeled. A radiofrequency (RF) pulse to invert or saturate the longitudinal magnetization does this.[38] The labeled blood flows through the vascular network into the muscle and is extracted from the microvascular bed to join a larger volume of nonlabeled water. After a specified time, known as the *arterial transit time*, the tagged water induces a measurable change in the apparent tissue T1 signal and the tissue magnetization is detected by an MR sequence. A control image must be created to subtract from the labeled image, which results in a signal difference allowing visualization of the tagged blood that was delivered to the image slice in the tissue of interest.[39] The approach is depicted in **Fig. 4.** The signal is directly related to the quantitative local perfusion, which is derived from the original Bloch equations.

Theoretically the ASL signal is proportional to the difference in longitudinal magnetization compared with the control in the target tissue. However, during the transit time, signal decay occurs, which can result in underestimation of the muscle perfusion. The measured ASL signal, therefore, needs to be corrected and compensated for this loss.

The advantage of the technique is the noninvasive characterization of perfusion and microcirculation; thus, it provides complementary information to MR angiography.[40–42]

The disadvantages of the technique include poor signal-to-noise ratio, the multiple images that must be acquired leading to increased acquisition times, and the difficulty with perfusion quantification in resting states.

Other limitations of the technique include motion artifact caused by the long acquisition time,[43–46] magnetization transfer (ASL images affecting the tissues other than blood),[47,48] transit time delay nonuniformity,[49,50] application in large vessels,[39] labeling efficiency issues, and the venous outflow effect. This venous outflow effect applies to situations of fast flow or anemia in which the tagged blood may leave the ROI before data acquisition.[49]

Several different techniques are commonly used as discussed later: (1) continuous ASL (CASL), (2) pulsed ASL (PASL), and (3) pseudocontinuous ASL (pCASL).

Continuous Arterial Spin Labeling

With CASL the blood is continuously labeled within multiple slices by the RF field, which inverts the longitudinal magnetization of the protons of the water in the blood with a long RF pulse.[50]

Pulsed Arterial Spin Labeling

With PASL, the blood is instantaneously labeled within a thick slice with a short RF pulse (~10–20 milliseconds). PASL is based on flow-sensitive alternating inversion recovery sequences. In this sequence, inversion recovery sequences are performed twice: labeled one with slice-selective inversion and a control with nonselective inversion. After each inversion, imaging is performed.[51–53]

Pseudocontinuous Arterial Spin Labeling

pCASL is a hybrid of PASL and CASL. The pCASL component provides an increase in SNR and higher tagging efficiency compared with CASL.[54]

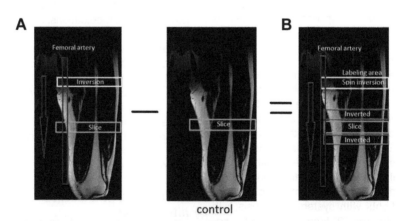

Fig. 4. The principle behind ASL perfusion imaging. (*A*) Blood is the endogenous contrast agent, which is magnetically labeled by an inversion pulse outside the imaging slice and then flows (femoral artery in this case) into the imaging slice. (*B*) The control (without labeled blood) is subtracted from the labeled image resulting in an image with signal only from inflowing blood and suppression of background signal creating a perfusion-weighted ASL image.

Specific Techniques

MR imaging protocol

There are many variations of the ASL protocol depending on the technique. A generally easy-to-follow protocol as done by Wu and colleagues[49] has been shown to provide reliable results.

One of the CASL sequences tailored for muscle perfusion is the flow-drive arterial water stimulation with elimination of tissue signal technique. In this technique, the labeled hydrogen consists of flow-driven adiabatic excitation instead of saturation or inversion. The need to compensate for magnetization transfer and arterial transit times is not required, and the temporal resolution is improved.[53,55,56]

Another CASL sequence variant has been used to quantify muscle perfusion using a standard 1.5-T imaging system fitted with a local gradient self-designed knee coil. The modified CASL technique has been applied to spatially and temporally examine perfusion in exercising human skeletal muscles. These studies demonstrate spatial heterogeneity of perfusion within different muscle groups of the lower extremity as well as perfusion changes to muscle workload.[50,57,58]

Saturation inversion recovery is a PASL sequence applied to quantification of muscle perfusion. Perfusion calculation is independent of T2 variations in exercising muscles. The sequence has been used to study muscle physiology at both stress and rest.[59–61]

The CASL technique of lower extremity studies can be performed on a standard 3-T MR scanner with a transmit-receive knee coil. The labeling slice is 6 cm proximal to the target slice in the tagging acquisition and 6 cm distal in the control acquisition. Imaging parameters can be as follows: TR = 4 seconds, TE = 17 milliseconds, tagging duration of 2 seconds, FOV = 22 cm, slice thickness = 1 cm, matrix size = 64 × 64, single-shot gradient-echo echo-planar sequence. A high-resolution magnetization-prepared rapid gradient echo is acquired for vascular and muscle quantitative flow evaluation.[49]

An ischemia-hyperemia paradigm can be applied during ASL data acquisition. Patients are placed supine for this technique and flexed in their knees for studies of the mid calf or foot. A tourniquet is placed on the thigh and inflated above the systolic blood pressure for several minutes to create ischemia, and then the tourniquet is released for the hyperemia period. Image acquisition starts at the final 2 minutes of tourniquet inflation and ends 3 to 5 minutes after tourniquet release.[62]

Postprocessing

Postprocessing is performed using VoxBo software (which is available as freeware) and software written in Interactive Data Language (RSI, Boulder, Colorado). The software includes motion correction using hand-drawn ROIs of the soleus muscle or foot plantar flexors. The flow is directly proportional and calculated by subtracting tagged from control images. The T_1 of blood chosen is approximately 1600 milliseconds.

Peak and mean hyperemic flow (milliliters per 100 g per minute), hyperemic blood volume (milliliters per 100 g), TTP (seconds), and hyperemic flow duration (seconds) are computed for each anatomic ROI. Initial positive deflection more than zero following cuff deflation to the return to the same level was calculated to be the hyperemic flow duration.[46]

Clinical Applications

Peripheral arterial occlusive disease

A study investigated peak exercise calf muscle blood flow in healthy individuals and patients with PAOD with ASL. The patients performed plantar flexion in a 3-T MR scanner and were imaged at peak exercise. Peak exercise calf perfusion was found to be higher in the healthy individuals versus the patients with PAOD (Fig. 5).[63] Thus, measurement of perfusion in skeletal muscle with the ASL technique is applicable for evaluation of PAOD.

Assessment after peripheral arterial angioplasty

Grözinger and colleagues[64] evaluated patients with PAOD before and after PTA during reactive hyperemia. They used a pCASL technique to assess perfusion in the soleus and tibialis anterior muscles in 10 patients. Mean perfusion value, TTP, and duration of hyperemia were measured. Reactive hyperemia was induced by cuff compression of the thigh. The compression was applied during the ischemic phase of 300 seconds. MR measurements began 60 seconds before cuff inflation and continued until 200 seconds after deflation. The mean perfusion value improved after PTA. The TTP and duration of hyperemia both decreased after PTA. This study showed that pCASL is an interesting tool for assessing the magnitude of improvement after PTA.

Validation by venous occlusion plethysmography

A study was performed comparing PASL with venous occlusion plethysmography as a reference standard. The results revealed that PASL agreed with occlusion plethysmography with a correlation coefficient of 0.87 to 0.92. Based on this study, PASL seems to assess muscle perfusion with relatively high accuracy.[65]

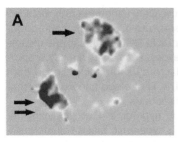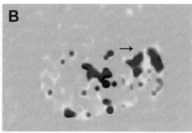

Fig. 5. Postexercise ASL skeletal muscle perfusion demonstrated in a healthy volunteer and a patient with PAOD. Axial image of the calf belonging to the healthy volunteer (*A*) with increased skeletal muscle blood flow seen in red for both the anterior tibialis (*arrow*) and gastrocnemius muscles (*double arrow*). For the patient with PAOD (*B*), the axial image reveals increased skeletal muscle blood flow in the gastrocnemius (*thin arrow*). (*From* Pollak AW, Meyer CH, Epstein FH, et al. Arterial spin labeling MR imaging reproducibly measures peak-exercise calf muscle perfusion: a study in patients with peripheral arterial disease and healthy volunteers. JACC Cardiovasc Imaging 2012;5(12):1227; with permission.)

Clinical Perspectives

Diabetes and peripheral arterial disease are widespread diseases leading to vascular and tissue compromise. In these cohorts of patients, administration of intravenous contrast is not always a feasible option because of secondary renal insufficiency. Therefore, perfusion and vascular studies with exogenous contrast agents are limited; but ASL is useful to overcome this limitation.

In addition, ASL can perform dynamic perfusion measurements of skeletal muscles in response to exercise and ischemia. In patients undergoing peripheral arterial angioplasty, ASL may be helpful to assess the treatment response by demonstrating changes in muscle perfusion and can also help evaluate the need for further intervention. Larger studies are needed to demonstrate its value.

DIFFUSION-WEIGHTED IMAGING
Introduction

Diffusion-weighted imaging (DWI) is a technique that is sensitive to cellularity and structural architecture. The physics behind DWI has been described in detail.[66,67] In brief, DWI provides qualitative and quantitative information about the random motion of water molecules in biological tissues and is able to give functional insights into tissue architecture and pathologic changes on a cellular level. Translation into the musculoskeletal arena became feasible with the advent of DWI with background body signal suppression.[68] The combination of being a fast, robust, and widely available sequence on standard clinical 1.5-T and 3.0-T MR systems makes DWI attractive for musculoskeletal imaging. It is a complementary imaging technique with a relatively short image acquisition time, adding a functional component to the established morphologic information in musculoskeletal imaging. Besides vendor-specific acquisition details,[69,70] institutional decisions have

resulted in the variability of the DWI protocols in musculoskeletal imaging. Clear guidelines including standardization of the technique are required to achieve superior qualitative and quantitative results and also to enable comparisons across scanners and institutions.

Several musculoskeletal pathologies have been evaluated by DWI, including vertebral fractures, hematoma, bone marrow infections, primary bone and soft-tissue tumors, as well as posttreatment follow-up.[71–74] Differentiation between benign and malignant vertebral fractures and monitoring of the therapy response by DWI in primary bone tumors have demonstrated promising results.[75] Differentiation of benign versus malignant tumors is not supported based on the current research data.

MR Imaging Protocol

MR imaging parameters and processing steps are summarized in Table 1. The range of imaging techniques includes conventional spin-echo (SE) and stimulated echo, fast SE, gradient-echo (eg, steady-state free precession), echo planar imaging (EPI) as well as line scan diffusion imaging.[66,67,72]

Currently, the most common way of acquiring local DWI for musculoskeletal imaging is via single-shot EPI (SS-EPI) sequences, which offer fast acquisition times while still offering a relatively high SNR. DWI should be acquired before intravenous administration of contrast medium. The b values in the published literature vary. To choose 3 to 4 b values covering low, middle, and high values have been shown to minimize apparent diffusion coefficient (ADC) misinterpretation.[69,74]

The authors perform DWI with the following parameters: TR = 6400; TE = 48; matrix = 512 × 512; flip angle = 90; slice thickness = 5 mm; b values = 50, 300, and 800.

Table 1
Protocol for diffusion-weighted MR imaging

Parameters	1.5 T	3.0 T
Acquisition plane	Axial (focal); coronal (WB)	
b values (s/mm^2)	0/50, 300, 800–1000	0/50, 400, 800–1000, 1400^a
Slice thickness/ gap (mm)	4–6/0	
Parallel imaging	Yes	Yes
Acquisition time (TA, min)	3–5 (focal)	2–3 (focal)
FOV (mm)	260–300	
Matrix	128–256	
Fat suppression	eg, STIR, SPAIR	
Sequence	eg, SS-EPI	
Parallel imaging	Yes	
Averaging/NEX	Yes	
Distortion correction	Yes	
Image processing		
Qualitative	ADC and DWI maps, coronal MIP/MPR, image fusion	
Quantitative	ROI analysis (ADC); histogram	

Abbreviations: ADC, apparent diffusion coefficient; MIP, maximum intensity projection; MPR, multiplanar reformation; SPAIR, spectral selection attenuated inversion recovery; SS-EPI, single-shot echo planar imaging; NEX, number of excitations; STIR, short tau inversion recovery; WB, whole body.
^{a} Whole-body bone marrow.

Postprocessing

Currently, some commercial picture archiving and communication systems (PACS) do not offer sufficient DWI processing tools. Although ADC maps are being calculated at the scanner, there is a lack of usable tools within the PACS that would allow sufficient analysis. Therefore, dedicated processing software often needs to be implemented in addition to providing state-of-the-art quantitative ADC analysis, including ROI and volume of interest (VOI) measurements, image registration, statistics, and motion correction (eg, Olea Medical, La Ciotat, France or noncommercial solutions like ImageJ, NIH, Bethesda, MD).

DWI and ADC maps can be analyzed qualitatively providing a quick overview for areas of restricted diffusion.[76] Visualization is facilitated by creating 3-dimensional (3D)–like images including maximum intensity projection and multiplanar reformation.[77] Image fusion can also be used to combine morphologic and functional information[78] as demonstrated in **Fig. 6**. Image fusion can be performed by combining DWI with a T2- or T1-weighted morphologic image. An ADC value (seconds per square millimeter) is a quantitative measure of restriction to diffusion and a promising biomarker. It can be assessed by ROI[72] or VOI analysis. Measurement of minimum and mean ADC values including hotspot analysis has been performed.[74]

Clinical Applications

Soft-tissue tumors

Soft-tissue tumors are often indeterminate based on MR imaging. Some benign lesions usually can be diagnosed with a high certainty based on conventional MR imaging protocols as cysts and ganglia. However, the differentiation between multiple other benign and malignant lesions based on morphologic MR imaging alone can be challenging. It was suggested that malignant lesions would express lower ADC values because of a high cellularity leading to a restriction in free-water diffusion. However, one study detected no significant difference between the ADC values of benign and malignant soft-tissue tumors.[79] Another study revealed the highest ADC values in a myxoid liposarcoma.[80] This entity is considered a lower-grade sarcoma. It was thought that such high values were caused by low collagen and high mucin content in myxoid tumors. In a larger number of benign and malignant lesions, an overall accuracy of 91% was found to differentiate between benign and malignant lesions when using an ADC cutoff value of 1.34×10^{-3} mm^2/s. In this study, b values of 500 s/mm^2 and 1000 s/mm^2 were used.[81] Although study results are heterogeneous and somehow controversial so far, ADC is helpful in discriminating cysts and solid soft-tissue tumors when intravenous contrast medium cannot be administered.[82] Moreover, it provides useful information about areas with high cellularity (hot spots), which should be chosen for image-guided biopsy to achieve adequate grading based on histopathology as demonstrated in **Fig. 7**. A quantitative analysis of DWI with an ADC map is demonstrated in **Fig. 8**.

Therapy Monitoring

Because of the known limitations of static contrast-enhanced T1-weighted imaging for therapy monitoring, DWI is being explored as a tool for monitoring the therapy response. As therapy monitoring requires information on tumor necrosis and viable tumor, morphologic information is often not sufficient. The expected response during or after tumor therapy would be an increase in ADC values, consistent with a decrease in cellularity.[75] In a study of patients with osteosarcoma and Ewing sarcoma, a significant increase in the ADC

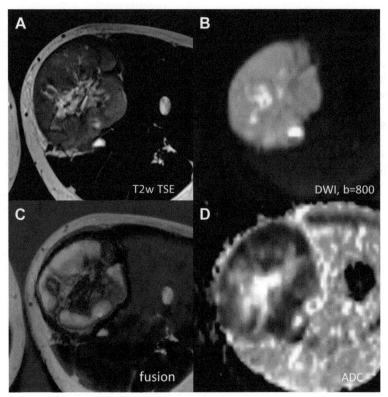

Fig. 6. A 23-year-old woman with a synovial sarcoma. Axial T2-weighted (T2w) turbo spin echo (TSE) (*A*) and DWI, b = 800 (*B*), fusion of T2w and DWI (*C*). The ADC map shows low signal intensity in the solid peripheral parts of the lesion containing high cellularity (*D*).

value was noted in patients with greater than 90% tumor necrosis after treatment.[83] In children with osteosarcomas, poor responders to neoadjuvant therapy demonstrated a minimal increase in the tumor mean ADC value.[84] In another study, it was shown that, after chemotherapy in patients with osteosarcoma, the good responders had a significantly higher minimum ADC ratio in comparison with the poor responders. When determining and comparing the average ADC ratio in good versus poor responders, there was no significant difference. Based on this study, the minimum ADC values have been recommended for the evaluation of the therapy response as opposed to average ADC values.[85]

In summary, ADC changes during therapy may help assess early treatment response.[86] Further studies are warranted to evaluate the role of ADC changes in different types of sarcomas for therapy monitoring.

Clinical Perspectives

We need to be aware of some imaging-related artifacts and pitfalls. One of the technical issues is the presence of susceptibility artifacts when scanning with field strengths greater than 1.5 T. Interpretation pitfalls include the so-called T2 shine-through effect caused by the inherent T2 weighting of DW sequences. This can be misinterpreted as diffusion restriction if DWIs are not evaluated along with the ADC map. Evaluation of a sclerotic lesion can also be misleading.[87] Because of the low water content in sclerotic lesions, low signal intensity similar to the usual low signal intensity of bone marrow may lead to false-negative results.[88] Furthermore, there may be false-positive results caused by postinterventional changes like inflammation or interstitial edema, which appear as high signal intensity on DWI at a low b value. Hematomas may have low ADC values, so they may be misinterpreted as malignant lesions[16]; also soft-tissue abscesses may resemble neoplasms.[89] In the authors' opinion, comparison with a native morphologic T1- and T2-weighted sequence is helpful for the interpretation of DWI.

In summary, DWI provides additional functional information that can be complementary to conventional morphologic MR imaging. The authors expect DWI to play an important role in the early

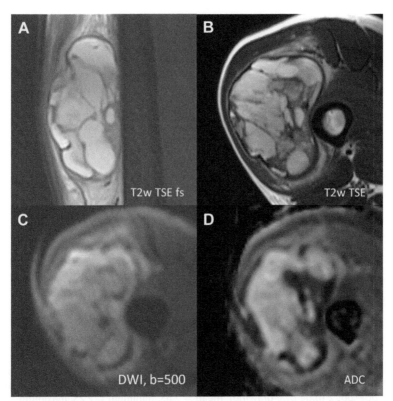

Fig. 7. A 57-year-old man with a myxoid liposarcoma. Large central parts of the tumor show a high signal in both T2-weighed (T2w) imaging (*A, B*) and DWI (*C*). The corresponding ADC map reveals that only some parts of the lesion have low ADC values (*D*). As these areas with low ADC values correspond to a high cellularity, these parts of the lesion should be chosen for biopsy. fs, fat saturation; TSE, turbo spin echo.

detection of therapy response in the future. However, DWI may have a limited value in differentiating benign from malignant lesions.

DIFFUSION TENSOR IMAGING
Introduction

Diffusion-tensor imaging (DTI) exploits the capability of MR imaging to obtain directional information of the diffusion process by taking advantage of magnetic field gradients in addition to those necessary to create the morphologic MR image. It can, therefore, be regarded as a preparation step in the MR imaging pulse sequence whereby the magnetization is manipulated so that the desired information (here the diffusion directionality) is accessible in the readout step of the sequence eventually creating the actual image. A multitude of studies have demonstrated the ability of DTI for tracing the direction of the large white matter fiber bundles in the brain,[90–93] but DTI has also been expanded to other areas of the body.[94–97] In particular, applications of DTI in musculoskeletal imaging have been reported to obtain insight into the organization of skeletal muscle.[98–112]

MR Imaging Protocol

DTI probes the strength of diffusion along different spatial directions by applying magnetic field gradients in these directions with the goal to derive the diffusion tensor, a 3×3 symmetric matrix, which characterizes the directional dependence of the diffusion process. In order to populate this matrix, the diffusion process in at least 6 noncollinear directions has to be probed in addition to one acquisition that is not sensitized to diffusion (b value = 0). In the authors' practice, 12 to 25 directions are commonly used. DTI is traditionally implemented with a SS-EPI readout. The TR for this readout is in the order of 3000 to 4500 milliseconds and is determined by the number of desired slices (anatomic coverage). The TE ranges from 40 milliseconds to 80 milliseconds, depending on the b value and the capabilities of the scanner, such as the gradient strength. The b value for musculoskeletal imaging varies from 400 s/mm^2 to 800 s/mm^2. The images are also acquired with a b value of 0, before the application of diffusion gradients, and, hence, are T2 weighted.

The FOV is adjusted to the anatomy to be covered, typically 140 mm × 140 mm to

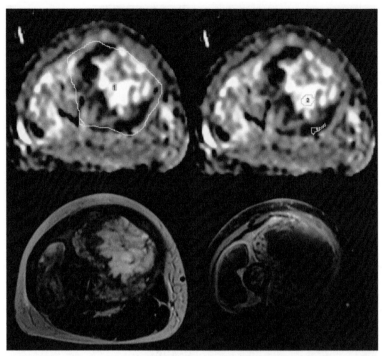

Fig. 8. A 24-year-old woman with osteosarcoma of the right distal femur. Total (*yellow drawing*): mean = 1.62, minimum = 0.009, maximum = 2.83; hot spot 1 (*blue irregular drawing*): mean = 0.915, minimum = 0.89, maximum = 1.08; hot spot 2 (*blue oval drawing*): mean = 2.65, minimum = 2.25, maximum = 2.79.

240 mm × 240 mm. The acquisition matrix is limited by the echo train of the EPI readout. Fast acquisitions can be achieved with a 64 × 64 matrix leading to a compromise of spatial resolution; therefore, acquisition matrices of 128 × 256 and 192 × 256 are more common where the zero filling is used in the phase encoding direction to arrive at a higher interpolated spatial resolution. Parallel imaging techniques with an acceleration factor of 2 or greater are commonly used in the authors' protocol. Recently, prototypes of multi-band methods for clinical imaging have been developed, which excite more than one slice, thereby even further reducing the total acquisition time.[113]

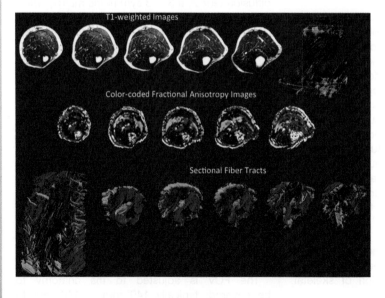

Fig. 9. Top: T1-weighted transversal sectional images of the calf muscle. Center: color-coded fractional anisotropy images at the same anatomic locations as slices shown on top. Color-coding scheme uses blue colors for fibers oriented superior-inferior, red for fibers oriented left-right, and green for fibers oriented anterior-superior. Other directions are combinations of these colors. Bottom: Fibers traced at the transverse locations shown on top using DTI information of the direction of the eigenvector with the largest eigenvalue of the tensor matrix. Lower left part of the image: All fibers traced in the entire imaging volume. Upper right part of the image: selected muscle fibers predominantly oriented superior-inferior.

Postprocessing

For every anatomic location or slice, the images for the different diffusion gradients are mathematically combined to yield the diffusion tensor. In the case of exactly 6 acquired directions, an analytical solution for this calculation exists; for more directions, nonweighted or weighted linear or nonlinear least-square methods are used.

From the diffusion tensor matrix, anisotropy of diffusion can be assessed; if present, the principal direction and strength of diffusion along this direction can be calculated (as the eigenvector and eigenvalue of this matrix, respectively).[114–116] The concept of the diffusion ellipsoid with the 3 eigenvalues determining the length of its 3 axis is introduced from this matrix.

Information obtained with DTI allows creating 2-dimensional (2D) images of fractional anisotropy, a scalar quantity valued from 0 to 1, which essentially quantifies the deviation of the diffusion ellipsoid from a regular spherical form. In addition, the ADC (so-called because its value depends on parameters of the DTI acquisition in addition to the underlying physiologic processes) is also visualized by 2D images. More importantly, DTI allows a true 3D reconstruction of the muscle fibers, along which the diffusion anisotropy is measured. The information content of these 3D reconstructions was greatly improved by introducing a consistent color scheme dependent on the directional information in the data.[117] In this color scheme, fibers extending superior-inferiorly are colored blue; those extending left-right are colored red; and those extending anterior-superiorly are colored green. Other directions are represented by a combination of these colors. Three-dimensional reconstructions created in this way are informative and support data visualization, which may have also contributed to its increasing popularity. Fig. 9 illustrates a reconstruction of muscle fibers using DTI acquired from the superior section of the human calf (Philips

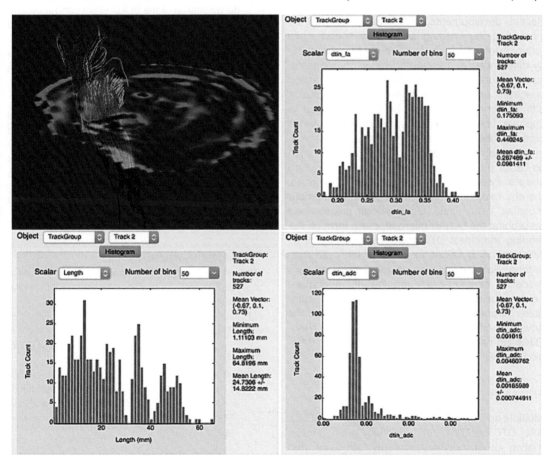

Fig. 10. Top left shows the ROI-based segmentation of a muscle fiber group (based on the tracts reconstructed with the DTI data). Directional color coding allows appreciating different fibers. Top right and lower panels: Statistical information of the fractional anisotropy (fa), fiber length, and ADC for the segmented fiber group on the left. Segmentation and statistical analysis were created with the TrackVis software (www.trackvis.org). dtin_fa, fractional anisotropy; dtin_adc, apparent diffusion coefficient.

Ingenia, 3.0 T, 15 gradient directions, b value 800 s/mm^2). In **Fig. 10**, seed-based extraction of a particular fiber group is illustrated together with the ability to obtain statistical information of the fractional anisotropy or ADC along the extracted fibers.

Clinical Applications

- Visualization of integrity and directionality of muscle fibers[98–112]
- Quantification of sex differences in skeletal muscle[118,119]
- Evaluation of injury or trauma[120–123]
- Assessment of ischemia induced damage[12]
- Quantification of degree of muscle regeneration[124,125]
- Demonstration of age-related changes[126]
- Development of imaging markers to assess the effects of exercise[122]

Clinical Perspectives

Recent developments in DTI have focused on increasing the imaging acquisition speed while reducing imaging artifacts adherent to susceptibility differences of muscle and other components, such as bone. Several methods, such as diffusion spectrum imaging and high angular resolution diffusion imaging,[93,127] are being investigated to improve fiber tractography, in particular when crossing fibers are present within a single voxel. In addition, using readouts other than EPI, such as SE or gradient-echo, may make the acquired images insensitive to susceptibility differences, thereby expanding areas of applications (lumbar muscles, extremities). Other efforts are focused on probing the cellular microstructure through extending traditional DTI model by measurements with various b values in low and high diffusion regime. Some examples include 2-compartment modeling of short-lived and long-lived components in the diffusion signal with the goal to distinguish intracellular and extracellular water and the advance diffusion model to assess the non-Gaussian nature of the diffusion signal with diffusion kurtosis imaging.[128]

SUMMARY

Multiple advanced MR sequences, such as BOLD, ASL, DTI, and DWI, can potentially provide information about muscle vascularity, structure, and function. When combined with traditional morphologic sequences, these techniques provide greater insights about structure and function of muscles in health and disease. Although many of these techniques are currently in the realm of research, larger studies documenting value of these techniques will aid in clinical translation and acceptance.

REFERENCES

1. Partovi S, Jacobi B, Rapps N, et al. Clinical standardized fMRI reveals altered language lateralization in patients with brain tumor. AJNR Am J Neuroradiol 2012;33(11):2151–7.
2. Partovi S, Konrad F, Karimi S, et al. Effects of covert and overt paradigms in clinical language fMRI. Acad Radiol 2012;19(5):518–25.
3. Gold GE. Dynamic and functional imaging of the musculoskeletal system. Semin Musculoskelet Radiol 2003;7(4):245–8.
4. Partovi S, Schulte AC, Jacobi B, et al. Blood oxygenation level-dependent (BOLD) MRI of human skeletal muscle at 1.5 and 3 T. J Magn Reson Imaging 2012;35(5):1227–32.
5. Li D, Dhawale P, Rubin PJ, et al. Myocardial signal response to dipyridamole and dobutamine: demonstration of the BOLD effect using a double-echo gradient-echo sequence. Magn Reson Med 1996;36(1):16–20.
6. Wigmore DM, Damon BM, Pober DM, et al. MRI measures of perfusion-related changes in human skeletal muscle during progressive contractions. J Appl Physiol (1985) 2004;97(6):2385–94.
7. Noseworthy MD, Kim JK, Stainsby JA, et al. Tracking oxygen effects on MR signal in blood and skeletal muscle during hyperoxia exposure. J Magn Reson Imaging 1999;9(6):814–20.
8. Weisskoff RM, Zuo CS, Boxerman JL, et al. Microscopic susceptibility variation and transverse relaxation: theory and experiment. Magn Reson Med 1994;31(6):601–10.
9. Yacoub E, Shmuel A, Pfeuffer J, et al. Imaging brain function in humans at 7 Tesla. Magn Reson Med 2001;45(4):588–94.
10. van der Zwaag W, Francis S, Head K, et al. fMRI at 1.5, 3 and 7 T: characterising BOLD signal changes. Neuroimage 2009;47(4):1425–34.
11. Heemskerk AM, Drost MR, van Bochove GS, et al. DTI-based assessment of ischemia-reperfusion in mouse skeletal muscle. Magn Reson Med 2006;56(2):272–81.
12. Lebon V, Brillault-Salvat C, Bloch G, et al. Evidence of muscle BOLD effect revealed by simultaneous interleaved gradient-echo NMRI and myoglobin NMRS during leg ischemia. Magn Reson Med 1998;40(4):551–8.
13. Duteil S, Wary C, Raynaud JS, et al. Influence of vascular filling and perfusion on BOLD contrast during reactive hyperemia in human skeletal muscle. Magn Reson Med 2006;55(2):450–4.
14. Ranft J, Heidrich H, Peters A, et al. Laser-Doppler examinations in persons with healthy vasculature

and in patients with peripheral arterial occlusive disease. Angiology 1986;37(11):818–27.

15. Feuerlein S, Pauls S, Juchems MS, et al. Pitfalls in abdominal diffusion-weighted imaging: how predictive is restricted water diffusion for malignancy. AJR Am J Roentgenol 2009;193(4):1070–6.

16. Bunt TJ, Holloway GA. TcPO2 as an accurate predictor of therapy in limb salvage. Ann Vasc Surg 1996;10(3):224–7.

17. Ledermann HP, Heidecker HG, Schulte AC, et al. Calf muscles imaged at BOLD MR: correlation with TcPO2 and flowmetry measurements during ischemia and reactive hyperemia–initial experience. Radiology 2006;241(2):477–84.

18. Partovi S, Aschwanden M, Jacobi B, et al. Correlation of muscle BOLD MRI with transcutaneous oxygen pressure for assessing microcirculation in patients with systemic sclerosis. J Magn Reson Imaging 2013;38(4):845–51.

19. Partovi S, Schulte AC, Staub D, et al. Correlation of skeletal muscle blood oxygenation level-dependent MRI and skin laser Doppler flowmetry in patients with systemic sclerosis. J Magn Reson Imaging 2013;40:1408–13.

20. Schulte AC, Aschwanden M, Bilecen D. Calf muscles at blood oxygen level-dependent MR imaging: aging effects at postocclusive reactive hyperemia. Radiology 2008;247(2):482–9.

21. Kos S, Klarhofer M, Aschwanden M, et al. Simultaneous dynamic blood oxygen level-dependent magnetic resonance imaging of foot and calf muscles: aging effects at ischemia and postocclusive hyperemia in healthy volunteers. Invest Radiol 2009;44(11):741–7.

22. Towse TF, Slade JM, Meyer RA. Effect of physical activity on MRI-measured blood oxygen level-dependent transients in skeletal muscle after brief contractions. J Appl Physiol (1985) 2005;99(2):715–22.

23. Zierath JR, Hawley JA. Skeletal muscle fiber type: influence on contractile and metabolic properties. PLoS Biol 2004;2(10):e348.

24. Jacobi B, Bongartz G, Partovi S, et al. Skeletal muscle BOLD MRI: from underlying physiological concepts to its usefulness in clinical conditions. J Magn Reson Imaging 2012;35(6):1253–65.

25. Toivonen J, Merisaari H, Pesola M, et al. Mathematical models for diffusion-weighted imaging of prostate cancer using b values up to 2000 s/mm: correlation with Gleason score and repeatability of region of interest analysis. Magn Reson Med 2014. [Epub ahead of print].

26. Bulte DP, Alfonsi J, Bells S, et al. Vasomodulation of skeletal muscle BOLD signal. J Magn Reson Imaging 2006;24(4):886–90.

27. Hirsch AT, Haskal ZJ, Hertzer NR, et al. ACC/AHA 2005 practice guidelines for the management of patients with peripheral arterial disease (lower extremity, renal, mesenteric, and abdominal aortic): a collaborative report from the American Association for Vascular Surgery/Society for Vascular Surgery, Society for Cardiovascular Angiography and Interventions, Society for Vascular Medicine and Biology, Society of Interventional Radiology, and the ACC/AHA Task Force on Practice Guidelines (Writing Committee to Develop Guidelines for the Management of Patients With Peripheral Arterial Disease): endorsed by the American Association of Cardiovascular and Pulmonary Rehabilitation; National Heart, Lung, and Blood Institute; Society for Vascular Nursing; TransAtlantic Inter-Society Consensus; and Vascular Disease Foundation. Circulation 2006;113(11):e463–654.

28. Aschwanden M, Partovi S, Jacobi B, et al. Assessing the end-organ in peripheral arterial occlusive disease-from contrast-enhanced ultrasound to blood-oxygen-level-dependent MR imaging. Cardiovasc Diagn Ther 2014;4(2):165–72.

29. Partovi S, Karimi S, Jacobi B, et al. Clinical implications of skeletal muscle blood-oxygenation-level-dependent (BOLD) MRI. MAGMA 2012;25(4):251–61.

30. Ledermann HP, Schulte AC, Heidecker HG, et al. Blood oxygenation level-dependent magnetic resonance imaging of the skeletal muscle in patients with peripheral arterial occlusive disease. Circulation 2006;113(25):2929–35.

31. Potthast S, Schulte A, Kos S, et al. Blood oxygenation level-dependent MRI of the skeletal muscle during ischemia in patients with peripheral arterial occlusive disease. Rofo 2009;181(12):1157–61.

32. Huegli RW, Schulte AC, Aschwanden M, et al. Effects of percutaneous transluminal angioplasty on muscle BOLD-MRI in patients with peripheral arterial occlusive disease: preliminary results. Eur Radiol 2009;19(2):509–15.

33. Versluis B, Backes WH, van Eupen MG, et al. Magnetic resonance imaging in peripheral arterial disease: reproducibility of the assessment of morphological and functional vascular status. Invest Radiol 2011;46(1):11–24.

34. Gabrielli A, Avvedimento EV, Krieg T. Scleroderma. N Engl J Med 2009;360(19):1989–2003.

35. Walker UA, Tyndall A, Czirjak L, et al. Clinical risk assessment of organ manifestations in systemic sclerosis: a report from the EULAR Scleroderma Trials And Research group database. Ann Rheum Dis 2007;66(6):754–63.

36. Partovi S, Schulte AC, Aschwanden M, et al. Impaired skeletal muscle microcirculation in systemic sclerosis. Arthritis Res Ther 2012;14(5):R209.

37. Jacobi B, Schulte AC, Partovi S, et al. Alterations of skeletal muscle microcirculation detected by blood

oxygenation level-dependent MRI in a patient with granulomatosis with polyangiitis. Rheumatology (Oxford) 2013;52(3):579–81.

38. Detre JA, Leigh JS, Williams DS, et al. Perfusion imaging. Magn Reson Med 1992;23(1):37–45.

39. Buxton RB, Frank LR, Wong EC, et al. A general kinetic model for quantitative perfusion imaging with arterial spin labeling. Magn Reson Med 1998;40(3): 383–96.

40. Katoh M, Spuentrup E, Barmet C, et al. Local re-inversion coronary MR angiography: arterial spin-labeling without the need for subtraction. J Magn Reson Imaging 2008;27(4):913–7.

41. Rehwald WG, Chen EL, Kim RJ, et al. Noninvasive cineangiography by magnetic resonance global coherent free precession. Nat Med 2004;10(5): 545–9.

42. Wheaton AJ, Miyazaki M. Non-contrast enhanced MR angiography: physical principles. J Magn Reson Imaging 2012;36(2):286–304.

43. Frouin F, Duteil S, Lesage D, et al. An automated image-processing strategy to analyze dynamic arterial spin labeling perfusion studies. Application to human skeletal muscle under stress. Magn Reson Imaging 2006;24(7):941–51.

44. Wong EC, Cronin M, Wu WC, et al. Velocity-selective arterial spin labeling. Magn Reson Med 2006; 55(6):1334–41.

45. Garcia DM, Duhamel G, Alsop DC. Efficiency of inversion pulses for background suppressed arterial spin labeling. Magn Reson Med 2005;54(2):366–72.

46. Norris DG, Schwarzbauer C. Velocity selective radiofrequency pulse trains. J Magn Reson 1999; 137(1):231–6.

47. Niemi PT, Komu ME, Koskinen SK. Tissue specificity of low-field-strength magnetization transfer contrast imaging. J Magn Reson Imaging 1992; 2(2):197–201.

48. Zhu XP, Zhao S, Isherwood I. Magnetization transfer contrast (MTC) imaging of skeletal muscle at 0.26 Tesla–changes in signal intensity following exercise. Br J Radiol 1992;65(769):39–43.

49. Wu WC, Wang J, Detre JA, et al. Transit delay and flow quantification in muscle with continuous arterial spin labeling perfusion-MRI. J Magn Reson Imaging 2008;28(2):445–52.

50. Detre JA, Alsop DC. Perfusion magnetic resonance imaging with continuous arterial spin labeling: methods and clinical applications in the central nervous system. Eur J Radiol 1999;30(2):115–24.

51. Kim SG. Quantification of relative cerebral blood flow change by flow-sensitive alternating inversion recovery (FAIR) technique: application to functional mapping. Magn Reson Med 1995;34(3): 293–301.

52. Kwong KK, Belliveau JW, Chesler DA, et al. Dynamic magnetic resonance imaging of human

brain activity during primary sensory stimulation. Proc Natl Acad Sci U S A 1992;89(12):5675–9.

53. Schwarzbauer C, Morrissey SP, Haase A. Quantitative magnetic resonance imaging of perfusion using magnetic labeling of water proton spins within the detection slice. Magn Reson Med 1996;35(4): 540–6.

54. Pollock JM, Tan H, Kraft RA, et al. Arterial spin-labeled MR perfusion imaging: clinical applications. Magn Reson Imaging Clin N Am 2009; 17(2):315–38.

55. Marro KI, Hyyti OM, Vincent MA, et al. Validation and advantages of FAWSETS perfusion measurements in skeletal muscle. NMR Biomed 2005; 18(4):226–34.

56. Marro KI, Hyyti OM, Kushmerick MJ. FAWSETS perfusion measurements in exercising skeletal muscle. NMR Biomed 2005;18(5):322–30.

57. Frank LR, Wong EC, Haseler LJ, et al. Dynamic imaging of perfusion in human skeletal muscle during exercise with arterial spin labeling. Magn Reson Med 1999;42(2):258–67.

58. Richardson RS, Haseler LJ, Nygren AT, et al. Local perfusion and metabolic demand during exercise: a noninvasive MRI method of assessment. J Appl Physiol (1985) 2001;91(4):1845–53.

59. Baligand C, Wary C, Menard JC, et al. Measuring perfusion and bioenergetics simultaneously in mouse skeletal muscle: a multiparametric functional-NMR approach. NMR Biomed 2011;24(3): 281–90.

60. Bertoldi D, Parzy E, Fromes Y, et al. New insight into abnormal muscle vasodilatory responses in aged hypertensive rats by in vivo nuclear magnetic resonance imaging of perfusion. J Vasc Res 2006; 43(2):149–56.

61. Menard JC, Giacomini E, Baligand C, et al. Non-invasive and quantitative evaluation of peripheral vascular resistances in rats by combined NMR measurements of perfusion and blood pressure using ASL and dynamic angiography. NMR Biomed 2010;23(2):188–95.

62. Wu WC, Mohler E, Ratcliffe SJ, et al. Skeletal muscle microvascular flow in progressive peripheral artery disease: assessment with continuous arterial spin-labeling perfusion magnetic resonance imaging. J Am Coll Cardiol 2009;53(25):2372–7.

63. Pollak AW, Meyer CH, Epstein FH, et al. Arterial spin labeling MR imaging reproducibly measures peak-exercise calf muscle perfusion: a study in patients with peripheral arterial disease and healthy volunteers. JACC Cardiovasc Imaging 2012; 5(12):1224–30.

64. Grözinger G, Pohmann R, Schick F, et al. Perfusion measurements of the calf in patients with peripheral arterial occlusive disease before and after percutaneous transluminal angioplasty using MR

arterial spin labeling. J Magn Reson Imaging 2014; 40(4):980–7.

65. Raynaud JS, Duteil S, Vaughan JT, et al. Determination of skeletal muscle perfusion using arterial spin labeling NMRI: validation by comparison with venous occlusion plethysmography. Magn Reson Med 2001;46(2):305–11.

66. White NS, McDonald CR, Farid N, et al. Diffusion-weighted imaging in cancer: physical foundations and applications of restriction spectrum imaging. Cancer Res 2014;74(17):4638–52.

67. Lenz C, Klarhofer M, Scheffler K, et al. Assessing extracranial tumors using diffusion-weighted whole-body MRI. Z Med Phys 2011;21(2):79–90.

68. Wilhelm T, Stieltjes B, Schlemmer HP. Whole-body-MR-diffusion weighted imaging in oncology. Rofo 2013;185(10):950–8.

69. Padhani AR, Liu G, Koh DM, et al. Diffusion-weighted magnetic resonance imaging as a cancer biomarker: consensus and recommendations. Neoplasia 2009;11(2):102–25.

70. Donati OF, Chong D, Nanz D, et al. Diffusion-weighted MR imaging of upper abdominal organs: field strength and intervendor variability of apparent diffusion coefficients. Radiology 2014; 270(2):454–63.

71. Khoo MM, Tyler PA, Saifuddin A, et al. Diffusion-weighted imaging (DWI) in musculoskeletal MRI: a critical review. Skeletal Radiol 2011; 40(6):665–81.

72. Costa FM, Ferreira EC, Vianna EM. Diffusion-weighted magnetic resonance imaging for the evaluation of musculoskeletal tumors. Magn Reson Imaging Clin N Am 2011;19(1):159–80.

73. Oka K, Yakushiji T, Sato H, et al. Ability of diffusion-weighted imaging for the differential diagnosis between chronic expanding hematomas and malignant soft tissue tumors. J Magn Reson Imaging 2008;28(5):1195–200.

74. Subhawong TK, Jacobs MA, Fayad LM. Diffusion-weighted MR imaging for characterizing musculoskeletal lesions. Radiographics 2014;34(5):1163–77.

75. Dietrich O, Biffar A, Reiser MF, et al. Diffusion-weighted imaging of bone marrow. Semin Musculoskelet Radiol 2009;13(2):134–44.

76. Lichy MP, Aschoff P, Plathow C, et al. Tumor detection by diffusion-weighted MRI and ADC-mapping–initial clinical experiences in comparison to PET-CT. Invest Radiol 2007;42(9):605–13.

77. Takahara T, Imai Y, Yamashita T, et al. Diffusion weighted whole body imaging with background body signal suppression (DWIBS): technical improvement using free breathing, STIR and high resolution 3D display. Radiat Med 2004;22(4): 275–82.

78. Giesel FL, Mehndiratta A, Locklin J, et al. Image fusion using CT, MRI and PET for treatment planning, navigation and follow up in percutaneous RFA. Exp Oncol 2009;31(2):106–14.

79. Nagata S, Nishimura H, Uchida M, et al. Diffusion-weighted imaging of soft tissue tumors: usefulness of the apparent diffusion coefficient for differential diagnosis. Radiat Med 2008;26(5):287–95.

80. Einarsdottir H, Karlsson M, Wejde J, et al. Diffusion-weighted MRI of soft tissue tumours. Eur Radiol 2004;14(6):959–63.

81. Razek A, Nada N, Ghaniem M, et al. Assessment of soft tissue tumours of the extremities with diffusion echoplanar MR imaging. Radiol Med 2012;117(1): 96–101.

82. Subhawong TK, Durand DJ, Thawait GK, et al. Characterization of soft tissue masses: can quantitative diffusion weighted imaging reliably distinguish cysts from solid masses? Skeletal Radiol 2013;42(11):1583–92.

83. Hayashida Y, Yakushiji T, Awai K, et al. Monitoring therapeutic responses of primary bone tumors by diffusion-weighted image: initial results. Eur Radiol 2006;16(12):2637–43.

84. Uhl M, Saueressig U, Koehler G, et al. Evaluation of tumour necrosis during chemotherapy with diffusion-weighted MR imaging: preliminary results in osteosarcomas. Pediatr Radiol 2006;36(12): 1306–11.

85. Oka K, Yakushiji T, Sato H, et al. The value of diffusion-weighted imaging for monitoring the chemotherapeutic response of osteosarcoma: a comparison between average apparent diffusion coefficient and minimum apparent diffusion coefficient. Skeletal Radiol 2010;39(2):141–6.

86. Fayad LM, Jacobs MA, Wang X, et al. Musculoskeletal tumors: how to use anatomic, functional, and metabolic MR techniques. Radiology 2012;265(2): 340–56.

87. Eiber M, Holzapfel K, Ganter C, et al. Whole-body MRI including diffusion-weighted imaging (DWI) for patients with recurring prostate cancer: technical feasibility and assessment of lesion conspicuity in DWI. J Magn Reson Imaging 2011;33(5): 1160–70.

88. Byun WM, Shin SO, Chang Y, et al. Diffusion-weighted MR imaging of metastatic disease of the spine: assessment of response to therapy. AJNR Am J Neuroradiol 2002;23(6):906–12.

89. Soldatos T, Durand DJ, Subhawong TK, et al. Magnetic resonance imaging of musculoskeletal infections: systematic diagnostic assessment and key points. Acad Radiol 2012;19(11):1434–43.

90. Assaf Y, Alexander DC, Jones DK, et al. The CONNECT project: combining macro- and micro-structure. Neuroimage 2013;80:273–82.

91. Basser PJ, Mattiello J, LeBihan D. MR diffusion tensor spectroscopy and imaging. Biophys J 1994;66(1):259–67.

92. Bardin J. Neuroscience: making connections. Nature 2012;483(7390):394–6.

93. Wedeen VJ, Wang RP, Schmahmann JD, et al. Diffusion spectrum magnetic resonance imaging (DSI) tractography of crossing fibers. Neuroimage 2008;41(4):1267–77.

94. Kido A, Kataoka M, Yamamoto A, et al. Diffusion tensor MRI of the kidney at 3.0 and 1.5 Tesla. Acta Radiol 2010;51(9):1059–63.

95. Finley DS, Ellingson BM, Natarajan S, et al. Diffusion tensor magnetic resonance tractography of the prostate: feasibility for mapping periprostatic fibers. Urology 2012;80(1):219–23.

96. Nath K, Saraswat VA, Krishna YR, et al. Quantification of cerebral edema on diffusion tensor imaging in acute-on-chronic liver failure. NMR Biomed 2008;21(7):713–22.

97. Stoeck CT, Kalinowska A, von Deuster C, et al. Dual-phase cardiac diffusion tensor imaging with strain correction. PLoS One 2014;9(9):e107159.

98. van Doorn A, Bovendeerd PH, Nicolay K, et al. Determination of muscle fibre orientation using diffusion-weighted MRI. Eur J Morphol 1996; 34(1):5–10.

99. Van Donkelaar CC, Kretzers LJ, Bovendeerd PH, et al. Diffusion tensor imaging in biomechanical studies of skeletal muscle function. J Anat 1999; 194(Pt 1):79–88.

100. Napadow VJ, Chen Q, Mai V, et al. Quantitative analysis of three-dimensional-resolved fiber architecture in heterogeneous skeletal muscle tissue using nmr and optical imaging methods. Biophys J 2001;80(6):2968–75.

101. Sinha U, Yao L. In vivo diffusion tensor imaging of human calf muscle. J Magn Reson Imaging 2002; 15(1):87–95.

102. Damon BM, Ding Z, Anderson AW, et al. Validation of diffusion tensor MRI-based muscle fiber tracking. Magn Reson Med 2002;48(1):97–104.

103. Bonny JM, Renou JP. Water diffusion features as indicators of muscle structure ex vivo. Magn Reson Imaging 2002;20(5):395–400.

104. Galban CJ, Maderwald S, Uffmann K, et al. Diffusive sensitivity to muscle architecture: a magnetic resonance diffusion tensor imaging study of the human calf. Eur J Appl Physiol 2004;93(3):253–62.

105. Heemskerk AM, Strijkers GJ, Vilanova A, et al. Determination of mouse skeletal muscle architecture using three-dimensional diffusion tensor imaging. Magn Reson Med 2005;53(6):1333–40.

106. Sinha S, Sinha U, Edgerton VR. In vivo diffusion tensor imaging of the human calf muscle. J Magn Reson Imaging 2006;24(1):182–90.

107. Lansdown DA, Ding Z, Wadington M, et al. Quantitative diffusion tensor MRI-based fiber tracking of human skeletal muscle. J Appl Physiol (1985) 2007;103(2):673–81.

108. Kermarrec E, Budzik JF, Khalil C, et al. In vivo diffusion tensor imaging and tractography of human thigh muscles in healthy subjects. AJR Am J Roentgenol 2010;195(5):W352–6.

109. Froeling M, Nederveen AJ, Heijtel DF, et al. Diffusion-tensor MRI reveals the complex muscle architecture of the human forearm. J Magn Reson Imaging 2012;36(1):237–48.

110. Schenk P, Siebert T, Hiepe P, et al. Determination of three-dimensional muscle architectures: validation of the DTI-based fiber tractography method by manual digitization. J Anat 2013;223(1):61–8.

111. Elzibak AH, Kumbhare DA, Harish S, et al. Diffusion tensor imaging of the normal foot at 3 T. J Comput Assist Tomogr 2014;38(3):329–34.

112. Sinha U, Sinha S, Hodgson JA, et al. Human soleus muscle architecture at different ankle joint angles from magnetic resonance diffusion tensor imaging. J Appl Physiol (1985) 2011;110(3):807–19.

113. Chang HC, Guhaniyogi S, Chen NK. Interleaved diffusion-weighted improved by adaptive partial-Fourier and multiband multiplexed sensitivity-encoding reconstruction. Magn Reson Med 2014. [Epub ahead of print].

114. Kingsley PB. Introduction to diffusion tensor imaging mathematics: part II. Anisotropy, diffusion-weighting factors, and gradient encoding schemes. Concept Magn Reson A 2006;28A(2): 123–54.

115. Kingsley PB. Introduction to diffusion tensor imaging mathematics: part III. Tensor calculation, noise, simulations, and optimization. Concept Magn Reson A 2006;28A(2):155–79.

116. Kingsley PB. Introduction to diffusion tensor imaging mathematics: part I. Tensors, rotations, and eigenvectors. Concept Magn Reson A 2006;28A(2): 101–22.

117. Pajevic S, Pierpaoli C. Color schemes to represent the orientation of anisotropic tissues from diffusion tensor data: application to white matter fiber tract mapping in the human brain. Magn Reson Med 1999;42(3):526–40.

118. Okamoto Y, Kunimatsu A, Kono T, et al. Gender differences in MR muscle tractography. Magn Reson Med Sci 2010;9(3):111–8.

119. Galbán CJ, Maderwald S, Uffmann K, et al. A diffusion tensor imaging analysis of gender differences in water diffusivity within human skeletal muscle. NMR Biomed 2005;18(8):489–98.

120. Zaraiskaya T, Kumbhare D, Noseworthy MD. Diffusion tensor imaging in evaluation of human skeletal muscle injury. J Magn Reson Imaging 2006;24(2): 402–8.

121. Zeng H, Zheng JH, Zhang JE, et al. Grading of rabbit skeletal muscle trauma by diffusion tensor imaging and tractography on magnetic resonance imaging. Chin Med Sci J 2006;21(4):276–80.

122. Cermak NM, Noseworthy MD, Bourgeois JM, et al. Diffusion tensor MRI to assess skeletal muscle disruption following eccentric exercise. Muscle Nerve 2012;46(1):42–50.

123. Jiang K, Wang X, Lei H, et al. Investigation of muscle degeneration process in young rats with ischemia injury using MR diffusion tensor imaging. Conf Proc IEEE Eng Med Biol Soc 2013; 2013:81–4.

124. Heemskerk AM, Strijkers GJ, Drost MR, et al. Skeletal muscle degeneration and regeneration after femoral artery ligation in mice: monitoring with diffusion MR imaging. Radiology 2007;243(2): 413–21.

125. Lehmann HC, Zhang J, Mori S, et al. Diffusion tensor imaging to assess axonal regeneration in peripheral nerves. Exp Neurol 2010;223(1):238–44.

126. Galban CJ, Maderwald S, Stock F, et al. Age-related changes in skeletal muscle as detected by diffusion tensor magnetic resonance imaging. J Gerontol A Biol Sci Med Sci 2007;62(4):453–8.

127. Yamabe E, Nakamura T, Oshio K, et al. Line scan diffusion spectrum of the denervated rat skeletal muscle. J Magn Reson Imaging 2007;26(6):1585–9.

128. Marschar AM, Kuder TA, Stieltjes B, et al. In vivo imaging of the time-dependent apparent diffusional kurtosis in the human calf muscle. J Magn Reson Imaging 2014. [Epub ahead of print].

Advances in Diffusion-Weighted Imaging

Lorenzo Mannelli, MD, PhD[a], Stephanie Nougaret, MD[a,b], Hebert A. Vargas, MD[a], Richard K.G. Do, MD, PhD[a,*]

KEYWORDS

- Diffusion-weighted imaging • IVIM • Reproducibility • Apparent diffusion coefficient • MR imaging

KEY POINTS

- Intravoxel incoherent motion is a methodology to evaluate diffusion-weighted imaging (DWI) with the use of multiple *b* values, to separate the contribution of perfusion from tissue diffusion.
- DWI has been applied to the detection and characterization of tumors from multiple organs.
- DWI has been used to predict and evaluate response to treatment for a number of different tumors and treatment modalities.
- Reproducibility of apparent diffusion coefficients (ADC) measurements from DWI is limited by variability in imaging techniques and methods of ADC analysis.

INTRODUCTION

Diffusion-weighted imaging (DWI) has become an increasingly routine component of clinical MR imaging. Its unique soft tissue contrast mechanism exploits differences in the motion of water molecules in vivo at a biologically meaningful scale. The clinical potential of DWI in lesion detection, characterization, and response assessment has been explored in multiple organs and for multiple tumors.[1,2] This review briefly covers basic principles of DWI and introduces some recent advances in the field, specifically for abdominopelvic organs. For additional introductory review articles, several excellent references are available.[3–5]

BASIC PRINCIPLES OF DIFFUSION-WEIGHTED IMAGING

DWI is based on the use of single shot echoplanar imaging sequence with a long time to echo (TE) (60–100 ms), fat suppression, and the addition of motion-probing gradient pulses. When turned on, these gradients are used to decrease the signal intensity (SI) of moving water molecules during image acquisition. The SI of water molecules within each tissue decreases exponentially with the magnitude of their motion and with the strength of the motion-probing gradients (Equation 1).

$$S_b = S_0 \exp (-b \times ADC) \qquad (1)$$

In this monoexponential equation, the strength of the motion-probing gradients is summarized in a *b* value that reflects the amplitude, duration, and interval between the gradients. The magnitude of the water diffusion is described by the apparent diffusion coefficient, or ADC, measured in mm^2/s. S_0 and S_b are the baseline SI (before a motion probing-gradient is applied) and the SI at a prescribed *b* value. Thus, various tissues lose their SI at different rates governed by their baseline SI, their ADC, and the choice of *b* value.

Intravoxel Incoherent Motion

DWI performed in body imaging quickly revealed a non-monoexponential behavior of ADC as a function of the *b* value. That is, the choice of *b* value influenced the calculated ADC of tissue (Fig. 1).

Disclosures: no relevant disclosures (L. Mannelli, S. Nougaret, and H.A. Vargas); Dr R.K.G. Do is a consultant/advisor for Merck & Co., Inc.
[a] Department of Radiology, Memorial Sloan Kettering Cancer Center, 1275 York Avenue, New York, NY 10065, USA; [b] St Eloi Hospital, CHU Montpellier, Montpellier, France
* Corresponding author. 1275 York Avenue, C-278D, New York, NY 10065.
E-mail address: dok@mskcc.org

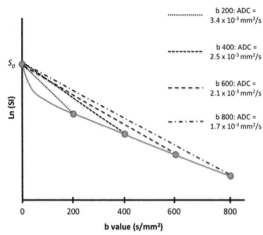

Fig. 1. Dependence of apparent diffusion coefficients (ADC) on *b* value used in single *b* value diffusion-weighted image (DWI). On a logarithmic scale, the signal intensity of soft tissue is usually observed to decrease more rapidly at lower *b* values (<200 s/mm^2) than at higher *b* values (>200 s/mm^2). When DWI is limited to a single *b* value, the calculated ADC can vary from 3.4×10^{-3} mm^2/s ($b = 200$) to 1.7×10^{-3} mm^2/s ($b = 800$).

This observation was explained in part by work from Le Bihan and colleagues,[6,7] recognizing that the motion of water molecules contributing to the signal in DWI arise from different compartments: extracellular space diffusion, intracellular space diffusion, and intravascular space diffusion (or perfusion).[8] Separating the motion of water molecules owing to perfusion in the microcirculation from that owing to diffusion in the extravascular space is summarized by the methodology of intravoxel incoherent motion (IVIM) imaging (Equation 2).

$$S_b = S_0 [(1 - f) \exp(-b \times D) + f \exp(-b \times D^*)] \quad (2)$$

Where S_0 and S_b represent the SI at baseline and at a specified *b* value, *f* represents the perfusion fraction (or the contribution of water moving in capillaries), *D* represents the tissue diffusion coefficient, and D^* represents the pseudodiffusion coefficient (or diffusion within the microcirculation). Because D^* is greater than *D* by several orders of magnitude, its contribution is negligible at higher *b* values (typically above $b = 200$ s/mm^2). At higher *b* values, the relationship between S_b and *b* again approximates a monoexponential equation dependent on *D* (Fig. 2). This limitation led to the 2009 consensus statement on the use of DWI as an imaging biomarker, emphasizing the role of multiple *b* values for measurement of ADC, and the possibility of calculating ADC$_{high}$, a surrogate for *D*, using only high *b* value DWI.[9]

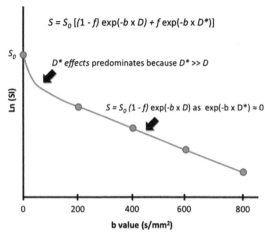

Fig. 2. Intravoxel incoherent motion (IVIM) parameters contribution to tissue signal intensity (SI). The rapid loss in SI of soft tissue, *S*, at lower *b* values is partly explained by the contribution of water signal from the intravascular space, which is defined by the perfusion fraction (*f*) and the pseudodiffusion coefficient D^*. Because D^* is usually several orders of magnitude larger than *D*, its contribution approaches zero as *b* increases above 100 to 200 s/mm^2. Thus, at higher *b* values (>200 s/mm^2), a monoexponential behavior is observed from the extravascular fraction of moving water molecules $(1 - f)$, which is governed by the tissue diffusion coefficient *D*.

Treatment Response

Much excitement has been generated from the use of DWI in oncologic imaging because of its potential to monitor treatment response in vivo.[4] The ability of DWI to evaluate oncologic outcomes can generally be separated into a pretreatment prediction of response, and the prediction of the response during or following treatment, such as chemotherapy or radiotherapy. The cellularity and vascularity of tumors are often affected by oncologic treatments, with potential changes affecting all 3 IVIM components, which are quantifiable by analysis of diffusion weighted images.

Diffusion-Weighted Imaging Reproducibility

Several barriers to the widespread adoption of DWI, especially in abdominal imaging, have included technical challenges to ensure a high-quality scan for every patient, and reproducible measurements of ADC. Quantifying the reproducibility of ADC and IVIM parameters is necessary before its use in clinical practice, and has been proposed by a panel of experts in the 2009 consensus statement.[9] The challenges in generating reproducible ADC and IVIM parameters is highlighted in selected studies.

ADVANCES IN LIVER DIFFUSION-WEIGHTED IMAGING

In the last decade, the use of DWI in liver MR imaging has been focused on improving lesion detection, lesion characterization, and tumor response.[10–12] In addition, DWI has also been used to evaluate the liver parenchyma as a predictor of fibrosis and cirrhosis,[13–17] a topic that is beyond the scope of this review. More recently, applications of IVIM in liver imaging and attempts at quantifying the reproducibility of DWI have been investigated.

Intravoxel Incoherent Motion in Liver Lesion Characterization

Distinguishing between benign and malignant liver lesion remains an important clinical challenge for radiologists. Initial studies with liver DWI were promising, showing differences in the ADC of benign and malignant lesions, although most studies included hepatic cysts and hemangiomas (with their corresponding high ADC values), entities that are often diagnosed easily with conventional T1 and T2 weighted imaging. The use of ADC to distinguish between solid benign and malignant liver lesions, such as hepatocellular carcinoma (HCC), focal nodular hyperplasia, or hepatocellular adenoma was not as promising.[18]

As multiple b value DWI became available on clinical scanners, several groups investigated the potential of IVIM parameters for improved characterization of focal liver lesions. Similar to prior studies evaluating ADC of liver lesions, Ichikawa and colleagues[19] found that D was lower for malignant compared with benign lesions; however, it was not useful for distinguishing benign lesions that were not hemangiomas or cysts. Similarly, Yoon and colleagues[20] compared the diagnostic performance of ADC and D for distinguishing benign and malignant focal liver lesions in 142 patients. A higher area under the curve was found by receiving operating characteristic analysis for D compared with ADC, although this study also included 23 hemangiomas. Thus, the diagnostic utility of the IVIM parameter D in characterizing a solid hypervascular liver lesion as malignant or benign remains uncertain.

Several studies have explored the utility of IVIM in further characterizing specific liver malignancies. The correlation between the ADC and D of HCC with its histologic grade was investigated, demonstrating a higher accuracy for distinguishing high-grade from low-grade HCC by D compared with ADC by receiving operating characteristic analysis. A stronger correlation between HCC tumor grade and D ($r = -0.604$) was found

compared with ADC ($r = -0.448$). The relatively modest sensitivity (88.9%) and specificity (78.3%) in distinguishing low-grade and high-grade HCC suggest that further refinement in IVIM technique and analysis, or combination with other MR imaging parameter, is needed before clinical application. For patients with colorectal cancer liver metastases on chemotherapy, both ADC and D values on whole tumor region of interest (ROI) were correlated with percent tumor necrosis on pathology.[21] On the other hand, a lack of correlation between necrosis with D^* and f was attributed to the general difficulty in fitting these parameters in the liver.

Reproducibility in the Liver

Despite the advances obtained from IVIM over single b value ADC measurements, the optimal DWI technique for clinical liver imaging remains unclear. The liver also poses additional challenges compared with other organs, because of its proximity to the diaphragm and heart, with related respiratory and cardiac motions. Several recent studies have investigated the reproducibility of DWI measurements, evaluating the impact of different b values, as well as respiratory schemes, including breath hold (BH), free breathing (FB), respiratory triggering (RT), and navigator triggering (NT).[22–24]

For focal liver lesions, Choi and colleagues[22] investigated potential differences in ADC measurements using BH, RT, and FB techniques. For focal liver lesions, excellent agreement in ADC (intraclass correlation = 0.952) were found at 3.0 T. In contrast, ADC of liver parenchyma had lower reproducibility with BH versus FB, RT, and NT respiratory techniques, although the results were possibly because of the lower number of excitations (NE_x) used for BH ($NE_x = 2$) versus other techniques ($NE_x = 4$).[24] Chen and colleagues[24] also found lesser ADC reproducibility and greater ADC mean values for the left compared with the right hepatic lobe, and decreasing ADC values as one measures from the superior to inferior left hepatic lobe, findings that reflect the potential effects of cardiac motion. These results further reinforce the suggestion by the consensus statement on DWI to measure ADC of focal liver lesions only in the right hepatic lobe.[9] Based on the limits of agreement for ADC measurements, the authors recommend a threshold of a 30% difference when using ADC as a biomarker, on baseline and follow-up studies. In a study of 20 patients with liver metastases, the potential use of ADC was investigated to predict treatment response to chemotherapy.[25] A similar repeatability coefficient of plus or minus 28% was found for ADC of liver metastases when limited to right hepatic lobe.

The choice of b values can influence the reproducibility of ADC measurements across various respiratory techniques, as demonstrated in a study that included 10 volunteers and 11 patients with focal liver lesions.[26] For example, higher maximal b values included in the ADC calculations led to higher reproducibility for FB and RT techniques. This study further highlights the difficulty in comparing the reproducibility of ADC measurements across various studies using different acquisition techniques and methods of ADC analysis. Future studies will need to demonstrate consistent DWI technique when using ADC as a biomarker for treatment response of liver malignancies.

The reproducibility of IVIM parameters for liver DWI has been more challenging, as illustrated in several recent works. There was good to excellent reproducibility for D, but moderate to good and poor to moderate reproducibility for f and D*, respectively, in a prospective study evaluating FB and RT DWI in volunteers and patients for evaluation of liver fibrosis.[23] Similarly, there was poor reproducibility of f and D*, and good reproducibility for D and ADC for HCC in a study of 10 patients with DWI performed on 2 separate MR imagings.[27] Despite the excitement surrounding IVIM in liver MR imaging, refinements in this technique and greater consensus on optimal techniques for clinical sites are needed to ascertain a baseline reproducibility in IVIM parameters.

At our own institution, we routinely use a BH DWI technique with multiple b values, and for patients with limited BH capacity, NT is available. With BH techniques, acquisition times are limited to 20 to 25 seconds, with the NE_x consequently limited to 2. Higher NE_x are possible with NT, but with longer resulting acquisition times (Table 1).

ADVANCES IN PANCREAS DIFFUSION-WEIGHTED IMAGING

Improvements in DWI techniques have also advanced the potential clinical applications in pancreatic imaging. Several studies are available on pancreatic lesion detection[28,29] and characterization,[30–32] normal pancreatic parenchyma,[33,34] and pancreatic function.[35,36]

Pancreatic tumors can be categorized into 4 main groups: cystic tumors, neuroendocrine tumors (NETs), solid nonendocrine neoplasms, and pseudotumors (chronic or acute inflammatory changes). Some of these lesions have overlapping clinical presentations and imaging is often requested to detect, characterize, and eventually stage these lesions. Some of the common clinical questions include how to differentiate indolent from malignant NETs, how to distinguish between tumors and pseudotumors, and how to identify benign from malignant cystic tumors. The potential utility of DWI and IVIM has been explored to address these clinical challenges.[28–32,37–47]

Diffusion-Weighted Imaging in Pancreatic Lesion Detection and Characterization

Normal pancreatic parenchyma is characterized by high ADC values with a mild gradient from the head toward the tail.[33,44] Noncystic pancreatic tumors demonstrate typically lower ADC values than normal parenchyma, and have higher SI compared with adjacent pancreatic parenchyma on DWI, making this technique a potentially useful tool for pancreatic tumor detection.

The relationship between tumor ADC and histologic grade has been explored for both cystic and

Table 1
Diffusion weighted imaging acquisition parameters

	Liver	Pancreas with Small FOV	Rectum	Prostate	Prostate with Small FOV
TR (ms)	3000	7500 (NT)	3500	3500	6000
TE (ms)	60	60	80	75	75
Slice thickness (mm)	7	6	5	4	3
Gap (mm)	1	0	1	0	0
FOV (cm)	40	24	22	16	16
Matrix size	128 × 128	160 × 80	128 × 128	128 × 128	160 × 80
NE_x	1, 2, 3, 4	6, 16	4	4	16
b Values	50, 250, 350, 500	50, 500	400, 800	400, 700, 1000	1000

Abbreviations: FOV, field of view; NE_x, number of excitations; NT, navigator triggering; TE, time to echo; TR, time to repetition.

solid pancreatic tumors. Two studies have investigated the potential prognostic significance of ADC values for pancreatic NETs. In the first, an inverse correlation was found between the cellular marker for proliferation Ki-67 and ADC values, that is, a lower ADC would indicate a more rapidly proliferating tumor,[39] whereas in the second study, when an ADC ratio between NETs and adjacent pancreatic parenchyma was calculated, a cutoff value of 1.03 could discriminate between benign and nonbenign NETs with a sensitivity of 92.9% and a specificity of 84.6%.[31]

Conflicting data have been published on the correlation between pancreatic adenocarcinoma pathologic grade and ADC values. Wang and colleagues[48] and Hayano and colleagues[49] demonstrated that the tumor ADC values correlate with their pathologic grade of differentiation: high-grade adenocarcinomas with limited glandular formation and dense fibrosis had lower ADC values than low-grade adenocarcinomas. However, Rosenkrantz and colleagues[50] found no such a correlation in 30 patients with adenocarcinoma. Significant differences exist between these studies with respect to the DWI sequences, b values, ROI placement, and type of ADC analysis. For example, Hayano and colleagues used minimum ADC values, whereas the other 2 studies used mean ADC values. In addition, Rosenkrantz and colleagues included the whole lesion in the ROI and the other 2 studies included only the solid and homogeneous portions of the tumor. The variability in how similar DWI datasets can be analyzed remains an obstacle for the widespread adoption of this technique for clinical use.

Differentiating between benign and malignant intraductal papillary mucinous neoplasms (IPMN) remains challenging for clinicians who are increasingly following patients with cystic pancreatic lesions. Although a consensus statement is available to guide the selection of IPMN for surgery, the guidelines remain imperfect.[51,52] In a cohort of 52 patients with cystic IPMN, Kang and colleagues[53] demonstrated lower ADC in malignant IPMN compared with benign IPMN. In this study, adding DWI to conventional MR cholangiopancreatography, 3 observers were able to differentiate between benign and malignant IPMN with a sensitivity ranging between 76% and 100% and a specificity between 84% and 97%. In a group of 50 patients, Fatima and colleagues[54] were able to define a 2.4 × 10^{-3} mm^2/s cutoff ADC value to differentiate between IPMN and MCN with a sensitivity of 98% and a specificity of 88%. Schraibman and colleagues[38] compared ADC values of serous cystadenoma and mucinous cystic tumors in 45 subjects and showed that mucinous tumors have lower ADCs. They proposed a greater restricted diffusion of water in the presence of mucin. Whether ADC measurements may be useful in cystic pancreatic lesions in a prospective setting remains to be seen.

Intravoxel Incoherent Motion in Pancreatic Lesion Characterization

At this time, only 4 groups have evaluated IVIM in pancreas imaging.[30,43–45,55,56] The evidence thus far suggests that normal pancreatic tissue demonstrates higher IVIM parameters D and f than noncystic pancreatic lesions. In a group of 71 patients, Lee and colleagues[45] also reported 87.2% sensitivity and 61.5% specificity when using D to differentiate pseudotumors from solid nonendocrine neoplasms. In the same study, solid nonendocrine neoplasms had significantly higher f compared with pseudotumors, and f could be used with a 92.3% specificity and 42.6% sensitivity in differentiating the same entities using 23.91% as cutoff value. In a smaller group of patients, Concia and colleagues[44] confirmed significant f values differences between neoplastic lesions and pseudotumors, but reported overlap of D values between the same entities. Kang and colleagues[30] in a group of 46 patients also demonstrated significantly lower f values in neoplastic lesions compared with pseudotumors with a sensitivity of 84% and a specificity of 100% in differentiating these 2 entities. In the same study, the authors analyzed fast and slow water molecules diffusion and found that no differences in D between pseudotumors and neoplastic lesions; however, it was possible to differentiate these 2 pathologic processes using D* measurements with a sensitivity of 94.9% and a specificity of 85.7%. In 37 patients with IPMN, Kang and colleagues were able differentiate between benign and malignant IPMN analyzing D and f values of the solid portions of these lesions. With f, a sensitivity of 93.3% and a specificity of 77.3% was achieved in differentiating benign versus malignant IPMN, whereas slow D had a sensitivity of 93.3% and a specificity 63.6%. No differences were found between these 2 entities when using analyzing D* values.

In summary, the initial experiences with IVIM for pancreatic pathologies are promising in their potential to discriminate between carcinoma of the pancreas and chronic pancreatitis, and between malignant and benign IPMN. However, the pulse sequences and methods for quantitative analysis differ between the different experiments and further studies are needed to validate these results.

Reproducibility in the Pancreas

Few studies have investigated the reproducibility of DWI for the pancreas. Ye and colleagues[57] found negligible (<5%) differences in ADC measurements of the pancreas in 24 healthy volunteers; these subjects were imaged during 2 different session using 2 different 1.5-T scanners and a 3-T scanner. No differences in normal pancreas ADC values were found before and after injection of intravenous gadolinium contrast agents[58]; similar results were demonstrated in pancreatic ductal adenocarcinoma.[59] The lack of differences in ADC before and after contrast should allow for some flexibility in pancreas MR protocol design, with the implementation of DWI sequences before or after contrast administration. Herrmann and colleagues[34] reported ADC values differences related to subjects age and sex; this observation may affect the use of ADC ratios to normal pancreas when characterizing focal pancreatic lesions. To date, no reproducibility study on IVIM parameters in pancreas DWI have been published.

At our own institution, during MR cholangiopancreatography studies, we currently perform both large field of view (FOV) DWI, as done for the liver DWI, and a small FOV DWI. Small, or reduced, FOV DWI is a recently available technique on GE scanners that allows for higher resolution imaging with reduced artifacts (Fig. 3). With the smaller voxel size, however, NT is required to achieve sufficient signal to noise (see Table 1).

ADVANCES IN RECTAL DIFFUSION-WEIGHTED IMAGING

Dramatic advances in image quality over the past few years have made DWI a promising tool for rectal lesion evaluation. As such, recent guidelines for rectal cancer imaging recommend DWI as part of a standard MR imaging protocol for preoperative restaging of rectal cancers after neoadjuvant chemoradiotherapy (CRT).[60]

Diffusion-Weighted Imaging for Initial Evaluation: Rectal Cancer Detection, Characterization, and Staging

Rectal cancer detection relies on clinical examination and endoscopy. However, in some cases DWI helps to locate very small rectal tumors during primary staging.[61] For characterization, several studies have demonstrated lower ADC values in rectal adenocarcinoma compared with normal rectal wall.[61] Curvo-Semedo and colleagues[62] also reported lower ADC values in more aggressive tumors. The added value of DWI for primary rectal cancer staging is still debated. DWI can facilitate lymph node detection, but alone it is not reliable for differentiating between benign and malignant lymph nodes.[63]

Evaluating the Response to Neoadjuvant Treatment with Diffusion-Weighted Imaging

The treatment of locally advanced rectal cancer has shifted in recent years from a standard

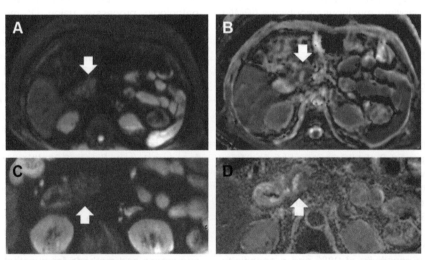

Fig. 3. Diffusion-weighted image (DWI) of the pancreas with large and small fields of view (FOV). Large FOV (*A*) and small FOV DWI (*C*) were obtained of the pancreas, with corresponding apparent diffusion coefficient maps (*B*, *D*). Finer details can be seen in the pancreatic head (*arrow*) with the small FOV DWI, which has a higher in plane resolution of 1.6×1.6 mm^2 (compared with 3.1×3.1 mm^2).

treatment for all patients including neoadjuvant CRT followed by operative resection to a more conservative approach. Response evaluation of locally advanced rectal cancer after CRT is thus emerging as a critical issue. Recent studies have illustrated the added value of DWI to differentiate viable tumor from fibrosis and to allow prediction of complete response.[64–70] Areas of fibrosis typically have a low cellular density, which results in low SI on high *b* value DWI. In contrast, residual tumor areas have a relatively high cellular density

and show high SI on DWI images that stands out against the low SI of the surrounding tissue and fibrosis. As such, small areas of residual tumor are better depicted on DWI images (**Fig. 4**). More recently, tumor volumetry with DWI has demonstrated highly accurate results in prediction of complete tumor response.[70]

The results from studies evaluating pre-CRT ADC values to predict rectal tumor response to neoadjuvant treatment are somewhat conflicting. Some authors have suggested that initial ADC

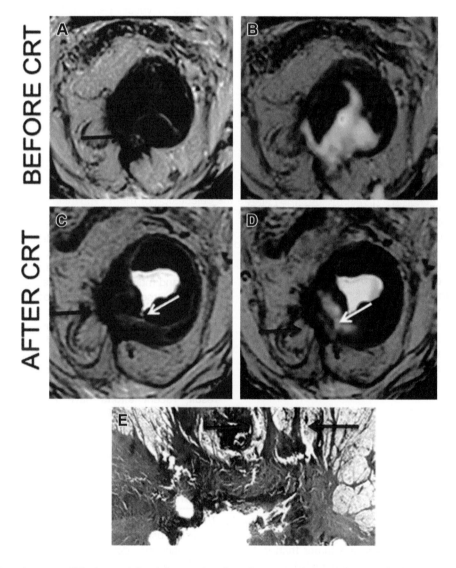

Fig. 4. Rectal cancer diffusion-weighted image (DWI). Before neoadjuvant chemoradiotherapy (CRT), T2WI sequence (*A*; *arrow*) and fused T2WI/DWI (*B*) image demonstrate T3c tumor extending thorough the mesorectal fascia. After CRT, the T2WI (*C*) demonstrate residual tumor (*white arrow*) but also T2 hypointense area (*black arrow*) in the muscularis propria with speculation extending thorough the mesorectal fascia. This could either represent fibrotic scar or residual tumor. Adding DWI to T2WI (*D*) enables to distinction of residual tumor (*white arrow*) from fibrotic scar (*black arrow*) confirmed on pathology (*E*) (*arrow*; original magnification, ×4; stain, hematoxylin-eosin).

values might predict tumor response to CRT[71–73] and others have demonstrated significantly lower pre-CRT ADC values in good responders compared with poor responders.[64,71] Conversely, other authors found no difference in the pre-CRT distribution of ADC values between nonresponders and responders.[70,74,75] Likewise, results concerning post CRT tumor response lack agreement: several studies have demonstrated significantly higher mean post-treatment ADC values in the complete responder group,[66,74,76] whereas others reported no difference.[70]

Reproducibility in the Rectum

ADC values often show great variability and are difficult to compare owing to differences in methodology. Most studies with ADC measurements have been conducted on selected ROIs placed on a representative image of the rectal tumor for analysis.[64,74,76,77] Thus, these techniques do not assess the problem of variable ROI size and positioning. In a study performed by Lambregts and colleagues,[78] the authors found that ADCs acquired from the whole tumor volume were more reproducible than those obtained from single-slice or small sample measurements.

Although normalized ADC values have been suggested, in pancreas ADC, for example, no similar studies have ever been performed in rectal DWI.[79] One study analyzed the repeatability of rectal tumor ADC at 1.5 T.[80] In this study, 18 patients with rectal cancer underwent a rectal MR imaging on 5 consecutive days with 2 identical DWI sequences. The repeatability coefficient of the ADC value was 9.8%, which is in the range of previous reported study of ADC value in the abdomen.[80]

Intravoxel Incoherent Motion in Rectal Cancer

To date, only preliminary results are available from a single study on the use of IVIM for rectal cancer. Bauerle and colleagues[81] compared the IVIM parameters (f and D) with histologic data (vascular area fraction and vessel diameter). First, although f was found to be significantly higher in the normal rectal wall of patients than in the tumor, histologic results showed significantly higher vascular area fractions in the tumor than in the rectum. The authors attributed their findings to the irregular morphology of tumor vasculature that led to a moderate perfusion in small and tortuous vessels. This paradoxic result has already been observed in some other tissues, such as prostate cancers versus surrounding normal tissues[39] and lung cancer versus

consolidation.[40] Moreover in this study, the parameters D and f were correlated with the vascular area fraction in patients without CRT.

The negative correlation found between D and the vascular area fraction in these patients could be an indicator that D is associated with tumor tissue, which is often strongly vascularized. In contradistinction, in patients who received CRT, the absence of correlations in rectal carcinoma between DWI and histologic parameters suggests that therapy induced inhomogeneous changes, such as focal fibrosis and necrosis, as well as changes in vessel permeability. Further studies are needed to validate prospectively the utility of IVIM parameters such as D, as a noninvasive imaging biomarker in rectal cancer.

At our own institution, we routinely use BH DWI technique with multiple b values (see **Table 1**). It is critical that the DWI sequence matches the oblique T2W axial sequence perpendicular to the tumor to assess correctly tumor response and to perform fused imaging.

ADVANCES IN PROSTATE DIFFUSION-WEIGHTED IMAGING

The use of DWI in prostate cancer has been the subject of extensive research in the literature and is now included most clinical prostate MR imaging protocols. Simple DWI-derived quantitative metrics such as the ADC have been used to differentiate benign and malignant prostate tissue.[82] Also, significant inverse correlations have been reported between ADC values and prostate cancer Gleason score as well as tumor proliferation markers such as Ki-67.[82–84] Despite these significant differences, substantial overlap exists between the ADC values of prostate cancer and benign conditions such as prostatitis and biopsy-induced changes. As a result, recent efforts have focused on more advanced methods for DWI acquisition, processing, and interpretation, with the aim of consolidating and further developing its well-established role in prostate cancer assessment.

Choice of b Values in Prostate Diffusion-Weighted Imaging

The optimal choice and number of b values that should be used to acquire prostate DWI is a matter of continuous debate. Absolute ADC values strongly depend on the choice of b values and therefore should be used with caution, particularly when attempting to establish "thresholds" for diagnosing disease states.[85] Higher b values offer the theoretic advantage of increased tumor to normal tissue contrast, at the expense of a decreased signal-to-noise ratio. One study reported higher lesion conspicuity and tumor–normal SI ratio when DWI was acquired with *b* values of 0 and 2000 s/mm^2 compared with 0 and 1000 s/mm^2.[86] Others suggest that, rather than acquiring high *b* value images, these can be "computed" by voxelwise fitting from a set of acquired lower *b* value images. Using numerical simulations, Maas and colleagues[86] reported comparable noise and the contrast-to-noise ratios between "calculated" and "acquired" DWI at a *b* value of 1400 s/mm^2 ($P = .395$). Another study reported the best diagnostic performance for prostate tumor detection when T2 weighted images were evaluated in conjunction with b2000 DWI, regardless of whether a set of "measured" or "calculated" b2000 images were used.[87]

Intravoxel Incoherent Motion in Prostate Cancer

The number of *b* values used in prostate DWI is also controversial. A minimum of 2 *b* values are required for monoexponential calculation of ADC. The use of 3 or more *b* values can better account for the non-monoexponential behavior of ADC as a function of *b* value and the influence of perfusion at low *b* values. There is evidence that IVIM parameters, including *D*, *D** and *f*, differ significantly between cancerous and normal peripheral zone prostatic tissue cancer.[88,89] Others have questioned the incremental value IVIM over simple monoexponential ADC measurements in prostate cancer, with some issues being raised about the influence of the *b* values used for acquisition and ideal method for calculating IVIM parameters.[90,91] One of these studies found significant differences in IVIM parameters using 2 different methods for calculation.[90] Despite this, the IVIM parameter *D* (but not *f* or *D**) was able to discriminate between tumor and normal areas with an area under the curve of 0.90 or greater in this study, regardless of the calculation method.[90] Further research into prostate IVIM is needed, with a focus on standardization of image acquisition techniques and approaches to fit the IVIM parameters from the measured DWI data.

At our own institution, we use a non-BH DWI technique with multiple *b* values (b 0, 400, 700, 1000). As described for the pancreas, we also use large and reduced FOV DWI for prostate imaging, which allows for higher resolution imaging with decreased artifacts. A summary of the DWI acquisition parameters is shown in **Table 1**.

SUMMARY

Exciting developments in DWI, both in imaging techniques and applications, have improved our ability to detect and characterize benign and malignant neoplasms. Predicting the histologic grade of malignancies and their response to treatment continue to be active areas of research. Multiple challenges remain, such as the standardization of acquisition parameters and DWI analysis across sites, to further the adoption of advanced methodologies, such as IVIM, to clinical practice.

REFERENCES

1. Moore WA, Khatri G, Madhuranthakam AJ, et al. Added value of diffusion-weighted acquisitions in MRI of the abdomen and pelvis. AJR Am J Roentgenol 2014;202(5):995–1006.
2. Rosenkrantz AB, Oei M, Babb JS, et al. Diffusion-weighted imaging of the abdomen at 3.0 Tesla: image quality and apparent diffusion coefficient reproducibility compared with 1.5 Tesla. J Magn Reson Imaging 2011;33(1):128–35.
3. Bonekamp S, Corona-Villalobos CP, Kamel IR. Oncologic applications of diffusion-weighted MRI in the body. J Magn Reson Imaging 2012;35(2):257–79.
4. Koh DM, Collins DJ. Diffusion-weighted MRI in the body: applications and challenges in oncology. AJR Am J Roentgenol 2007;188(6):1622–35.
5. Qayyum A. Diffusion-weighted imaging in the abdomen and pelvis: concepts and applications. Radiographics 2009;29(6):1797–810.
6. Le Bihan D, Breton E, Lallemand D, et al. Separation of diffusion and perfusion in intravoxel incoherent motion MR imaging. Radiology 1988;168(2):497–505.
7. Le Bihan D, Breton E, Lallemand D, et al. MR imaging of intravoxel incoherent motions: application to diffusion and perfusion in neurologic disorders. Radiology 1986;161(2):401–7.
8. Dixon WT. Separation of diffusion and perfusion in intravoxel incoherent motion MR imaging: a modest proposal with tremendous potential. Radiology 1988;168(2):566–7.
9. Padhani AR, Liu G, Koh DM, et al. Diffusion-weighted magnetic resonance imaging as a cancer biomarker: consensus and recommendations. Neoplasia 2009;11(2):102–25.
10. Coenegrachts K, Delanote J, Ter Beek L, et al. Improved focal liver lesion detection: comparison of single-shot diffusion-weighted echoplanar and single-shot T2 weighted turbo spin echo techniques. Br J Radiol 2007;80(955):524–31.
11. Galea N, Cantisani V, Taouli B. Liver lesion detection and characterization: role of diffusion-weighted imaging. J Magn Reson Imaging 2013;37(6):1260–76.
12. Parikh T, Drew SJ, Lee VS, et al. Focal liver lesion detection and characterization with diffusion-weighted MR imaging: comparison with standard

breath-hold T2-weighted imaging. Radiology 2008; 246(3):812–22.

13. Do RK, Chandarana H, Felker E, et al. Diagnosis of liver fibrosis and cirrhosis with diffusion-weighted imaging: value of normalized apparent diffusion coefficient using the spleen as reference organ. AJR Am J Roentgenol 2010;195(3):671–6.

14. Girometti R, Furlan A, Esposito G, et al. Relevance of b-values in evaluating liver fibrosis: a study in healthy and cirrhotic subjects using two single-shot spin-echo echo-planar diffusion-weighted sequences. J Magn Reson Imaging 2008;28(2):411–9.

15. Razek AA, Khashaba M, Abdalla A, et al. Apparent diffusion coefficient value of hepatic fibrosis and inflammation in children with chronic hepatitis. Radiol Med 2014;119:903–9.

16. Taouli B, Chouli M, Martin AJ, et al. Chronic hepatitis: role of diffusion-weighted imaging and diffusion tensor imaging for the diagnosis of liver fibrosis and inflammation. J Magn Reson Imaging 2008; 28(1):89–95.

17. Chandarana H, Do RK, Mussi TC, et al. The effect of liver iron deposition on hepatic apparent diffusion coefficient values in cirrhosis. AJR Am J Roentgenol 2012;199(4):803–8.

18. Taouli B. Diffusion-weighted MR imaging for liver lesion characterization: a critical look. Radiology 2012;262(2):378–80.

19. Ichikawa S, Motosugi U, Ichikawa T, et al. Intravoxel incoherent motion imaging of focal hepatic lesions. J Magn Reson Imaging 2013;37(6):1371–6.

20. Yoon JH, Lee JM, Yu MH, et al. Evaluation of hepatic focal lesions using diffusion-weighted MR imaging: comparison of apparent diffusion coefficient and intravoxel incoherent motion-derived parameters. J Magn Reson Imaging 2014;39(2):276–85.

21. Chiaradia M, Baranes L, Van Nhieu JT, et al. Intravoxel incoherent motion (IVIM) MR imaging of colorectal liver metastases: are we only looking at tumor necrosis? J Magn Reson Imaging 2014;39(2):317–25.

22. Choi JS, Kim MJ, Chung YE, et al. Comparison of breathhold, navigator-triggered, and free-breathing diffusion-weighted MRI for focal hepatic lesions. J Magn Reson Imaging 2013;38(1):109–18.

23. Dyvorne HA, Galea N, Nevers T, et al. Diffusion-weighted imaging of the liver with multiple b values: effect of diffusion gradient polarity and breathing acquisition on image quality and intravoxel incoherent motion parameters–a pilot study. Radiology 2013;266(3):920–9.

24. Chen X, Qin L, Pan D, et al. Liver diffusion-weighted MR imaging: reproducibility comparison of ADC measurements obtained with multiple breath-hold, free-breathing, respiratory-triggered, and navigator-triggered techniques. Radiology 2014;271(1):113–25.

25. Deckers F, De Foer B, Van Mieghem F, et al. Apparent diffusion coefficient measurements as very early predictive markers of response to chemotherapy in hepatic metastasis: a preliminary investigation of reproducibility and diagnostic value. J Magn Reson Imaging 2014;40:448–56.

26. Larsen NE, Haack S, Larsen LP, et al. Quantitative liver ADC measurements using diffusion-weighted MRI at 3 Tesla: evaluation of reproducibility and perfusion dependence using different techniques for respiratory compensation. MAGMA 2013;26(5): 431–42.

27. Kakite S, Dyvorne H, Besa C, et al. Hepatocellular carcinoma: short-term reproducibility of apparent diffusion coefficient and intravoxel incoherent motion parameters at 3.0T. J Magn Reson Imaging 2015;41: 149–56.

28. Wiggermann P, Grutzmann R, Weissenbock A, et al. Apparent diffusion coefficient measurements of the pancreas, pancreas carcinoma, and mass-forming focal pancreatitis. Acta Radiol 2012;53(2):135–9.

29. Mannelli L, Yeh MM, Wang CL. A pregnant patient with hypoglycemia. Gastroenterology 2012;143(4): e3–4.

30. Kang KM, Lee JM, Yoon JH, et al. Intravoxel incoherent motion diffusion-weighted MR imaging for characterization of focal pancreatic lesions. Radiology 2014;270(2):444–53.

31. Jang KM, Kim SH, Lee SJ, et al. The value of gadoxetic acid-enhanced and diffusion-weighted MRI for prediction of grading of pancreatic neuroendocrine tumors. Acta Radiol 2014;55(2):140–8.

32. Ma X, Zhao X, Ouyang H, et al. Quantified ADC histogram analysis: a new method for differentiating mass-forming focal pancreatitis from pancreatic cancer. Acta Radiol 2014;55:785–92.

33. Schoennagel BP, Habermann CR, Roesch M, et al. Diffusion-weighted imaging of the healthy pancreas: apparent diffusion coefficient values of the normal head, body, and tail calculated from different sets of b-values. J Magn Reson Imaging 2011;34(4): 861–5.

34. Herrmann J, Schoennagel BP, Roesch M, et al. Diffusion-weighted imaging of the healthy pancreas: ADC values are age and gender dependent. J Magn Reson Imaging 2013;37(4):886–91.

35. Balci NC, Momtahen AJ, Akduman EI, et al. Diffusion-weighted MRI of the pancreas: correlation with secretin endoscopic pancreatic function test (ePFT). Acad Radiol 2008;15(10):1264–8.

36. Wathle GK, Tjora E, Ersland L, et al. Assessment of exocrine pancreatic function by secretin-stimulated magnetic resonance cholangiopancreaticography and diffusion-weighted imaging in healthy controls. J Magn Reson Imaging 2014;39(2):448–54.

37. Muraoka N, Uematsu H, Kimura H, et al. Apparent diffusion coefficient in pancreatic cancer: characterization and histopathological correlations. J Magn Reson Imaging 2008;27(6):1302–8.

38. Schraibman V, Goldman SM, Ardengh JC, et al. New trends in diffusion-weighted magnetic resonance imaging as a tool in differentiation of serous cystadenoma and mucinous cystic tumor: a prospective study. Pancreatology 2011;11(1):43–51.

39. Wang Y, Chen ZE, Yaghmai V, et al. Diffusion-weighted MR imaging in pancreatic endocrine tumors correlated with histopathologic characteristics. J Magn Reson Imaging 2011;33(5):1071–9.

40. Barral M, Sebbag-Sfez D, Hoeffel C, et al. Characterization of focal pancreatic lesions using normalized apparent diffusion coefficient at 1.5-Tesla: preliminary experience. Diagn Interv Imaging 2013; 94(6):619–27.

41. Kamisawa T, Takuma K, Anjiki H, et al. Differentiation of autoimmune pancreatitis from pancreatic cancer by diffusion-weighted MRI. Am J Gastroenterol 2010;105(8):1870–5.

42. Kartalis N, Lindholm TL, Aspelin P, et al. Diffusion-weighted magnetic resonance imaging of pancreas tumours. Eur Radiol 2009;19(8):1981–90.

43. Klauss M, Lemke A, Grunberg K, et al. Intravoxel incoherent motion MRI for the differentiation between mass forming chronic pancreatitis and pancreatic carcinoma. Invest Radiol 2011;46(1): 57–63.

44. Concia M, Sprinkart AM, Penner AH, et al. Diffusion-weighted magnetic resonance imaging of the pancreas: diagnostic benefit from an intravoxel incoherent motion model-based 3 b-value analysis. Invest Radiol 2014;49(2):93–100.

45. Lee SS, Byun JH, Park BJ, et al. Quantitative analysis of diffusion-weighted magnetic resonance imaging of the pancreas: usefulness in characterizing solid pancreatic masses. J Magn Reson Imaging 2008;28(4):928–36.

46. Lalwani N, Mannelli L, Ganeshan DM, et al. Uncommon pancreatic tumors and pseudo-tumors. Abdom Imaging 2014;40:167–80.

47. Colagrande S, Belli G, Politi LS, et al. The influence of diffusion- and relaxation-related factors on signal intensity: an introductive guide to magnetic resonance diffusion-weighted imaging studies. J Comput Assist Tomogr 2008;32(3):463–74.

48. Wang Y, Chen ZE, Nikolaidis P, et al. Diffusion-weighted magnetic resonance imaging of pancreatic adenocarcinomas: association with histopathology and tumor grade. J Magn Reson Imaging 2011; 33(1):136–42.

49. Hayano K, Miura F, Amano H, et al. Correlation of apparent diffusion coefficient measured by diffusion-weighted MRI and clinicopathologic features in pancreatic cancer patients. J Hepatobiliary Pancreat Sci 2013;20(2):243–8.

50. Rosenkrantz AB, Matza BW, Sabach A, et al. Pancreatic cancer: lack of association between apparent diffusion coefficient values and adverse pathological features. Clin Radiol 2013;68(4): e191–7.

51. Tanaka M, Fernandez-del Castillo C, Adsay V, et al. International consensus guidelines 2012 for the management of IPMN and MCN of the pancreas. Pancreatology 2012;12(3):183–97.

52. Tanaka M. International consensus guidelines for the management of IPMN and MCN of the pancreas. Nihon Shokakibyo Gakkai Zasshi 2007;104(9): 1338–43.

53. Kang KM, Lee JM, Shin CI, et al. Added value of diffusion-weighted imaging to MR cholangiopancreatography with unenhanced MR imaging for predicting malignancy or invasiveness of intraductal papillary mucinous neoplasm of the pancreas. J Magn Reson Imaging 2013;38(3):555–63.

54. Fatima Z, Ichikawa T, Motosugi U, et al. Magnetic resonance diffusion-weighted imaging in the characterization of pancreatic mucinous cystic lesions. Clin Radiol 2011;66(2):108–11.

55. Re TJ, Lemke A, Klauss M, et al. Enhancing pancreatic adenocarcinoma delineation in diffusion derived intravoxel incoherent motion f-maps through automatic vessel and duct segmentation. Magn Reson Med 2011;66(5):1327–32.

56. Lemke A, Laun FB, Klauss M, et al. Differentiation of pancreas carcinoma from healthy pancreatic tissue using multiple b-values: comparison of apparent diffusion coefficient and intravoxel incoherent motion derived parameters. Invest Radiol 2009;44(12): 769–75.

57. Ye XH, Gao JY, Yang ZH, et al. Apparent diffusion coefficient reproducibility of the pancreas measured at different MR scanners using diffusion-weighted imaging. J Magn Reson Imaging 2014;40:1375–81.

58. Wang CL, Chea YW, Boll DT, et al. Effect of gadolinium chelate contrast agents on diffusion weighted MR imaging of the liver, spleen, pancreas and kidney at 3 T. Eur J Radiol 2011;80(2):e1–7.

59. Liu K, Peng W, Zhou Z. The effect of gadolinium chelate contrast agent on diffusion-weighted imaging of pancreatic ductal adenocarcinoma. Acta Radiol 2013;54(4):364–8.

60. Beets-Tan RG, Lambregts DM, Maas M, et al. Magnetic resonance imaging for the clinical management of rectal cancer patients: recommendations from the 2012 European Society of Gastrointestinal and Abdominal Radiology (ESGAR) consensus meeting. Eur Radiol 2013;23(9):2522–31.

61. Soyer P, Lagadec M, Sirol M, et al. Free-breathing diffusion-weighted single-shot echo-planar MR imaging using parallel imaging (GRAPPA 2) and high b value for the detection of primary rectal adenocarcinoma. Cancer Imaging 2010;10:32–9.

62. Curvo-Semedo L, Lambregts DM, Maas M, et al. Diffusion-weighted MRI in rectal cancer: apparent diffusion coefficient as a potential noninvasive

marker of tumor aggressiveness. J Magn Reson Imaging 2012;35(6):1365–71.

63. Heijnen LA, Lambregts DM, Mondal D, et al. Diffusion-weighted MR imaging in primary rectal cancer staging demonstrates but does not characterise lymph nodes. Eur Radiol 2013;23(12):3354–60.

64. Lambregts DM, Vandecaveye V, Barbaro B, et al. Diffusion-weighted MRI for selection of complete responders after chemoradiation for locally advanced rectal cancer: a multicenter study. Ann Surg Oncol 2011;18(8):2224–31.

65. Jang KM, Kim SH, Choi D, et al. Pathological correlation with diffusion restriction on diffusion-weighted imaging in patients with pathological complete response after neoadjuvant chemoradiation therapy for locally advanced rectal cancer: preliminary results. Br J Radiol 2012;85(1017):e566–72.

66. Song I, Kim SH, Lee SJ, et al. Value of diffusion-weighted imaging in the detection of viable tumour after neoadjuvant chemoradiation therapy in patients with locally advanced rectal cancer: comparison with T2 weighted and PET/CT imaging. Br J Radiol 2012;85(1013):577–86.

67. Genovesi D, Filippone A, Ausili Cefaro G, et al. Diffusion-weighted magnetic resonance for prediction of response after neoadjuvant chemoradiation therapy for locally advanced rectal cancer: preliminary results of a monoinstitutional prospective study. Eur J Surg Oncol 2013;39(10):1071–8.

68. Andreano A, Rechichi G, Rebora P, et al. MR diffusion imaging for preoperative staging of myometrial invasion in patients with endometrial cancer: a systematic review and meta-analysis. Eur Radiol 2014;24(6):1327–38.

69. Carbone SF, Pirtoli L, Ricci V, et al. Diffusion-weighted MR volumetry for assessing the response of rectal cancer to combined radiation therapy with chemotherapy. Radiology 2012;263(1):311.

70. Curvo-Semedo L, Lambregts DM, Maas M, et al. Rectal cancer: assessment of complete response to preoperative combined radiation therapy with chemotherapy–conventional MR volumetry versus diffusion-weighted MR imaging. Radiology 2011; 260(3):734–43.

71. Sun YS, Zhang XP, Tang L, et al. Locally advanced rectal carcinoma treated with preoperative chemotherapy and radiation therapy: preliminary analysis of diffusion-weighted MR imaging for early detection of tumor histopathologic downstaging. Radiology 2010;254(1):170–8.

72. Jung SH, Heo SH, Kim JW, et al. Predicting response to neoadjuvant chemoradiation therapy in locally advanced rectal cancer: diffusion-weighted 3 Tesla MR imaging. J Magn Reson Imaging 2012;35(1):110–6.

73. Lambrecht M, Vandecaveye V, De Keyzer F, et al. Value of diffusion-weighted magnetic resonance imaging for prediction and early assessment of response to neoadjuvant radiochemotherapy in rectal cancer: preliminary results. Int J Radiat Oncol Biol Phys 2012;82(2):863–70.

74. Kim SH, Lee JY, Lee JM, et al. Apparent diffusion coefficient for evaluating tumour response to neoadjuvant chemoradiation therapy for locally advanced rectal cancer. Eur Radiol 2011;21(5):987–95.

75. Kim YC, Lim JS, Keum KC, et al. Comparison of diffusion-weighted MRI and MR volumetry in the evaluation of early treatment outcomes after preoperative chemoradiotherapy for locally advanced rectal cancer. J Magn Reson Imaging 2011;34(3):570–6.

76. Kim SH, Lee JM, Hong SH, et al. Locally advanced rectal cancer: added value of diffusion-weighted MR imaging in the evaluation of tumor response to neoadjuvant chemo- and radiation therapy. Radiology 2009;253(1):116–25.

77. Park MJ, Kim SH, Lee SJ, et al. Locally advanced rectal cancer: added value of diffusion-weighted MR imaging for predicting tumor clearance of the mesorectal fascia after neoadjuvant chemotherapy and radiation therapy. Radiology 2011;260(3):771–80.

78. Lambregts DM, Beets GL, Maas M, et al. Tumour ADC measurements in rectal cancer: effect of ROI methods on ADC values and interobserver variability. Eur Radiol 2011;21(12):2567–74.

79. Soyer P, Kanematsu M, Taouli B, et al. ADC normalization: a promising research track for diffusion-weighted MR imaging of the abdomen. Diagn Interv Imaging 2013;94(6):571–3.

80. Intven M, Reerink O, Philippens ME. Repeatability of diffusion-weighted imaging in rectal cancer. J Magn Reson Imaging 2014;40:146–50.

81. Bäuerle T, Seyler L, Münter M, et al. Diffusion-weighted imaging in rectal carcinoma patients without and after chemoradiotherapy: a comparative study with histology. Eur J Radiol 2013;82(3):444–52.

82. Vargas HA, Akin O, Franiel T, et al. Diffusion-weighted endorectal MR imaging at 3 T for prostate cancer: tumor detection and assessment of aggressiveness. Radiology 2011;259(3):775–84.

83. Turkbey B, Shah VP, Pang Y, et al. Is apparent diffusion coefficient associated with clinical risk scores for prostate cancers that are visible on 3-T MR images? Radiology 2011;258(2):488–95.

84. Zhang J, Jing H, Han X, et al. Diffusion-weighted imaging of prostate cancer on 3T MR: relationship between apparent diffusion coefficient values and Ki-67 expression. Acad Radiol 2013;20(12):1535–41.

85. Thormer G, Otto J, Reiss-Zimmermann M, et al. Diagnostic value of ADC in patients with prostate cancer: influence of the choice of b values. Eur Radiol 2012;22(8):1820–8.

86. Tamada T, Kanomata N, Sone T, et al. High b value (2,000 s/mm^2) diffusion-weighted magnetic resonance imaging in prostate cancer at 3 Tesla: comparison with 1,000 s/mm^2 for tumor conspicuity and discrimination of aggressiveness. PLoS One 2014;9(5):e96619.

87. Ueno Y, Takahashi S, Kitajima K, et al. Computed diffusion-weighted imaging using 3-T magnetic resonance imaging for prostate cancer diagnosis. Eur Radiol 2013;23(12):3509–16.

88. Shinmoto H, Tamura C, Soga S, et al. An intravoxel incoherent motion diffusion-weighted imaging study of prostate cancer. AJR Am J Roentgenol 2012; 199(4):W496–500.

89. Dopfert J, Lemke A, Weidner A, et al. Investigation of prostate cancer using diffusion-weighted intravoxel incoherent motion imaging. Magn Reson Imaging 2011;29(8):1053–8.

90. Kuru TH, Roethke MC, Stieltjes B, et al. Intravoxel incoherent motion (IVIM) diffusion imaging in prostate cancer - what does it add? J Comput Assist Tomogr 2014;38(4):558–64.

91. Pang Y, Turkbey B, Bernardo M, et al. Intravoxel incoherent motion MR imaging for prostate cancer: an evaluation of perfusion fraction and diffusion coefficient derived from different b-value combinations. Magn Reson Med 2013;69(2): 553–62.

Advances in T1-Weighted and T2-Weighted Imaging in the Abdomen and Pelvis

 CrossMark

Justin M. Ream, MD*, Andrew B. Rosenkrantz, MD

KEYWORDS

- Abdominal MR imaging • T1-weighted imaging • T2-weighted imaging • Radial imaging
- Dixon technique • 3D imaging

KEY POINTS

- Non-Cartesian T1-weighted acquisitions provide high spatial and high temporal resolution data acquisition during free-breathing without sacrificing image quality. These sequences' resistance to motion degradation makes them ideal for patient populations in whom compliance with breath-holding instructions is limited.
- Non-Cartesian T2-weighted acquisitions are relatively motion resistant, although they have slightly increased acquisition time.
- Several advances in Dixon imaging have helped to improve the separation of signal from water and fat protons and achieve superior fat suppression compared with prior techniques.
- Three-dimensional volumetric T2-weighted acquisitions may allow for a reduction in overall examination length by eliminating the need for separate multiplanar 2-dimensional acquisitions, but they have variable effects on tissue contrast.

INTRODUCTION

Utilization of MR imaging for applications in the abdomen and pelvis continues to increase and gain widespread clinical acceptance, owing to MR imaging's excellent inherent tissue contrast and ability to derive functional information in addition to morphologic and anatomic information. However, abdominopelvic imaging must cope with several important issues that are less relevant in other modalities and organ systems. For example, respiratory motion, which has minimal impact in the extremities or central nervous system, can profoundly impact MR image quality, particularly of upper abdominal organs in close proximity to the diaphragm, such as the liver. In addition, as the number of available MR sequences expands, and the ability and desire to extract an increasing amount of anatomic and functional information from routine MR scans increase, a balance is needed between such ability and desire to acquire more information from the scans and the practical consequences of doing so, particularly the increased time needed for both scanning and interpretation of abdominopelvic MR imaging.

T1-weighted and T2-weighted sequences remain the mainstay sequences for providing MR tissue contrast. This article discusses several recent advances in T1-weighted and T2-weighted imaging. As these advances transition from the investigational phase to routine clinical

Disclosures: None.
Department of Radiology, NYU School of Medicine, NYU Langone Medical Center, 660 First Avenue, New York, NY 10016, USA
* Corresponding author. Department of Radiology, Center for Biomedical Imaging, NYU Langone Medical Center, 660 First Avenue, 3rd Floor, New York, NY 10016.
E-mail address: Justin.Ream@nyumc.org

Radiol Clin N Am 53 (2015) 583–598
http://dx.doi.org/10.1016/j.rcl.2015.01.003
0033-8389/15/$ – see front matter © 2015 Elsevier Inc. All rights reserved.

usage, it is hoped that this article will provide a guide for evaluating current knowledge of these sequences, including their advantages and disadvantages over the widely used clinical imaging sequences that they may replace.

ADVANCES IN T1-WEIGHTED IMAGING
Non-Cartesian K-Space Acquisition

MR imaging data acquisition is a multistep process in which a 2-dimensional (2D) or 3-dimensional (3D) array of spatial frequency data ("k-space") is initially acquired and then converted into image data ("image space") via a Fourier transform.[1,2] Traditionally, acquisition of k-space data has been performed with a rectilinear or Cartesian scheme,[3] in which k-space is filled via a line-by-line sampling of spatial frequency data. This method of data acquisition has several important limitations in abdominopelvic imaging. First, because of respiratory motion, many clinical sequences are acquired during breath-holding, which limits the amount of time available for the acquisition and still incurs a large risk of respiratory motion artifact when patients are unable to follow breath-holding instructions. Second, because of the rectilinear acquisition, artifacts that occur despite the use of breath-holding are distributed in a coherent fashion that frequently significantly hampers image quality.

Several acquisition schema have been developed that sample k-space in a non-Cartesian manner. Such acquisitions offer several advantages over traditional rectilinear k-space acquisition.[4] Non-Cartesian acquisition allows for a motion-robust acquisition during free-breathing, limiting the need for patient compliance with breath-holding instructions. This benefit is especially important in scans in which sustained breath-holding is difficult, such as in the pediatric population[5–7] or in the setting of gadoxetic acid intravenous contrast administration for hepatobiliary imaging (Eovist; Bayer Pharmaceuticals, Wayne, NJ, USA),[8–10] because this agent has been shown to cause transient dyspnea and therefore increased respiratory motion artifact, shortly after injection.[11] In addition, as opposed to the coherent artifact in the phase encoding direction observed for traditional rectilinear acquisitions, non-Cartesian k-space sampling distributes motion-related artifact in a less coherent manner, which generally produces a less noticeable effect on diagnostic image quality (**Fig. 1**).[12] Finally, the oversampling the center of k-space that is possible with non-Cartesian acquisitions confers a theoretic gain in image contrast.

There are multiple general methods of performing non-Cartesian T1-weighted acquisition that involve the same general principle of k-space acquisitions that rotate in a non-Cartesian fashion with repeated sampling of the center of k-space. One of the more widely used acquisition methods is a radial acquisition in which k-space is acquired in multiple radial spokes, all of which cross the center of k-space (eg, Radial VIBE[13] or Star VIBE, *Volume Interpolated Breath hold Examination*; Siemens Healthcare, Erlangen, Germany). This sequence is a modification of the standard rectilinear VIBE sequence, but does not actually require breath-holding given the non-Cartesian approach. Spiral acquisition, in which k-space is filled by multiple spiral arcs, all of which cross the center of k-space, is an additional method (eg, Spiral LAVA,[14] or *Liver Acquisition with Volume Acceleration*; GE Medical Systems,

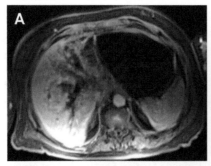 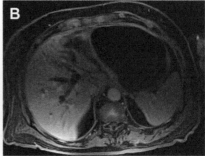

Fig. 1. An 81-year-old man with a history of Parkinson disease and new onset jaundice. (A) Axial breath-hold T1-weighted fat-saturated gradient-echo image of the liver obtained with rectilinear k-space filling (axial VIBE) exhibits extensive artifact from motion, which causes indistinctness of the liver edge and of the dilated intrahepatic biliary tree. (B) Axial free-breathing T1-weighted fat-saturated gradient-echo image at the same level obtained with radial filling of k-space (radial VIBE) shows improved sharpness and overall image quality, although radial streak artifact is present.

Milwaukee, WI, USA). Many of the non-Cartesian acquisition schema have been combined with other MR imaging techniques for reducing scan time, including parallel imaging[15–17] and compressed sensing,[15,18] to achieve a combination of both high spatial resolution and high temporal resolution. A summary of abdominopelvic applications of non-Cartesian T1-weighted acquisitions is listed in **Table 1**.

The major disadvantage of the non-Cartesian acquisition relative to the standard rectilinear acquisition is increased time of acquisition. However, it is important to note that although the total acquisition time is longer, all of the non-Cartesian sequences can be acquired with free-breathing and thus require less patient compliance with instructions. In addition, with advanced post-processing, many of the non-Cartesian acquisitions, if originally acquired using appropriate sequence modifications, can be parsed into multiple shorter temporal blocks. For example, the sequence GRASP (Golden angle RAdial Sparse Parallel acquisition) can be acquired using the similar parameters as radial VIBE[15,17] and then be reconstructed at a higher effective temporal resolution relative to standard breath-hold acquisitions, despite this sequence's relatively longer scan time. In addition, although non-Cartesian acquisitions tend to reduce artifact related to motion, several studies report the introduction of radially oriented streak artifacts.

Clinical Summary: Non-Cartesian T1-Weighted Acquisition

- Non-Cartesian T1-weighted acquisition is less sensitive to motion than standard acquisition and allows for acquisition during free-breathing.
- Studies have shown improved image quality[5,6,8,10,21,22] and decreased motion-related artifact[5,10,13,20–22,24,25] in abdominopelvic applications.
- The major downside is the increase in time of acquisition,[5,8,10,13,21,22,24] precluding rapid dynamic imaging for currently available commercial implementations, and the introduction of streak artifact,[22,24,25] although these generally do not significantly affect image quality.
- Non-Cartesian T1-weighted acquisitions should be considered in studies in which motion artifact is common and breath-holding is difficult, and when precise timing of postcontrast sequences is not necessary. One common application is pediatric imaging,[5,6] in which gross patient motion and respiratory motion are difficult to control. In addition, by combining non-Cartesian acquisitions with

novel reconstructions schemes, including compressed sensing, this technique can be applied to situations in which breath-holding is difficult but timing of scans is also critical, such as in hepatic imaging using gadoxetic acid (Eovist/Primovist, Bayer Pharmaceuticals).[8,10,17,20]

- Clinical implementation example: using standard scanning parameters for radial VIBE, a scan covering the upper abdomen with a 1.6 × 1.6 × 3 mm spatial resolution can be achieved in approximately 1 minute during free-breathing.[13]

Advanced Dixon Sequences

Dixon[26,27] first described the use of in-phase and opposed-phase echo time pairs for separation of signal from water and fat protons on T1-weighted images. As originally conceived, Dixon imaging involves the acquisition of paired spin-echo pulse sequences, one with water and fat protons precessing "in phase" (and thus having additive signal), and the second with water and fat protons precessing "opposed phase" (and thus having signal that cancels out). With this standard 2-point Dixon acquisition, "water only" and "fat only" sequences can be derived from in-phase and opposed-phase sequences using simple algebraic transformation (**Fig. 2**).

Traditional 2-point Dixon sequences have key limitations.[28] First, Dixon sequences are sensitive to B_0 field inhomogeneities, which can cause phase shifts that are indistinguishable from the chemical shift caused by the differences in precession of fat and water protons with the standard Dixon transformation. These errors can lead to unreliable separation of signal from fat and water protons. In addition, traditional Dixon sequences are hampered by relatively long acquisition times.[28,29]

Several modifications have been proposed to address the limitations of standard 2-point Dixon acquisitions. The "3-point Dixon technique"[30–33] acquires data with a third echo time in addition to the standard in-phase and opposed-phase sequences, which allows for determination of field inhomogeneity that can be incorporated into the Dixon modeling for more accurate fat and water separation. Several "extended 2-point Dixon techniques"[34,35] have also been developed, which apply sophisticated phase correction algorithms to achieve deconvolution of the previously noted phase error while still only requiring images obtained at 2 different echo times. Both the 3-point Dixon and the extended 2-point Dixon techniques provide improved separation of water

Table 1
Applications of non-Cartesian T1-weighted image acquisition in the abdomen and pelvis

Author, Year	Acquisition	Organ	Benefits	Disadvantages
Fujinaga et al,[8] 2014	Radial VIBE	Liver (gadoxetic acid)	• Improved overall image quality • Improved quantitative enhancement • Improved scan timing • Improved hepatic vessel clarity • Decreased artifact	• Increased acquisition time
Gomi et al,[19] 2014	RADAR-SE	Liver (gadoxetic acid)	• Increased contrast ratio • Increased liver signal intensity ratio	• Increased artifact
Cheng et al,[6] 2014	VDRad	Pediatric imaging	• Improved image quality • Decreased overall scan time	• None
Rosenkrantz et al,[20] 2014	Radial VIBE with GRASP	Prostate	• Improved spatial resolution • Improved capsular clarity • Improved clarity of boundary between peripheral and transition zones • Improved interreader lesion size correlation	• None
Chandarana et al,[5] 2014	Radial VIBE	Pediatric imaging	• Improved overall image quality • Improved hepatic vessel clarity • Improved hepatic edge sharpness • Improved lesion detection • Improved lesion conspicuity	• Increased acquisition time
Agrawal et al,[10] 2013	Spiral LAVA	Liver (gadoxetic acid)	• Improved overall image quality • Improved hepatic vessel clarity • Improved aorta-to-liver signal ratio • Improved bolus timing	• Increased total acquisition time
Reiner et al,[21] 2013	Radial 3D-GRE	Liver (gadoxetic acid)	• Improved overall image quality • Improved liver edge sharpness • Improved lesion conspicuity	• Increased acquisition time
Bamrungchart et al,[22] 2013	Radial 3D-GRE	Pancreas	• Improved image quality and decreased artifact in noncooperative patients	• Increased acquisition time • Increased streak artifact • Decreased pancreatic edge sharpness • Decreased pancreatic ductal clarity • Decreased lesion conspicuity • Decreased confidence in lesion detection
Kim et al,[23] 2013	Radial VIBE	Abdomen and chest	• Improved spatial resolution	• Slightly worse overall image quality

(continued on next page)

Table 1
(continued)

Author, Year	Acquisition	Organ	Benefits	Disadvantages
Chandarana et al,[13] 2011	Radial VIBE	Liver	• Decreased pulsation artifact • Improvement in multiple image quality parameters	• Decreased hepatic vessel clarity • Increased acquisition time
Azevedo et al,[24] 2011	Radial 3D-GRE	Liver Pancreas	• Decreased motion related artifact • Increased homogeneity of fat signal • Decreased "pixel graininess"	• Increased acquisition time • Increased streak artifact • Decreased overall image quality for post-contrast acquisition • Decreased sharpness of liver, pancreas, and vessels • Decreased lesion conspicuity • Decreased confidence of lesion detection for small (<1 cm) lesions
Hattori et al,[25] 2009	RADAR-SE	Female pelvis	• Decreased motion artifact	• Increased streak artifact • Decreased sharpness

Abbreviations: RADAR-SE, *RAD*ial *A*cquisition *R*egime, *S*pin *E*cho; VDRad, *V*ariable *D*ensity sampling and *Rad*ial view-ordering.

and fat protons. These sequences have been used not only for quantification of fat content in tissues[36,37] but also for improving the quality of background fat suppression.[38,39] Nonetheless, these sequences still suffer from imperfections related to the magnitude of the phase error induced by field inhomogeneity and have some difficulty in voxels in which fat and water coexist.[28]

A refinement of the 3-point Dixon technique for water and fat separation called IDEAL (*I*terative *D*ecomposition of water and fat with *E*cho *A*symmetry and *L*east squares estimation)[40,41] uses selected echo times to optimize signal-to-noise ratio and further improve fat and water signal separation. IDEAL can theoretically be applied to any sequence.

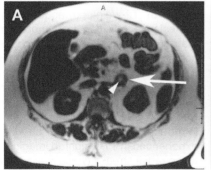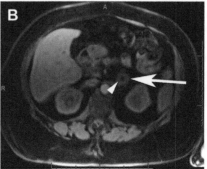

Fig. 2. A 73-year-old woman with incidental suprarenal lesion noted on ultrasound. (*A*) Fat-only and (*B*) water-only images from 3D 2-point Dixon acquisition show a rounded left adrenal lesion (*arrow*) with a central focus of increased signal on the fat-only image (*arrowhead*), compatible with a benign myelolipoma. Note the excellent suppression of subcutaneous fat, visceral fat, and the central fat within the myelolipoma (*arrowhead*) on the water-only image.

Clinical Summary: Advanced Dixon Sequences

- Advances in acquisition and postprocessing of Dixon sequences provide excellent separation of water and fat signal in T1-weighted imaging.
- These techniques may be applied to virtually any T1-weighted acquisition, although details of the actual implementation vary by scanner and vendor.
- Consider implementation of advanced Dixon sequences when there is a need for assessment of fat content within lesions, such as adrenal imaging[36,42] or imaging of renal masses.[42,43] In addition, advanced Dixon sequences may be applied for robust fat suppression in precontrast and postcontrast imaging.[44,45]
- Clinical implementation example: an extended 2-point 3D Dixon sequence of the upper abdomen with 1.4 × 1.1 × 3.0 mm spatial resolution can be obtained during a single breath-hold in approximately 20 seconds.[43]

ADVANCES IN T2-WEIGHTED IMAGING
Non-Cartesian T2-Weighted Imaging

Similar to the previously described challenges in T1-weighted imaging, diaphragmatic motion from respiration also poses a key challenge for the acquisition of high-quality images of the abdomen and pelvis for T2-weighted imaging. Abdominopelvic T2-weighted imaging, most commonly performed using turbo spin-echo acquisitions, has involved either a breath-hold or a respiratory-triggered sequence. Breath-hold T2-weighted imaging is often performed using multiple separate breath-hold acquisitions[46–48] given the extended time needed for turbo spin-echo sequences. Although the multiple breath-hold approach increases signal and significantly decreases respiratory motion artifact compared with free-breathing, this method significantly increases the time of acquisition and, even with optimal patient compliance with breath-holding, is still susceptible to nonrespiratory motion-related artifact from bulk patient motion, vascular pulsation, and bowel peristalsis. Although the half-Fourier acquisition turbo spin-echo T2-weighted sequence may be rapid enough to fit into a single breath-hold,[49,50] this sequence suffers from a blurring of T2 contrast given the extended echo train and consequent suboptimal lesion characterization.[51] In comparison, respiratory triggering can be performed physically using external bellows placed over the patient's abdomen[52] or in a virtual fashion based on rapid "navigator" MR acquisitions that continuously monitor the position of the patient's diaphragm and triggers actual image acquisition when the diaphragm is in an appropriate acceptance window.[53] Although respiratory triggering improves image quality of T2-weighted imaging in some patients, this approach can greatly prolong acquisition times in patients with an irregular respiratory pattern, does not fully eliminate respiratory artifact, and does not compensate for nonrespiratory sources of motion.[54]

Similar to the non-Cartesian sampling used in T1-weighted imaging, several methods for motion-robust non-Cartesian acquisition of T2-weighted images have been developed. The most commonly implemented acquisition has been alternatively named PROPELLER (Periodically Rotated Overlapping ParallEL Lines with Enhanced Reconstruction; GE Medical Systems) or BLADE (Siemens Healthcare). PROPELLER and BLADE both involve the acquisition of multiple slabs of k-space data that are oriented in a radial fashion. Each slab includes the center of k-space. This rotating k-space acquisition provides similar advantages as in non-Cartesian T1-weighted acquisition, most notably a dispersion of artifacts in the phase-encoding direction in a nonlinear (in this case, radial) fashion[55] as well as oversampling of the center of k-space. These effects can lead to a virtual elimination of artifacts from bulk patient motion as well as from other sources (Fig. 3). Non-Cartesian T2-weighted acquisitions have proven to be effective in multiple different abdominopelvic applications (Table 2).

Although non-Cartesian T2-weighted acquisitions have gained wide acceptance, there are several disadvantages, as summarized in Table 3. The major disadvantage is increased acquisition time; in all studies that reported acquisition times of Cartesian versus non-Cartesian T2-weighted acquisitions, the non-Cartesian acquisition was more time-intensive than the standard turbo spin-echo T2-weighted acquisition, albeit typically a difference of less than 1 minute of added time within the context of a 3- to 4-minute scan. In addition, although overall artifact was reduced using a non-Cartesian acquisition, this approach may introduce radially oriented streak artifact, as experienced in T1-weighted imaging.[58] However, these radial streaks typically are most prominent along the periphery of the image, manifesting for instance within the patient's superficial soft tissues, if not the air outside the patient and thus may have only minimal impact on overall image quality.

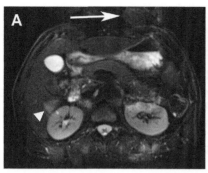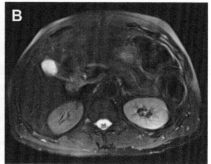

Fig. 3. A 57-year-old man undergoing surveillance MR imaging for Crohn disease. (*A*) Axial fat-suppressed turbo spin-echo T2-weighted image performed with standard rectilinear acquisition shows extensive ghosting artifact (*arrow*) related to motion from bowel peristalsis as well as ghosting artifact from the gallbladder (*arrowhead*), which obscures a portion of the liver. (*B*) Axial fat-suppressed turbo spin-echo T2-weighted image in the same patient performed using BLADE acquisition scheme shows near-elimination of these artifacts.

Clinical Summary: Non-Cartesian T2-Weighted Imaging

- Non-Cartesian T2-weighted acquisitions allow for T2-weighted imaging with decreased sensitivity to motion.
- Studies have shown improved image quality[57,60,62–65] and decreased motion-related artifact.[56–59,64,65]
- The qualitative improvement in imaging comes with a penalty of increased acquisition time.[58,63–65]
- Non-Cartesian T2-weighted imaging is best applied in situations in which breath-holding is difficult or patient motion may be problematic. Clinically, the technique has been most commonly applied to liver imaging,[59,61–63,65] in which respiratory motion from the diaphragm is problematic, and in imaging of the female pelvis,[57,58] in which adjacent bowel peristalsis may cause motion-related artifact.
- Clinical implementation example: Using standard parameters for T2-weighted imaging using the BLADE technique, a 1.7 × 1.2 × 4.0 mm spatial resolution sequence of the upper abdomen can be obtained in approximately 75 seconds during multiple breath-holds or using a respiratory-triggered acquisition.[59]

3-Dimensional Volumetric T2-Weighted Imaging

Traditional 2D T2-weighted MR acquisition involves the serial excitation of multiple discrete nonoverlapping slices acquired in a single imaging plane. With 2D acquisition, if additional imaging planes are required, they must be acquired in a separate scan because the relatively thick slices used in standard 2D acquisitions preclude the creation of diagnostic quality multiplanar reformatted images. 3D T2-weighted sequences with isotropic or nearly isotropic voxels overcome this limitation. Briefly, such methods use a second phase-encoding direction to acquire either multiple contiguous or overlapping "slabs" of data, or a single volumetric slab encompassing the entire volume of acquisition. 3D T2-weighted sequences have historically had prohibitively long acquisition times, which limited implementation into routine clinical practice. More recently, however, modifications to the extended echo-trains of these sequences have been developed that led to reduced interecho spacing and allow for performing 3D T2-weighted imaging in a time-efficient, clinically acceptable manner. Commercially available versions of such sequences include SPACE (*S*ampling *P*erfection with *A*pplication optimized *C*ontrasts using different flip angle *E*volution; Siemens Healthcare), VISTA (*V*olumetric *IS*otropic *T*SE *A*cquisition; Phillips Healthcare, Best, the Netherlands), XETA (e*X*tended *E*cho *T*rain *A*cquisition; GE Healthcare), and CUBE (GE Healthcare).

The major advantage of 3D T2-weighted acquisitions over traditional 2D acquisitions arises from the ability to acquire high-resolution isotropic data. Isotropic voxel acquisition allows for the creation of multiplanar reformatted images in any imaging plane from a single acquisition (**Fig. 4**). Thus, although the acquisition of volumetric 3D T2-weighted sequences is greater than that of a single 2D T2-weighted acquisition, the total scan time can be reduced considerably by eliminating the need for multiple discrete 2D acquisitions in multiple planes.[73,75,77] In addition, for studies that require orientation of the imaging plane to specific anatomic landmarks rather than the conventional axial, sagittal, or coronal planes (for example, imaging of congenital uterine anomalies,[81] rectal cancer,[82] and female pelvic

Table 2
Applications of non-Cartesian T2-weighted acquisitions (BLADE/PROPELLER) in the abdomen and pelvis

Author, Year	Organ	Benefits	Disadvantages
Rosenkrantz et al,[56] 2014	Prostate	• Reduced motion artifact • Improved EPE detection	• Reduced image contrast
Fujimoto et al,[57] 2011	Female pelvis	• Improved lesion detection • Higher image quality • Decreased artifact	• None
Lane et al,[58] 2011	Female pelvis	• Improved junctional zone evaluation • Improved fibroid detection • Improved ovarian follicle detection and ovarian edge sharpness • Decreased motion artifact	• Increased acquisition time • Introduction of "radial artifact"
Rosenkrantz et al,[59] 2011	Liver	• Decreased motion artifact • Improved lesion detection	• None
Haneder et al,[60] 2011	General abdominopelvic imaging	• Improved image quality and decreased artifact in the pelvis only	• No image quality or artifact benefits in the abdomen
Hirokawa et al,[61] 2010	Liver	• Improved detection of hepatic metastases after SPIO administration	• None
Bayramoglu et al,[62] 2010	Liver Pancreas Gallbladder Spleen	• Improved organ edge sharpness • Improved overall image quality • Improved SNR	• None
Nanko et al,[63] 2009	Liver	• Improved image quality	• Increased acquisition time
Michaely et al,[64] 2008	Kidneys	• Improved image quality • Decreased artifact	• Increased acquisition time
Hirokawa et al,[65] 2008	Liver	• Improved image quality • Decreased artifact	• Increased acquisition time

Abbreviations: SNR, signal-to-noise ratio; SPIO, superparamagnetic iron oxide.

cancers[83]), 3D T2-weighted acquisitions allow for reconstructing these alternate orientations following the acquisition, rather than relying solely on prospective identification of the relevant anatomic landmarks by the technologist at the time of the examination. Finally, the high resolution and near-isotropic nature of the 3D data set as well as ability to manipulate these images in real-time, including viewing in any orientation, may facilitate evaluation of complex pathologic processes, such as congenital uterine anomalies[79] and prostate cancer extraprostatic extension.[72] **Table 3** presents abdominopelvic applications and their advantages and disadvantages relative to standard 2D T2-weighted acquisitions.

The most commonly reported disadvantage of the 3D T2-weighted acquisition is this sequence's long acquisition time given the time required to perform phase-encoding in 2 different directions. In studies that compared a single 2D acquisition with a 3D acquisition, the 3D acquisition was uniformly reported to be longer. However, as discussed above, a key advantage of 3D acquisition, if not a primary motivation for this technique, is the potential ability to replace multiplanar 2D acquisitions with a single isotropic

Table 3
Applications of time-efficient 3-dimensional volumetric T2-weighted imaging in the abdomen and pelvis

Author, Year	Organ	Benefits	Disadvantages
Takayama et al,[66] 2014	Liver	• Improved lesion detection • Improved lesion characterization • Improved suppression of signals from hepatic vessels ("black-blood" effect)	• Increased acquisition time (vs a single 2D acquisition)
Bazot et al,[67] 2013	Female pelvis	• Decreased total acquisition time (vs 3 multiplanar 2D acquisitions)	• Lower overall image quality
Denoiseux et al,[68] 2013	Liver	• Improved lesion detection • Improved reader confidence • Improved interreader correlation	• Lower overall image quality • Increased artifact • Increased acquisition time (vs a single 2D acquisition)
Shin et al,[69] 2013	Uterus	• Decreased total acquisition time (vs 3 multiplanar 2D acquisitions)	• Decreased sharpness of tumor margin
Dohan et al,[70] 2013	Liver	• Improved contrast-to-noise ratio for liver lesions • Decreased motion artifact from respiratory, cardiac, and vascular motion	• Increased acquisition time (vs a single 2D acquisition)
Watanabe et al,[71] 2012	Liver	• Improved lesion conspicuity • Improved detection of small (<10 mm) lesions	• Increased susceptibility artifact • Decreased sharpness of the left hepatic lobe
Cornud et al,[72] 2012	Prostate	• Improved detection of extracapsular extension of prostate cancer	• None
Hecht et al,[73] 2011	Female pelvis	• Decreased total acquisition time (vs 3 multiplanar 2D acquisitions)	• Decreased contrast between fluid and fat
Hori et al,[74] 2011	Uterus	• Improved image quality • Increased conspicuity of endometrial cancer • Decreased total acquisition time (vs 2 multiplanar 2D acquisitions) • Increased myometrial SNR • Increased SI difference between endometrial and cervical cancer relative to normal muscle	• Decreased SI difference between uterine fibroids and normal myometrium
Rosenkrantz et al,[75] 2010	Prostate	• Improved peripheral to transition zone contrast • Improved tumor conspicuity • Decreased total acquisition time (vs 3 multiplanar 2D acquisitions)	• Lower SNR in the normal peripheral zone

(continued on next page)

Table 3
(continued)

Author, Year	Organ	Benefits	Disadvantages
Rosenkrantz et al,[76] 2010	Liver (respiratory triggered study)	• Improved image quality • Improved tissue contrast • Improved contrast between hepatic lesions and normal parenchyma • Decreased motion related artifact	• Increased acquisition time (vs a single 2D acquisition) • Increased B_1 inhomogeneity
Proscia et al,[77] 2010	Female pelvis	• Improved subjective contrast between cervical epithelium and stroma • Decreased respiratory motion artifact • Decreased artifact from bowel peristalsis • Decreased total acquisition time (vs 3 multiplanar 2D acquisitions)	• None
Kim et al,[78] 2010	Rectum	• Decreased total acquisition time (vs 4 multiplanar 2D acquisitions)	• Decreased tumor conspicuity
Agrawal et al,[79] 2009	Uterus	• Decreased total acquisition time (vs 3 multiplanar 2D acquisitions) • Improved overall image quality • Improved 3D reconstructions?	• None
Fütterer et al,[80] 2008	Rectum	• None	• Decreased area under the curve in detecting muscularis invasion • Increased acquisition time (vs a single sagittal 2D acquisition)

Abbreviations: SI, signal intensity; SNR, signal-to-noise ratio.

3D acquisition that can be reformatted into multiple different planes, thus obviating multiple separate acquisitions and decreasing the total time of acquisition. Even if the 3D T2-weighted sequence is used to replace multiplanar 2D scans and thereby reduce overall examination length, the prolonged acquisition time of the single 3D scan, often requiring more than 5 minutes, can contribute to greater artifact from patient motion in comparison with several shorter 2D scans. Another potential disadvantage of the 3D T2-weighted sequences stems from the fact that some of the commercially available 3D acquisition techniques use varying flip angles across the long echo train to facilitate feasibility of the rapid acquisition. This strategy may alter image contrast, for instance, by introducing a component of T1 weighting into the T2-weighted image. Indeed, several studies reported worse image contrast with 3D acquisitions relative to standard 2D acquisitions. Finally, there does not seem to be a clear advantage in image quality or lesion detection using 3D acquisitions across the peer-reviewed studies regarding this sequence, with different studies variously reporting improvement, worsening, or no significant difference between 3D and 2D acquisitions in various measures of image quality and lesion detection and conspicuity. Thus, the implementation of a 3D T2-weighted acquisition should be approached cautiously and take into account the specific organ or organ system being imaged, locally available sequences and scanners, and sequence optimization.

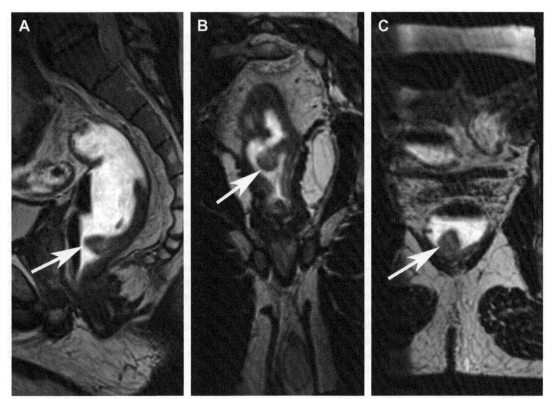

Fig. 4. A 38-year-old man with newly diagnosed rectal cancer. Turbo spin-echo T2-weighted images in the sagittal plane (*A*), coronal oblique plane parallel to the rectum (*B*), and axial oblique plane perpendicular to the rectum (*C*) show a polypoid mass in the rectum (*arrow*). All 3 planes were created from a single 3D T2-weighted SPACE acquisition that required approximately 5 minutes of acquisition time. Obtaining comparable separate 2D T2-weighted acquisitions in all 3 planes would have required a total of approximately 12 minutes of scan time.

Clinical Summary: 3-Dimensional Volumetric T2-Weighted Imaging

- 3D volumetric T2-weighted imaging allows for the acquisition of isotropic or near-isotropic T2-weighted images that can be reconstructed into any plane of imaging during postprocessing without the need for additional acquisitions.
- Although the most commonly reported downside is the increased acquisition time per scan,[66,68,70,76,80] the overall acquisition time can be reduced by using a single 3D volumetric T2-weighted acquisition to replace multiple 2D acquisitions performed in different imaging planes.[67,69,73–75,77,79]
- In addition, the imaging parameters used in time-efficient 3D acquisitions may cause slight loss of inherent T2 contrast and thus a decrease in perceived image quality.[67–69,71,73,74]
- 3D volumetric T2-weighted imaging is most useful in clinical situations in which multiple planes of imaging are required. Clinically,

these sequences should be considered for use in imaging protocols that require multiplanar T2-weighted imaging, particularly when the planes of acquisition are angled relative to anatomic landmarks rather than in standard axial, sagittal, and coronal planes. For example, it has been successfully applied to imaging of the female pelvis[67,69,73,74,77,79] and imaging of rectal cancer.[78,80]

- Clinical implementation example: Using standard scanning parameters for an SPACE sequence, a 3D T2-weighted acquisition through the entire pelvis with near isotropic 1.5 × 1.5 × 1.0 cm spatial resolution can be achieved in just less than 4 minutes and subsequently reconstructed in 3 different planes.[76]

SUMMARY

Recent advances in T1-weighted and T2-weighted imaging (**Tables 4** and **5**) hold promise for routine MR imaging of the abdomen and

Table 4
Representative scanning parameters for advanced T1-weighted and T2-weighted techniques

Sequence	TR (ms)	TE (ms)	Flip Angle	Slice Thickness (mm)	Matrix
Radial VIBE	3.3	1.6	12°	2	256 × 216
3-point Dixon T1WI	6.2	1.6/3.2/4.8	10°	3	128 × 100
BLADE T2WI	2710	112	150°	3	256 × 256
SPACE T2WI	1200	141	150°	3	192 × 123

Abbreviations: T1WI, T1-weighted imaging; T2WI, T2-weighted imaging.

pelvis. In particular, non-Cartesian T1-weighted and T2-weighted acquisitions reduce the need for patient compliance with breath-hold acquisitions and allow for motion robust free-breathing acquisitions. Furthermore, non-Cartesian T1-weighted acquisitions, when combined with other techniques such as compressed sensing and parallel imaging, achieve both high spatial and high temporal resolution while maintaining excellent diagnostic imaging quality. Advances in Dixon techniques for T1-weighted imaging improve the reliability of separation of water and fat signal within a relatively short acquisition time. 3D T2-weighted volumetric acquisitions have the potential to shorten overall examination length by reducing the need for acquisition of multiple discrete multiplanar 2D sequences. Each of these sequences also has tradeoffs and limitations, as discussed in this article. Awareness of these insights should help the practicing abdominal radiologist in effectively incorporating these new implementations of traditional MR sequences into routine clinical protocols.

Table 5
Summary of recent advances in T1-weighted and T2-weighted sequences in abdominopelvic imaging

Sequence	Examples	Major Advantages	Major Disadvantages
Non-Cartesian T1-weighted imaging	Radial VIBE; spiral	• Reduced artifact from patient motion and other sources of ghosting (ie, peristalsis, vascular pulsation) • Improved image sharpness • Very high temporal resolution achieved in combination with compressed-sensing	• Longer scan time • Radial streak artifacts
Non-Cartesian T2-weighted imaging	PROPELLER, BLADE	• Reduced artifact from patient motion and other sources of ghosting (ie, peristalsis, vascular pulsation) • Improved image sharpness	• Longer scan time • Radial streak artifacts
Advanced Dixon methods for T1-weighted imaging	"Extended" 2-point Dixon; IDEAL	• More reliable water/fat signal separation • Improved fat suppression	• Potential errors in water and fat signal separation (uncommon) • Potentially longer scan times for some acquisitions
3D volumetric T2-weighted imaging	SPACE; CUBE; XETA; VISTA	• Potential reduction in overall examination length • Thinner sections • Ability to reconstruct images in any orientation may aid assessment of complex pathology	• Altered image contrast • Longer scan time for a single acquisition, possibly increasing image artifacts

REFERENCES

1. Lee VS. Cardiovascular MRI: physical principles to practical protocols. Philadelphia: Lippincott Williams & Wilkins; 2006.
2. Brown MA, Semelka RC. MRI: basic principles and applications. Hoboken (NJ): John Wiley & Sons; 2011.
3. Paschal CB, Morris HD. K-space in the clinic. J Magn Reson Imaging 2004;19(2):145–59.
4. Wright KL, Hamilton JI, Griswold MA, et al. Non-Cartesian parallel imaging reconstruction. J Magn Reson Imaging 2014;40:1022–40.
5. Chandarana H, Block KT, Winfeld MJ, et al. Free-breathing contrast-enhanced T1-weighted gradient-echo imaging with radial k-space sampling for paediatric abdominopelvic MRI. Eur Radiol 2014; 24(2):320–6.
6. Cheng JY, Zhang T, Ruangwattanapaisarn N, et al. Free-breathing pediatric MRI with nonrigid motion correction and acceleration. J Magn Reson Imaging 2014. http://dx.doi.org/10.1002/jmri.24785.
7. Chavhan GB, Babyn PS, Vasanawala SS. Abdominal MR imaging in children: motion compensation, sequence optimization, and protocol organization. Radiographics 2013;33(3):703–19.
8. Fujinaga Y, Ohya A, Tokoro H, et al. Radial volumetric imaging breath-hold examination (VIBE) with k-space weighted image contrast (KWIC) for dynamic gadoxetic acid (Gd-EOB-DTPA)-enhanced MRI of the liver: advantages over Cartesian VIBE in the arterial phase. Eur Radiol 2014;24(6):1290–9.
9. Chandarana H, Block TK, Ream J, et al. Estimating liver perfusion from free-breathing continuously acquired dynamic gadolinium-ethoxybenzyl-diethylenetriamine pentaacetic acid-enhanced acquisition with compressed sensing reconstruction. Invest Radiol 2014. http://dx.doi.org/10.1097/RLI.0000000000000105.
10. Agrawal MD, Spincemaille P, Mennitt KW, et al. Improved hepatic arterial phase MRI with 3-second temporal resolution. J Magn Reson Imaging 2013; 37(5):1129–36.
11. Davenport MS, Viglianti BL, Al-Hawary MM, et al. Comparison of acute transient dyspnea after intravenous administration of gadoxetate disodium and gadobenate dimeglumine: effect on arterial phase image quality. Radiology 2013;266(2):452–61.
12. Glover GH, Pauly JM. Projection reconstruction techniques for reduction of motion effects in MRI. Magn Reson Med 1992;28(2):275–89.
13. Chandarana H, Block TK, Rosenkrantz AB, et al. Free-breathing radial 3D fat-suppressed T1-weighted gradient echo sequence: a viable alternative for contrast-enhanced liver imaging in patients unable to suspend respiration. Invest Radiol 2011; 46(10):648–53.
14. Kressler B, Spincemaille P, Nguyen TD, et al. Three-dimensional cine imaging using variable-density spiral trajectories and SSFP with application to coronary artery angiography. Magn Reson Med 2007; 58(3):535–43.
15. Chandarana H, Feng L, Block TK, et al. Free-breathing contrast-enhanced multiphase MRI of the liver using a combination of compressed sensing, parallel imaging, and golden-angle radial sampling. Invest Radiol 2013;48(1):10–6.
16. Deshmane A, Gulani V, Griswold MA, et al. Parallel MR imaging. J Magn Reson Imaging 2012;36(1):55–72.
17. Feng L, Grimm R, Block KT, et al. Golden-angle radial sparse parallel MRI: combination of compressed sensing, parallel imaging, and golden-angle radial sampling for fast and flexible dynamic volumetric MRI. Magn Reson Med 2014;72(3):707–17.
18. Vasanawala SS, Alley MT, Hargreaves BA, et al. Improved pediatric MR imaging with compressed sensing. Radiology 2010;256(2):607–16.
19. Gomi T, Nagamoto M, Hasegawa M, et al. Radial MRI during free breathing in contrast-enhanced hepatobiliary phase imaging. Acta Radiol 2014; 55(1):3–7.
20. Rosenkrantz AB, Geppert C, Grimm R, et al. Dynamic contrast-enhanced MRI of the prostate with high spatiotemporal resolution using compressed sensing, parallel imaging, and continuous golden-angle radial sampling: preliminary experience. J Magn Reson Imaging 2014. http://dx.doi.org/10.1002/jmri.24661.
21. Reiner CS, Neville AM, Nazeer HK, et al. Contrast-enhanced free-breathing 3D T1-weighted gradient-echo sequence for hepatobiliary MRI in patients with breath-holding difficulties. Eur Radiol 2013; 23(11):3087–93.
22. Bamrungchart S, Tantaway EM, Midia EC, et al. Free breathing three-dimensional gradient echo-sequence with radial data sampling (radial 3D-GRE) examination of the pancreas: comparison with standard 3D-GRE volumetric interpolated breathhold examination (VIBE). J Magn Reson Imaging 2013;38(6):1572–7.
23. Kim KW, Lee JM, Jeon YS, et al. Free-breathing dynamic contrast-enhanced MRI of the abdomen and chest using a radial gradient echo sequence with K-space weighted image contrast (KWIC). Eur Radiol 2013;23(5):1352–60.
24. Azevedo RM, de Campos RO, Ramalho M, et al. Free-breathing 3D T1-weighted gradient-echo sequence with radial data sampling in abdominal MRI: preliminary observations. AJR Am J Roentgenol 2011;197(3):650–7.
25. Hattori N, Senoo A, Gomi T, et al. T1-weighted MR imaging of the female pelvis using RADAR-FSE sequence. Magn Reson Med Sci 2009;8(4):175–80.
26. Dixon WT. Simple proton spectroscopic imaging. Radiology 1984;153(1):189–94.
27. Lee JK, Dixon WT, Ling D, et al. Fatty infiltration of the liver: demonstration by proton spectroscopic

imaging. Preliminary observations. Radiology 1984; 153(1):195–201.

28. Ma J. Dixon techniques for water and fat imaging. J Magn Reson Imaging 2008;28(3):543–58.

29. Low RN, Austin MJ, Ma J. Fast spin-echo triple echo Dixon: initial clinical experience with a novel pulse sequence for simultaneous fat-suppressed and nonfat-suppressed T2-weighted spine magnetic resonance imaging. J Magn Reson Imaging 2011; 33(2):390–400.

30. Glover GH, Schneider E. Three-point Dixon technique for true water/fat decomposition with B0 inhomogeneity correction. Magn Reson Med 1991; 18(2):371–83.

31. Glover GH. Multipoint Dixon technique for water and fat proton and susceptibility imaging. J Magn Reson Imaging 1991;1(5):521–30.

32. Szumowski J, Coshow W, Li F, et al. Double-echo three-point-Dixon method for fat suppression MRI. Magn Reson Med 1995;34(1):120–4.

33. Yeung HN, Kormos DW. Separation of true fat and water images by correcting magnetic field inhomogeneity in situ. Radiology 1986;159(3):783–6.

34. Coombs BD, Szumowski J, Coshow W. Two-point Dixon technique for water-fat signal decomposition with B0 inhomogeneity correction. Magn Reson Med 1997;38(6):884–9.

35. Skinner TE, Glover GH. An extended two-point Dixon algorithm for calculating separate water, fat, and B0 images. Magn Reson Med 1997;37(4):628–30.

36. Marin D, Dale BM, Bashir MR, et al. Effectiveness of a three-dimensional dual gradient echo two-point Dixon technique for the characterization of adrenal lesions at 3 Tesla. Eur Radiol 2012;22(1):259–68.

37. Marin D, Soher BJ, Dale BM, et al. Characterization of adrenal lesions: comparison of 2D and 3D dual gradient-echo MR imaging at 3 T–preliminary results. Radiology 2010;254(1):179–87.

38. Rosenkrantz AB, Mannelli L, Kim S, et al. Gadolinium-enhanced liver magnetic resonance imaging using a 2-point Dixon fat-water separation technique: impact upon image quality and lesion detection. J Comput Assist Tomogr 2011;35(1):96–101.

39. Cornfeld DM, Israel G, McCarthy SM, et al. Pelvic imaging using a T1W fat-suppressed three-dimensional dual echo Dixon technique at 3T. J Magn Reson Imaging 2008;28(1):121–7.

40. Reeder SB, McKenzie CA, Pineda AR, et al. Water-fat separation with IDEAL gradient-echo imaging. J Magn Reson Imaging 2007;25(3):644–52.

41. Reeder SB, Pineda AR, Wen Z, et al. Iterative decomposition of water and fat with echo asymmetry and least-squares estimation (IDEAL): application with fast spin-echo imaging. Magn Reson Med 2005;54(3):636–44.

42. Pokharel SS, Macura KJ, Kamel IR, et al. Current MR imaging lipid detection techniques for diagnosis of lesions in the abdomen and pelvis. Radiographics 2013;33(3):681–702.

43. Rosenkrantz AB, Raj S, Babb JS, et al. Comparison of 3D two-point Dixon and standard 2D dual-echo breath-hold sequences for detection and quantification of fat content in renal angiomyolipoma. Eur J Radiol 2012;81(1):47–51.

44. Clauser P, Pinker K, Helbich TH, et al. Fat saturation in dynamic breast MRI at 3 Tesla: is the Dixon technique superior to spectral fat saturation? A visual grading characteristics study. Eur Radiol 2014; 24(9):2213–9.

45. Lee MH, Kim YK, Park MJ, et al. Gadoxetic acid-enhanced fat suppressed three-dimensional T1-weighted MRI using a multiecho Dixon technique at 3 Tesla: emphasis on image quality and hepatocellular carcinoma detection. J Magn Reson Imaging 2013;38(2):401–10.

46. Augui J, Vignaux O, Argaud C, et al. Liver: T2-weighted MR imaging with breath-hold fast-recovery optimized fast spin-echo compared with breath-hold half-Fourier and non-breath-hold respiratory-triggered fast spin-echo pulse sequences. Radiology 2002;223(3):853–9.

47. Lee MG, Jeong YK, Kim JC, et al. Fast T2-weighted liver MR imaging: comparison among breath-hold turbo-spin-echo, HASTE, and inversion recovery (IR) HASTE sequences. Abdom Imaging 2000;25(1):93–9.

48. Reinig JW. Breath-hold fast spin-echo MR imaging of the liver: a technique for high-quality T2-weighted images. Radiology 1995;194(2):303–4.

49. Sasaki K, Ito K, Fujita T, et al. Small hepatic lesions found on single-phase helical CT in patients with malignancy: diagnostic capability of breath-hold, multisection fluid-attenuated inversion-recovery (FLAIR) MR imaging using a half-fourier acquisition single-shot turbo spin-echo (HASTE) sequence. J Magn Reson Imaging 2007;25(1):129–36.

50. Altbach MI, Outwater EK, Trouard TP, et al. Radial fast spin-echo method for T2-weighted imaging and T2 mapping of the liver. J Magn Reson Imaging 2002;16(2):179–89.

51. Herborn CU, Vogt F, Lauenstein TC, et al. MRI of the liver: can true FISP replace HASTE? J Magn Reson Imaging 2003;17(2):190–6.

52. Santelli C, Nezafat R, Goddu B, et al. Respiratory bellows revisited for motion compensation: preliminary experience for cardiovascular MR. Magn Reson Med 2011;65(4):1097–102.

53. Taylor AM, Jhooti P, Wiesmann F, et al. MR navigator-echo monitoring of temporal changes in diaphragm position: implications for MR coronary angiography. J Magn Reson Imaging 1997;7(4):629–36.

54. Choi JS, Kim MJ, Chung YE, et al. Comparison of breathhold, navigator-triggered, and free-breathing diffusion-weighted MRI for focal hepatic lesions. J Magn Reson Imaging 2013;38(1):109–18.

55. Pipe JG. Motion correction with PROPELLER MRI: application to head motion and free-breathing cardiac imaging. Magn Reson Med 1999;42(5):963–9.

56. Rosenkrantz AB, Bennett GL, Doshi A, et al. T2-weighted imaging of the prostate: impact of the BLADE technique on image quality and tumor assessment. Abdom Imaging 2014. http://dx.doi.org/10.1007/s00261-014-0225-7.

57. Fujimoto K, Koyama T, Tamai K, et al. BLADE acquisition method improves T2-weighted MR images of the female pelvis compared with a standard fast spin-echo sequence. Eur J Radiol 2011;80(3):796–801.

58. Lane BF, Vandermeer FQ, Oz RC, et al. Comparison of sagittal T2-weighted BLADE and fast spin-echo MRI of the female pelvis for motion artifact and lesion detection. AJR Am J Roentgenol 2011; 197(2):W307–13.

59. Rosenkrantz AB, Mannelli L, Mossa D, et al. Breath-hold T2-weighted MRI of the liver at 3T using the BLADE technique: impact upon image quality and lesion detection. Clin Radiol 2011;66(5):426–33.

60. Haneder S, Dinter D, Gutfleisch A, et al. Image quality of T2w-TSE of the abdomen and pelvis with Cartesian or BLADE-type k-space sampling: a retrospective interindividual comparison study. Eur J Radiol 2011;79(2):177–82.

61. Hirokawa Y, Isoda H, Okada T, et al. Improved detection of hepatic metastases from pancreatic cancer using periodically rotated overlapping parallel lines with enhanced reconstruction (PROPELLER) technique after SPIO administration. Invest Radiol 2010;45(3):158–64.

62. Bayramoglu S, Kilickesmez O, Cimilli T, et al. T2-weighted MRI of the upper abdomen: comparison of four fat-suppressed T2-weighted sequences including PROPELLER (BLADE) technique. Acad Radiol 2010;17(3):368–74.

63. Nanko S, Oshima H, Watanabe T, et al. Usefulness of the application of the BLADE technique to reduce motion artifacts on navigation-triggered prospective acquisition correction (PACE) T2-weighted MRI (T2WI) of the liver. J Magn Reson Imaging 2009; 30(2):321–6.

64. Michaely HJ, Kramer H, Weckbach S, et al. Renal T2-weighted turbo-spin-echo imaging with BLADE at 3.0 Tesla: initial experience. J Magn Reson Imaging 2008;27(1):148–53.

65. Hirokawa Y, Isoda H, Maetani YS, et al. MRI artifact reduction and quality improvement in the upper abdomen with PROPELLER and prospective acquisition correction (PACE) technique. AJR Am J Roentgenol 2008;191(4):1154–8.

66. Takayama Y, Nishie A, Asayama Y, et al. Three-dimensional T2-weighted imaging for liver MRI: clinical values of tissue-specific variable refocusing flip-angle turbo spin echo imaging. J Magn Reson Imaging 2014. http://dx.doi.org/10.1002/jmri.24554.

67. Bazot M, Stivalet A, Daraï E, et al. Comparison of 3D and 2D FSE T2-weighted MRI in the diagnosis of deep pelvic endometriosis: preliminary results. Clin Radiol 2013;68(1):47–54.

68. Denoiseux CC, Boulay-Coletta I, Nakache JP, et al. Liver T2-weighted MR imaging: assessment of a three-dimensional fast spin-echo with extended echo train acquisition sequence at 1.5 Tesla. J Magn Reson Imaging 2013;38(2):336–43.

69. Shin YR, Rha SE, Choi BG, et al. Uterine cervical carcinoma: a comparison of two- and three-dimensional T2-weighted turbo spin-echo MR imaging at 3.0 T for image quality and local-regional staging. Eur Radiol 2013;23(4):1150–7.

70. Dohan A, Gavini JP, Placé V, et al. T2-weighted MR imaging of the liver: qualitative and quantitative comparison of SPACE MR imaging with turbo spin-echo MR imaging. Eur J Radiol 2013;82(11):e655–61.

71. Watanabe H, Kanematsu M, Goshima S, et al. Detection of focal hepatic lesions with 3-T MRI: comparison of two-dimensional and three-dimensional T2-weighted sequences. Jpn J Radiol 2012;30(9): 721–8.

72. Cornud F, Rouanne M, Beuvon F, et al. Endorectal 3D T2-weighted 1mm-slice thickness MRI for prostate cancer staging at 1.5Tesla: should we reconsider the indirects signs of extracapsular extension according to the D'Amico tumor risk criteria? Eur J Radiol 2012;81(4):e591–7.

73. Hecht EM, Yitta S, Lim RP, et al. Preliminary clinical experience at 3 T with a 3D T2-weighted sequence compared with multiplanar 2D for evaluation of the female pelvis. AJR Am J Roentgenol 2011;197(2): W346–52.

74. Hori M, Kim T, Onishi H, et al. Uterine tumors: comparison of 3D versus 2D T2-weighted turbo spin-echo MR imaging at 3.0 T–initial experience. Radiology 2011;258(1):154–63.

75. Rosenkrantz AB, Neil J, Kong X, et al. Prostate cancer: comparison of 3D T2-weighted with conventional 2D T2-weighted imaging for image quality and tumor detection. AJR Am J Roentgenol 2010;194(2): 446–52.

76. Rosenkrantz AB, Patel JM, Babb JS, et al. Liver MRI at 3 T using a respiratory-triggered time-efficient 3D T2-weighted technique: impact on artifacts and image quality. AJR Am J Roentgenol 2010;194(3): 634–41.

77. Proscia N, Jaffe TA, Neville AM, et al. MRI of the pelvis in women: 3D versus 2D T2-weighted technique. AJR Am J Roentgenol 2010;195(1):254–9.

78. Kim H, Lim JS, Choi JY, et al. Rectal cancer: comparison of accuracy of local-regional staging with two- and three-dimensional preoperative 3-T MR imaging. Radiology 2010;254(2):485–92.

79. Agrawal G, Riherd JM, Busse RF, et al. Evaluation of uterine anomalies: 3D FRFSE cube versus standard

2D FRFSE. AJR Am J Roentgenol 2009;193(6): W558–62.

80. Fütterer JJ, Yakar D, Strijk SP, et al. Preoperative 3T MR imaging of rectal cancer: local staging accuracy using a two-dimensional and three-dimensional T2-weighted turbo spin echo sequence. Eur J Radiol 2008;65(1):66–71.

81. Yoo RE, Cho JY, Kim SY, et al. A systematic approach to the magnetic resonance imaging-based differential diagnosis of congenital Müllerian

duct anomalies and their mimics. Abdom Imaging 2014. http://dx.doi.org/10.1007/s00261-014-0195-9.

82. Kaur H, Choi H, You YN, et al. MR imaging for preoperative evaluation of primary rectal cancer: practical considerations. Radiographics 2012; 32(2):389–409.

83. Rauch GM, Kaur H, Choi H, et al. Optimization of MR imaging for pretreatment evaluation of patients with endometrial and cervical cancer. Radiographics 2014;34(4):1082–98.

Recent Advances in MR Hardware and Software

Andrea Kierans, MD, Nainesh Parikh, MD,
Hersh Chandarana, MD*

KEYWORDS

- Abdominal MRI • Non-Cartesian imaging techniques • Radial imaging • Spiral imaging
- Hybrid PET/MR imaging • PET/MR systems

KEY POINTS

- Non-Cartesian imaging techniques, including radial and spiral imaging, allow for increased motion robustness when compared to traditional Cartesian MRI.
- Radial T1-weighted GRE has recently become available for free-breathing imaging, and has shown major advantages in abdominal, pediatric, and head and neck imaging.
- Clinical hybrid PET/MR imaging was made possible by the technical development of avalanche photodiodes, although attenuation correction was and remains a technical challenge.
- There are number of different system designs that are either currently commercially available or are undergoing the US Food and Drug Administration approval process.
- PET/MRI will play an increasing role in clinical evaluation of oncologic and nononcologic diseases.

INTRODUCTION

Tremendous advances have been made in abdominopelvic MR imaging which continue to improve image quality, and make acquisitions faster and more robust. We briefly discuss the role of non-Cartesian acquisition schemes as well as dual parallel radiofrequency (RF) transmit systems in the article to further improve image quality of the abdominal MRI. Furthermore, the use of hybrid PET/MR systems has the potential to synergistically combine MR imaging with PET acquisition, and evolving role of hybrid PET/MRI is discussed.

MR imaging is being used increasingly for abdominal and pelvic imaging because it provides superior soft tissue contrast and lacks ionizing radiation.[1] However, several limitations persist, the most important of which are respiratory motion and long scan times. Respiratory and physiologic motion, including bowel and cardiac motion, often

lead to suboptimal image quality, rendering examinations nondiagnostic.[2,3] Over the past decade, several techniques have been applied to overcome motion-related artifact, such as suspended respiration, acquiring images with navigation triggering, and respiratory ordered phase encoding.[4,5] However, despite these efforts, respiratory motion is still problematic in elderly and pediatric patients, as well as debilitated patients with limited breath holding capacity. Furthermore, the need to obtain data during a breath hold limits the achievable in plane resolution and anatomic coverage.[6] To address these problems, several advances have been developed, including non-Cartesian acquisition MRI, which allows for increased motion robustness and superior image quality than conventional Cartesian imaging.[7–10]

Cartesian acquisition of k-space, in which the imaged body part is sampled along parallel lines, has been used in almost all conventional MR

Department of Radiology, New York University Langone Medical Center, 660 First Avenue, New York, NY 10016, USA
* Corresponding author.
E-mail address: hersh.chandarana@nyumc.org

Radiol Clin N Am 53 (2015) 599–610
http://dx.doi.org/10.1016/j.rcl.2015.02.002
0033-8389/15/$ – see front matter © 2015 Elsevier Inc. All rights reserved.

imaging techniques. Although non-Cartesian sequences were initially described in 1973,[11] they have not gained widespread clinical acceptance owing to various obstacles, including the need for higher field homogeneity, superior image reconstruction, and generation of more precise time-varying field gradients.[7] Through improvement in MR hardware design and algorithmic developments over the past several years, these technical challenges have been overcome, making it feasible to use non-Cartesian acquisition schemes.

Radial and spiral are 2 non-Cartesian imaging techniques. Radial imaging performs the "stack of stars" sampling in-plane and Cartesian sampling in the slice direction,[12,13] whereas spiral imaging covers k-space starting from the center of k-space.[14] In effect, radial and spiral imaging allow for reduced motion artifact compared with traditional Cartesian imaging.[14–16] Secondary to their motion robustness and improved spatial resolution, these non-Cartesian techniques have shown major advantage in abdominal, pediatric, cardiac and MR angiography imaging.[9,15–18]

In addition to motion artifact and long scan times, new technical challenges are arising as MRI is moving toward higher field strengths, including variations in specific absorption rate, as well as artifacts such as dielectric effect.[19,20] The recent implementation of parallel transmission with more than 1 radiofrequency (RF) source allows for adjustment of independent RF transmission, enabling B1 shimming and homogeneity.[20,21] This leads to decreased artifacts and improved spatial resolution. Both non-Cartesian imaging and parallel transmission are 2 recent advances in MR imaging allowing for faster acquisition and improved image quality.

RADIAL IMAGING

Radial sampling using the radial T1-weighted gradient echo (GRE) sequence has recently become available for routine imaging, (Star VIBE, Siemens Health Care, Germany). In this acquisition scheme, radial spokes are acquired along the k_x–k_y plane and conventional sampling is performed along the k_z dimension, resulting in a 3-dimensional (3D) "stack of stars."[16] The key advantage of radial imaging is its insensitivity to motion-induced distortions. Motion averaging is attained owing to overlapping spokes in the center of k-space. In addition, changing read-out directions prevents image shifting or "ghosting," as seen in Cartesian imaging.[7] Although radial imaging may lead to streak artifacts and object blurring that radiate from the motion-affected regions, this is usually minor and does not compromise diagnostic quality significantly. These artifacts appear as "texture" like on the underlying image, and are therefore less likely to cause lesion obscuration than traditional ghosting artifacts from Cartesian imaging.[7]

Radial T1-weighted GRE imaging has been in clinical use for free breathing imaging of the abdomen (**Fig. 1**). In addition to its motion robustness, radial T1-weighted GRE acquisition allows for superior spatial resolution. Unlike conventional imaging, which is limited to a breath hold of approximately 20 seconds, radial imaging allows sampling of data over several minutes, allowing for higher spatial resolution. Free-breathing radial T1-weighted GRE has been demonstrated to have similar overall image quality to standard breath hold T1-weighted GRE, and significantly better image quality compared with conventional free breathing T1-weighted GRE for contrast-enhanced imaging of the liver in adults.[16] Radial imaging has also shown to be of utility in pediatric imaging. Chandarana and colleagues[15] demonstrated significantly better overall image quality and increased lesion detection in the pediatric abdomen and pelvis using radial T1-weighted GRE acquisition, in which standard T1-weighted

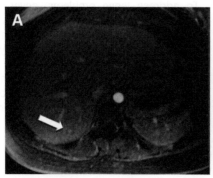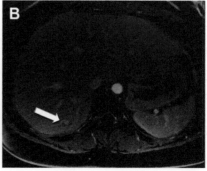

Fig. 1. A 48-year-old woman with right hepatic lobe focal nodular hyperplasia underwent postcontrast MRI with standard T1 weighted gradient echo (GRE; *A*) and radial T1 weighted-GRE (*B*) sequences. The lesion is more conspicuous on radial T1-weighted GRE sequence.

GRE was acquired using breath hold or free breathing schemes in patients who were unable to breath hold, and radial T1-weighted GRE was performed using free breathing. Similarly, Roque and colleagues[22] evaluated 3 T1-weighted sequences in pediatric patients; Cartesian T1-weighted GRE, T1-weighted magnetization-prepared gradient recalled echo technique, and radial T1-weighted GRE, demonstrating significantly higher overall image quality with radial T1-weighted GRE for sedated pediatric patients under 5 years old. Radial T1-weighted GRE imaging has also been evaluated in the pancreas, and was shown to demonstrate fair to good overall image quality in patients who were uncooperative with breath holding.[23]

The advantages of radial imaging, however, are not limited to the abdomen, and have found utility in neck and orbit imaging.[24,25] Conventional neck imaging consists of a fat suppressed postcontrast T1-weighted spin echo or turbo spin echo sequences. However, this sequence is especially sensitive to flow and motion, which can be detrimental to the evaluation of small structures within the neck. Furthermore, evaluation of the upper chest region is often severely limited with conventional MR imaging owing to marked flow artifact from the great vessels, as well as respiratory artifact. Wu and colleagues[24] demonstrated superior overall image quality, anatomic clarity, lesion clarity, and fat suppression with radial T1-weighted GRE compared with standard T1-weighted turbo spin echo for imaging of the neck. Orbit MRI is often prone to motion artifact secondary to patients moving of the eyes or blinking of the eyelids, leading to ghosting artifacts.[7] Radial T1-weighted GRE has been demonstrated to provide improved fat suppression, as well as superior depiction of the optic nerves compared with standard T1-weighted fat-suppressed imaging.[25]

A further application of radial imaging is in PET/MR imaging.[26,27] A known limitation in PET/CT is respiratory and motion artifact between the PET, which is obtained during free breathing and the CT, which is acquired during a specific stage of breathing or with shallow breathing.[27] Rakheja and colleagues[27] demonstrated more accurate spatial registration using simultaneous PET/MR with radial T1-weighted GRE than with PET/CT, for evaluation of multiple metastatic lesions. Similarly, although PET/MR has shown potential for superior oncologic evaluation, a concern of replacing the CT portion of PET/CT with MRI is in the detection of pulmonary nodules.[26] However, using PET/MR with simultaneously acquired radial T1-weighted GRE and PET data, Chandarana and colleagues[26] demonstrated a high sensitivity in the detection of FDG avid pulmonary nodules and

nodules with diameter of at least 0.5 cm. Therefore, radial T1-weighted GRE imaging has shown to have important and varied applications in abdominal and extraabdominal imaging.

Golden-Angle Radial Sparse Parallel MR Imaging

Despite the numerous advantages of radial imaging, disadvantages include a higher sampling requirement and lower scan efficiency, owing to less efficient coverage of k-space. This limits the ability to perform dynamic contrast-enhanced imaging, because the arterial and venous phases of contrast enhancement cannot be acquired. Reconstruction techniques aimed at improving temporal resolution, including golden-angle radial sparse parallel MR imaging (GRASP) and k-space weighted image contrast (KWIK), which acquire data continuously throughout the entire examination during contrast administration and retrospectively reconstruct different phases of enhancement, are under development.[7]

GRASP imaging, although not available commercially, has been investigated for several applications in research setting. In GRASP imaging, a compressed sensing reconstruction scheme is combined with parallel imaging for radial undersampled data. In effect, rapid continuous acquisition can be performed using a flexible temporal resolution.[28] Rosenkrantz and colleagues[29] demonstrated better clarity of prostate anatomic structures, as well as improved lesion detection on GRASP imaging (Fig. 2), compared with standard Cartesian dynamic contrast-enhanced imaging. Owing to its motion robustness, GRASP has also been used in the evaluation of inflammatory bowel disease, where increased vascularity in inflamed bowel segments can be identified, as well as evaluation of quantitative perfusion using signal enhancement curves generated from dynamic GRASP images can be performed.[17] This may be used to noninvasively predict disease status and treatment response. Additionally, the clinical use of GRASP has been extended to the head and neck, and has been used for dynamic imaging of the pituitary gland. This has proven advantageous secondary to its high spatial resolution, which is crucial in detecting small lesions such as mircroadenomas, in comparison to traditional 2-dimensional (2D) turbo spin-echo sequences.[30]

GRASP performs well with moderate motion in free breathing; however, in the presence of extensive motion, image quality is compromised severely. With varying motion, the data for each time point is affected by strong inconsistencies. However, techniques to compensate for this are

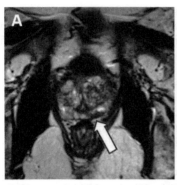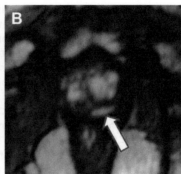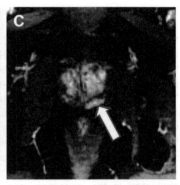

Fig. 2. A 71-year-old man with biopsy-proven Gleason 3 + 3 prostate cancer in the left posteromedial apex of the prostate. A nonspecific region of decreased T2 signal is present in this region (*A, arrow*). Early time-point from standard dynamic contrast-enhanced (DCE; *B*) and golden-angle radial sparse parallel (GRASP) DCE (*C*) MRI show corresponding focus of abnormal early enhancement in this region (*arrow, B, C*), which has sharper edges and is more clearly visualized using GRASP.

under development, including an approach called XD-GRASP. In this technique, a respiratory curve can be generated from the center of k-space, whereupon GRASP reconstruction can be extended to treat the respiratory state as an extra dimension, allowing sorting or compensation of respiration in the reconstructed images.[31,32]

Vastly Undersampled Isotropic Projection Reconstruction

Radial acquisition is shown to be advantageous in MR angiography imaging.[33,34] A 3D radially acquired sequence termed, vastly undersampled isotropic projection reconstruction (VIPR), allows for free-breathing, high-resolution MR angiography images in significantly reduced scan time,[35] and enables an acceleration factor of up to 61 relative to conventional Cartesian 3D phase contrast imaging.[8] The VIPR sequence samples data along radial lines evenly spaced through a spherical volume, each intersecting the origin of k-space.[8] Low spatial frequencies are sampled repeatedly in every projection with interleaving of these projections, so that all spatial frequency directions are coarsely sampled every few seconds. The temporal filter width and shape is then chosen retrospectively.[8] In addition to the motion robustness and increased temporal resolution inherent in radial imaging, advantages of phase-contrast VIPR include broader spatial coverage, isotropic spatial resolution, and smaller voxel sizes than those at conventional 3D Cartesian phase-contrast imaging,[34] which are crucial features for MR angiography imaging. Furthermore, sampling in 3D leads to greater dispersion of artifacts, which in effect are less pronounced than when using 2D sampling.[18]

This technique has been evaluated for iliac and intracranial MR angiography,[8,36] and when used with Navier–Stokes analysis,[37] has allowed for the measurements of vascular gradients and assessments of wall shear stress.[36,38,39] Lum and colleagues[36] demonstrated that phase-contrast MR angiography with VIPR enables reliable measurements of trans-stenotic pressure gradients in carotid and iliac lesions that are comparable to those obtained with endovascular pressure-sensing guidewires. Moftakhar and colleagues[38] obtained cardiac-gated velocity measurements in surgically created canine aneurysms, demonstrating high statistical correlation between phase-contrast VIPR aneurysmal pressures and microcatheter pressure measurements. In addition, by using continuously adapting respiratory gating, MR angiography for areas of respiratory motion, including abdominal and thoracic MR angiography, is now feasible.[34] Francois and colleagues[34] demonstrated no difference in image quality for proximal renal artery evaluation and greater quality scores for segmental renal artery evaluation, using phase contrast VIPR compared with contrast-enhanced MR renal angiography.

An additional technique based on a noniterative, unfiltered, constrained back-projection reconstruction to improve the achievable temporal resolution in radial MR imaging has been explored to achieve an additional acceleration factor beyond that provided by VIPR, and is applicable to time resolved acquisitions using arbitrary k-space trajectories, referred to as HighlY constrained back-Projection (HYPR). Acceleration factors of up to 1000 compared with traditional nonaccelerated Cartesian imaging have been achieved when HYPR is combined with VIPR acquisition.[18]

SPIRAL IMAGING

Spiral imaging, another form of non-Cartesian imaging, is also being investigated.[14] Similar to radial imaging, spiral trajectories sample the center of k-space more frequently than traditional Cartesian imaging, allowing increased temporal resolution with sliding window reconstruction.[10] In effect, major advantages of this acquisition include more effective coverage of k-space and higher signal-to-noise ratio.[14] In addition, variable density spirals, including oversampling of the k-space center, allow the trajectory to be less susceptible to motion artifacts, as well as reducing effects of residual aliasing from signal outside of the reconstructed field of view in each coil.[10] However, because spiral imaging has longer readout times than traditional Cartesian imaging, disadvantages include susceptibility to eddy currents and off-resonance artifact, which may lead to image blurring.[14] Reconstruction is typically performed by gridding, which convolves the data onto a rectilinear grid in k-space, so that the Fourier inversion can be performed rapidly using a 2D fast Fourier transform.[14]

Spiral imaging has been found to be of use in real-time cardiac[40–42] and coronary MRI,[10,43,44] by improving data acquisition efficiency and temporal resolution. Narayan and colleagues[40] demonstrated rapid and accurate assessment of right and left ventricular function in a single-breath hold using real time spiral steady-state free precession, which is especially prone to k-space inefficiencies and decreased temporal and spatial resolution using traditional Cartesian acquisition. In addition, Nayak and colleagues[41] used spiral GRE imaging sequences to achieve the necessary temporal resolution for real time cardiac and coronary imaging at 3 T. Spiral imaging has also shown to be of advantage in coronary artery MR angiography, which requires high temporal resolution and signal-to-noise ratio, and is also susceptible to artifact from physiologic motion.[44] Taylor and colleagues[44] demonstrated that spiral MR coronary angiogram images of the right coronary artery can be acquired in normal subjects and patients with coronary artery disease, during free respiration, and demonstrated superior image quality when compared with 2D segmented k-space fast low-angle shot images.

More recently, spiral imaging has been applied for dynamic contrast enhanced MRI of the liver using spiral liver acquisition with volume acceleration (LAVA). In spiral LAVA, 3 fully sampled 3D volumes are acquired, each requiring 10 seconds, with sliding reconstruction at every 3 seconds to reconstruct multiple arterial phases. Agrawal and colleagues[9] demonstrated superior bolus timing as well as superior overall image quality with spiral LAVA than standard Cartesian LAVA for dynamic contrast-enhanced liver MRI. Similar to radial T1-weighted GRE, artifacts secondary to motion and peristalsis can occur in spiral LAVA. However, the noise secondary to this artifact was not shown to cause significant difference in contrast-to-noise ratio between spiral LAVA and standard LAVA.[45]

As demonstrated, spiral imaging has the potential to improve clinical diagnostic imaging by reducing overall acquisition time, providing increased temporal and spatial resolution, as well as reducing motion artifact. However, its lack of mainstream clinical usage is owing to many factors, including challenges in gradient design, gradient deviations, and off-resonance artifacts.[14] Further developments each as adaptation of parallel imaging to spiral trajectory are underway, which will improve image quality and acquisition time and bring spiral imaging closer to routine clinical use.[14]

PARALLEL TRANSMISSION

Most clinical MRI examinations currently use a single channel volume transmit coil. With higher field strengths, this can lead to significant RF nonuniformity causing dielectric effect (ie, standing waves or B1 inhomogenieity artifacts), which occur when the wavelength of the RF reaches the dimension of the human head or body, creating destructive excitation field interference among sections of a conventional transmit coil.[20,46] This occurs especially in obese patients and those with ascites, rendering images diagnostically inadequate. The use of multiple RF transmit and receive coil elements in parallel can lead to significantly improved RF homogeneity at higher field strengths,[47–51] because the additional degrees of freedom provided by multiple transmit channel coils allow for B1 RF shimming, while maintaining low specific absorption rate.[47,52] Willinek and colleagues[21] demonstrated that liver MR imaging performed with dual source parallel RF excitation resulted in reduced dielectric shading, improved B1 homogeneity, and accelerated imaging at 3.0 T when compared with standard single-source RF imaging. In addition, Kukuk and colleagues[19] demonstrated improved liver lesion detection with dual source parallel RF transmission for liver lesion detection on 3.0 T T2-weighted single shot turbo spin echo when compared with single source RF transmission.

An additional function of the 2-channel parallel transmit systems is the ability to apply focused excitation of an inner volume of tissue using a 2D selective RF pulse, allowing for reduction in the field of view in the phase encoding direction, termed 'zoomed.' This reduction in phase field of view and phase encoding steps can lead to decreased phase-encoding artifacts, reduced geometric distortions, and increased spatial resolution.[53] In addition, the field of view does not need to be much larger than the tissue of interest, because specific RF excitation pulses prevent the occurrence of aliasing. This has found utility in diffusion-weighted imaging (DWI) of relatively small organs such as the pancreas and prostate,[54,55] because standard DWI has low in-plane resolution and is often prone to susceptibility artifact from adjacent structures such as loops of bowel. Riffel and colleagues[54] demonstrated significantly reduced blur, and increased diagnostic confidence for evaluation of the pancreas with zoomed DWI compared with single shot echo planar imaging. Thierfelder and colleagues[55,56] demonstrated superior overall image quality and detectability of small anatomic structures, with reduced artifact for accelerated zoomed echo planar imaging compared with standard DWI for evaluation of both the pancreas and prostate. Similar findings of improved imaging quality and reduced blur have also been demonstrated in the spine, as well as leading to faster acquisition and more detailed analysis of spinal lesions in patients with spinal cord ischemia, when compared with standard echo planar imaging.[57]

HYBRID PET/MR IMAGING

Positron emission tomography (PET) combined with magnetic resonance (MR) imaging is a recently introduced hybrid imaging modality that is increasingly being investigated for clinical application in the evaluation of oncologic and nononcologic pathologies. Although PET/CT (PET combined with CT) remains the workhorse for diagnosis and staging of oncologic pathology, PET/MR can add diagnostic value in areas where PET/CT may fall short. This section provides a brief overview on some of the potential applications of hybrid PET/MR imaging.

Until recently, PET/MR imaging has been performed as separate PET and MR examinations on separate systems with varying temporal delay between the acquisitions. Subsequently, the acquisitions are either fused cognitively through interpretation of the separate image sets by a radiologist or they are post-processed and fused with software with fused images available for interpretation. Vendors have been working on various implementations of PET and MR acquisitions, either sequentially or simultaneously to create a hybrid modality that is sustainable clinically. Several systems are recently approved by the US Food and Drug Administration (FDA; including the Siemens Biograph mMR and the Philips Ingenuity TF PET/MR imaging) or are currently under FDA review (from General Electric).

Hardware

System configuration: In general, 3 types of 'hybrid' PET/MR imaging systems are available.

Trimodality system: This technology employs separate PET/CT and MR systems with a shared bed, and therefore is termed a "trimodality" system. For accurate image registration, the patient remains on a multipurpose bed for both PET/CT and MR examinations while being transported between the systems.

Sequential system: This system represents modification upon the 'trimodality' system because it employs an MR scanner and PET scanner with a single, multipurpose bed that facilitates moving between the 2 systems which are in close proximity in one area, such that the patient is scanned through the PET/CT system and then sequentially scanned through the MR system.

Integrated simultaneous system: This system simultaneously acquires PET and MR data without acquiring CT information. MR images are utilized for attenuation correction in addition to anatomic information, thereby eliminating the need for CT acquisition.

Development of avalanche photodiodes has made it feasible to perform simultaneous acquisition of PET and MR using a single system.

Clinical Experience

The majority of experience with PET/MR systems can be divided into "oncologic" and "nononcologic" indications. The nononcologic experience is predominantly with neurodegenerative disorders and cardiovascular imaging. The oncologic indications include local and distant staging for lymphoma, breast cancer, head and neck cancer, and rectal and gynecologic malignancies, as well as bone and soft tissue tumors, to name a few. These areas are of interest because current imaging algorithms (PET/CT, MR alone, CT alone) are felt to be inadequate and many patients undergo multimodality examinations for assessment of full extent of the disease.

Nononcologic Neurologic Pathology

Dementia

Although MRI is the first step in the workup of dementia syndromes, PET/MRI represents a "1-stop" approach for advanced imaging evaluation. Structural etiologies such as tumors and hydrocephalus as well as atrophy can be identified. In addition, advanced techniques can be used to provide detailed metabolic, functional, and morphologic information for more specific diagnosis. Although this area has been an intense focus of investigation over the past several years, inaccurate attenuation correction of integrated data remains an unresolved issue and may lead to quantification errors. A recent study[58] evaluating PET/CT and PET/MRI in patients with dementia found considerable disagreement between the 2 modalities and their corresponding attenuation correction approaches, thereby potentially leading to an overestimation of cortical hypometabolism on PET/MRI. More work is needed to assess clinical utility of PET/MRI for dementia disorders.[59]

Epilepsy

Although MRI remains the first choice in the imaging evaluation of medically intractable temporal lobe epilepsy, it is generally well-accepted that in up to 20% of patients, MRI is nondiagnostic or MRI and electroencephalographic findings are discordant. A recent review demonstrated that the coregistration of PET and MRI enhances focus identification and improves the outcome of epilepsy surgery.[60] A handful of authors have demonstrated feasibility of hybrid PET/MRI for the detection of epileptogenic foci in small case series or single patient reports.[61–63] Added value of hybrid PET/MR imaging over current imaging techniques (eg, PET and PET/CT) will be the primary focus of further investigational studies.

Neurooncologic Pathology

Brain tumors

Although MRI remains the workhorse for imaging evaluation of tumors of the central nervous system, some recent publications demonstrate added diagnostic value of hybrid MR over the single modality approach and argue for its use in the primary work-up and staging of brain tumors.[64] There has been some recent investigation regarding diagnostic image quality, tumor concordance between PET/CT and PET/MR, and the added value of various advanced MRI techniques. The investigators agree on the convenience of obtaining all necessary imaging in 1 session with excellent spatial coregistration of MR and PET data.[59]

Head and neck cancer

Although PET/CT remains the workhorse for distant staging of metastatic disease, perhaps the most compelling indication for PET/MR is for local staging within the neck. For local staging, the high spatial and contrast resolution of MRI demarcates tumor extent and lymph node involvement, particularly in the context of the complex neck anatomy, which may lead to superior tumor staging and regional lymph node staging. Moreover, PET/MRI will likely prove useful for treatment planning.[65]

Cardiovascular Pathology

Cardiac imaging represents an exciting area for application of hybrid PET/MRI imaging because PET and MR imaging separately are routinely utilized in the workup and management of various cardiovascular disease, both benign and malignant. Although in theory there are numerous applications for hybrid PET/MR imaging in the assessment of cardiovascular diseases, published literature is limited.

Nononcologic Cardiac Diseases

Coronary artery disease

Currently, cardiac MRI is used to evaluate for myocardial infarctions and PET is used to evaluate perfusion and reversible ischemia and for assessing viable myocardium that could benefit from revascularization.[66–68] Hybrid PET/MRI imaging has the potential to combine the molecular information from PET with structural and functional information from MRI.

Sarcoidosis

Cardiac sarcoid may represent an important indication for hybrid PET/MRI.[69] Although cardiac MR is highly sensitive for revealing active inflammation and chronic fibrosis, simultaneously acquired PET information can improve both sensitivity and specificity. Furthermore, PET may help to discriminate between active inflammations versus fibrosis. Very early work suggests utility of imaging with hybrid modality.[70,71]

Cardiac Tumors

The evaluation of cardiac tumors may represent the most clinically applicable and simplest application of PET/MRI for cardiovascular diseases. Although MR provides a great deal of anatomic and structural information regarding cardiac tumors, PET is ideal for local and distant staging as well as for evaluating treatment response. Early work has demonstrated that PET/MR is similar or even superior to PET/CT for the evaluation of locoregional nodal and metastatic disease foci.[72]

Body Oncology

Breast oncology

Use of MR for local staging of breast cancer and PET for distant staging is a common practice.

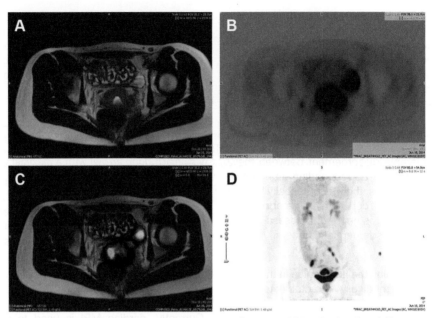

Fig. 3. A 38-year-old patient underwent simultaneous PET and MR acquisition for local and distant staging of the cervical cancer. (*A*) Standard axial T2-weighted single shot image demonstrates a cervical mass that is fluorodeoxyglucose avid on (*B*) attenuation-corrected axial PET. There is excellent coregisteration between MR and PET acquisition as seen on (*C*) fused attenuation-corrected PET and T2-weighted image. (*D*) Maximum intensity projection of the PET acquisition.

Combining PET/MR makes sense for simultaneous local and distant staging in selected subjects. Pacea and colleagues[73] have demonstrated that integrated whole body PET/MRI is feasible in a clinical setting and is comparable to whole body PET/CT for the qualitative detection of lesions. Furthermore, addition of PET to breast MRI, which is known to have relatively

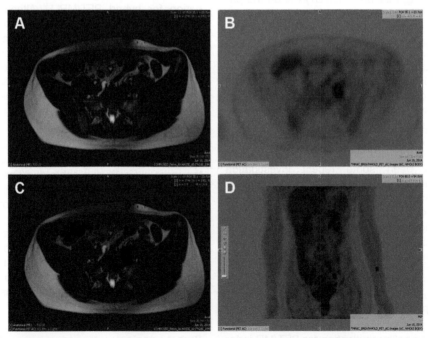

Fig. 4. In the same 38-year-old patient with cervical cancer, there is metastatic adenopathy as seen on (*A*) Standard axial T2-weighted single shot image. (*B*) Attenuation-corrected axial PET. (*C*) Fused attenuation-corrected PET and T2-weighted image and (*D*) maximum intensity projection of the PET acquisition.

low specificity, might potentially increase the specificity of MRI.

Abdominal and pelvic oncology

It has been demonstrated several times that PET/MR is comparable with PET/CT for anatomic lesion localization; however, there is improved soft tissue resolution, particularly for pelvis and colorectal cancers.[72,74] Although the superior soft tissue resolution of MR over CT is well-known, additional work is required to define the exact role of hybrid PET/MR. For pancreatic cancer, early research suggests that PET/MRI is helpful in attempting to differentiate posttreatment changes from residual/recurrent tumor.[75] Pelvic malignancies such as cervical cancer, ovarian cancer, prostate cancer, and rectal cancer in theory would benefit from the hybrid modality; current algorithms call for traditional MRI alone for locoregional staging, possibly in combination with whole body PET/CT for evaluating for distant disease (Figs. 3 and 4).

Although PET/CT remains the workhorse for the whole body evaluation of lymphoma, PET/MR has been shown to assess disease burden with similar sensitivity, and represents a viable alternative for lymphoma staging and follow-up. Multiple myeloma is another indication for which hybrid PET/MR imaging can potentially play an important role.

Pediatric oncology: Although it has not been studied on a large scale, it should be noted that, owing to the obvious reduction in ionizing radiation by using PET/MR rather than PET/CT, hybrid PET/MR represents an exciting area of investigation for pediatric tumor assessment (such as neuroblastoma staging). A "1-stop" approach can be used to minimize logistic, emotional, and physical discomfort. Performing MRI and PET examination with single induction of sedation is an additional and important benefit.

SUMMARY

Clinical hybrid PET/MRI was made possible by the technical development of avalanche photodiodes, although attenuation correction was and remains a technical challenge. Whereas Dixon T1-weighted sequences serve currently as the primary mode of attenuation correction in clinical PET/MRI, advanced techniques and algorithms are being investigated. There are a number of different system designs that are either currently commercially available or are undergoing the FDA approval process. PET/MRI thus will play an increasing role in clinical evaluation of oncologic and nononcologic diseases.

REFERENCES

1. Ahn S, Kim WY, Lim KS, et al. Advanced radiology utilization in a tertiary care emergency department from 2001 to 2010. PloS One 2014;9(11):e112650.
2. Maki JH, Chenevert TL, Prince MR. The effects of incomplete breath-holding on 3D MR image quality. J Magn Reson Imaging 1997;7(6):1132–9.
3. Paling MR, Brookeman JR. Respiration artifacts in MR imaging: reduction by breath holding. J Comput Assist Tomogr 1986;10(6):1080–2.
4. Nagle SK, Busse RF, Brau AC, et al. High resolution navigated three-dimensional T(1)-weighted hepatobiliary MRI using gadoxetic acid optimized for 1.5 Tesla. J Magn Reson Imaging 2012;36(4):890–9.
5. Young PM, Brau AC, Iwadate Y, et al. Respiratory navigated free breathing 3D spoiled gradient-recalled echo sequence for contrast-enhanced examination of the liver: diagnostic utility and comparison with free breathing and breath-hold conventional examinations. AJR Am J Roentgenol 2010; 195(3):687–91.
6. Chandarana H, Block TK, Ream J, et al. Estimating liver perfusion from free-breathing continuously acquired dynamic gadolinium-ethoxybenzyl-diethylenetriamine pentaacetic acid-enhanced acquisition with compressed sensing reconstruction. Invest Radiol 2014; 20:20.
7. Block TK, CHandarana H, Milla S. Towards routine clinical use of radial stack-of-stars 3d gradient-echo sequences for reducing motion sensitivity. J Korean Soc Magn Reson Med 2014;18(2):87–106.
8. Gu T, Korosec FR, Block WF, et al. PC VIPR: a high-speed 3D phase-contrast method for flow quantification and high-resolution angiography. AJNR Am J Neuroradiol 2005;26(4):743–9.
9. Agrawal MD, Spincemaille P, Mennitt KW, et al. Improved hepatic arterial phase MRI with 3-second temporal resolution. J Magn Reson Imaging 2013; 37(5):1129–36.
10. Kressler B, Spincemaille P, Nguyen TD, et al. Three-dimensional cine imaging using variable-density spiral trajectories and SSFP with application to coronary artery angiography. Magn Reson Med 2007; 58(3):535–43.
11. Lauterbur PD. Image formation by induced local interactions: examples employing nuclear magnetic resonance. Nature 1973;242:190–1.
12. Lin W, Guo J, Rosen MA, et al. Respiratory motion-compensated radial dynamic contrast-enhanced (DCE)-MRI of chest and abdominal lesions. Magn Reson Med 2008;60(5):1135–46.
13. Song HK, Dougherty L. Dynamic MRI with projection reconstruction and KWIC processing for simultaneous high spatial and temporal resolution. Magn Reson Med 2004;52(4):815–24.

14. Delattre BM, Heidemann RM, Crowe LA, et al. Spiral demystified. Magn Reson Imaging 2010;28(6): 862–81.

15. Chandarana H, Block KT, Winfeld MJ, et al. Free-breathing contrast-enhanced T1-weighted gradient-echo imaging with radial k-space sampling for paediatric abdominopelvic MRI. Eur Radiol 2014; 24(2):320–6.

16. Chandarana H, Block TK, Rosenkrantz AB, et al. Free-breathing radial 3D fat-suppressed T1-weighted gradient echo sequence: a viable alternative for contrast-enhanced liver imaging in patients unable to suspend respiration. Invest Radiol 2011; 46(10):648–53.

17. Ream JM, Doshi AM, Block KT, et al. High spatiotemporal dynamic contrast-enhanced MRI of the small bowel in active Crohn's terminal ileitis using compressed sensing, parallel imaging, and golden-angle radial sampling. In: Proc Intl Soc Mag Reson Med. 2014. 22:p. 4292.

18. Grist TM, Mistretta CA, Strother CM, et al. Time-resolved angiography: past, present, and future. J Magn Reson Imaging 2012;36(6):1273–86.

19. Kukuk GM, Gieseke J, Weber S, et al. Focal liver lesions at 3.0 T: lesion detectability and image quality with T2-weighted imaging by using conventional and dual-source parallel radiofrequency transmission. Radiology 2011;259(2):421–8.

20. Merkle EM, Dale BM. Abdominal MRI at 3.0 T: the basics revisited. AJR Am J Roentgenol 2006; 186(6):1524–32.

21. Willinek WA, Gieseke J, Kukuk GM, et al. Dual-source parallel radiofrequency excitation body MR imaging compared with standard MR imaging at 3.0 T: initial clinical experience. Radiology 2010; 256(3):966–75.

22. Roque A, Ramalho M, AlObaidy M, et al. Post-contrast T1-weighted sequences in pediatric abdominal imaging: comparative analysis of three different sequences and imaging approach. Pediatr Radiol 2014;44(10):1258–65.

23. Bamrungchart S, Tantaway EM, Midia EC, et al. Free breathing three-dimensional gradient echo-sequence with radial data sampling (radial 3D-GRE) examination of the pancreas: Comparison with standard 3D-GRE volumetric interpolated breathhold examination (VIBE). J Magn Reson Imaging 2013;38(6):1572–7.

24. Wu X, Raz E, Block TK, et al. Contrast-enhanced radial 3D fat-suppressed T1-weighted gradient-recalled echo sequence versus conventional fat-suppressed contrast-enhanced T1-weighted studies of the head and neck. AJR Am J Roentgenol 2014; 203(4):883–9.

25. Bangiyev L, Raz E, Block KT, et al. Contrast-enhanced radial 3D fat-suppressed T1-weighted gradient echo (radial-VIBE) sequence: a viable and potentially superior alternative to conventional T1-MPRAGE with water excitation and fat-suppressed contrast-enhanced T1W sequence for evaluation of the orbit. ASNR Annual Meeting. San Diego, May 20-23, 2013. p. O–413.

26. Chandarana H, Heacock L, Rakheja R, et al. Pulmonary nodules in patients with primary malignancy: comparison of hybrid PET/MR and PET/CT imaging. Radiology 2013;268(3):874–81.

27. Rakheja R, DeMello L, Chandarana H, et al. Comparison of the accuracy of PET/CT and PET/MRI spatial registration of multiple metastatic lesions. AJR Am J Roentgenol 2013;201(5):1120–3.

28. Chandarana H, Feng L, Block TK, et al. Free-breathing contrast-enhanced multiphase MRI of the liver using a combination of compressed sensing, parallel imaging, and golden-angle radial sampling. Invest Radiol 2013;48(1):10–6.

29. Rosenkrantz AB, Geppert C, Grimm R, et al. Dynamic contrast-enhanced MRI of the prostate with high spatiotemporal resolution using compressed sensing, parallel imaging, and continuous golden-angle radial sampling: Preliminary experience. J Magn Reson Imaging 2014;16(10):24661.

30. Espagnet CR, Bangiyev L, Block KT, et al. High resolution DCE MRI of the pituitary gland using radial K space aquisition with compressed sensing reconstruction. In: Proc Intl Soc Mag Reson Med. 2014. 22:p. 4669.

31. Grimm R, Block KT, Kiefer B, et al. Bias correction for respiration detection in radial 3D gradient-echo imaging. In: Proc Intl Soc Mag Reson Med. 2011. 19:p. 2677.

32. Feng L, Liu J, Block KT, et al. Compressed sensing reconstruction with an additional respiratory-phase dimension for free-breathing imaging. In: Proc Intl Soc Mag Reson Med. 2013. 21:p. 606.

33. Johnson KM, Lum DP, Turski PA, et al. Improved 3D phase contrast MRI with off-resonance corrected dual echo VIPR. Magn Reson Med 2008;60(6): 1329–36.

34. Francois CJ, Lum DP, Johnson KM, et al. Renal arteries: isotropic, high-spatial-resolution, unenhanced MR angiography with three-dimensional radial phase contrast. Radiology 2011;258(1):254–60.

35. Barger AV, Block WF, Toropov Y, et al. Time-resolved contrast-enhanced imaging with isotropic resolution and broad coverage using an undersampled 3D projection trajectory. Magn Reson Med 2002;48(2): 297–305.

36. Lum DP, Johnson KM, Paul RK, et al. Transstenotic pressure gradients: measurement in swine–retrospectively ECG-gated 3D phase-contrast MR angiography versus endovascular pressure-sensing guidewires. Radiology 2007;245(3):751–60.

37. Tyszka JM, Laidlaw DH, Asa JW, et al. Three-dimensional, time-resolved (4D) relative pressure mapping

using magnetic resonance imaging. J Magn Reson Imaging 2000;12(2):321–9.

38. Moftakhar R, Aagaard-Kienitz B, Johnson K, et al. Noninvasive measurement of intra-aneurysmal pressure and flow pattern using phase contrast with vastly undersampled isotropic projection imaging. AJNR Am J Neuroradiol 2007;28(9):1710–4.

39. Turk AS, Johnson KM, Lum D, et al. Physiologic and anatomic assessment of a canine carotid artery stenosis model utilizing phase contrast with vastly undersampled isotropic projection imaging. AJNR Am J Neuroradiol 2007;28(1):111–5.

40. Narayan G, Nayak K, Pauly J, et al. Single-breath-hold, four-dimensional, quantitative assessment of LV and RV function using triggered, real-time, steady-state free precession MRI in heart failure patients. J Magn Reson Imaging 2005;22(1):59–66.

41. Nayak KS, Cunningham CH, Santos JM, et al. Real-time cardiac MRI at 3 tesla. Magn Reson Med 2004; 51(4):655–60.

42. Ryf S, Kissinger KV, Spiegel MA, et al. Spiral MR myocardial tagging. Magn Reson Med 2004;51(2): 237–42.

43. Santos JM, Cunningham CH, Lustig M, et al. Single breath-hold whole-heart MRA using variable-density spirals at 3T. Magn Reson Med 2006; 55(2):371–9.

44. Taylor AM, Keegan J, Jhooti P, et al. A comparison between segmented k-space FLASH and interleaved spiral MR coronary angiography sequences. J Magn Reson Imaging 2000;11(4):394–400.

45. Xu B, Spincemaille P, Chen G, et al. Fast 3D contrast enhanced MRI of the liver using temporal resolution acceleration with constrained evolution reconstruction. Magn Reson Med 2013;69(2):370–81.

46. Kuhl CK, Kooijman H, Gieseke J, et al. Effect of B1 inhomogeneity on breast MR imaging at 3.0 T. Radiology 2007;244(3):929–30.

47. Katscher U, Bornert P. Parallel RF transmission in MRI. NMR Biomed 2006;19(3):393–400.

48. Vernickel P, Roschmann P, Findeklee C, et al. Eight-channel transmit/receive body MRI coil at 3T. Magn Reson Med 2007;58(2):381–9.

49. Ullmann P, Junge S, Wick M, et al. Experimental analysis of parallel excitation using dedicated coil setups and simultaneous RF transmission on multiple channels. Magn Reson Med 2005;54(4):994–1001.

50. Zhu Y. Parallel excitation with an array of transmit coils. Magn Reson Med 2004;51(4):775–84.

51. Mihara H, Iriguchi N, Ueno S. A method of RF inhomogeneity correction in MR imaging. MAGMA 1998; 7(2):115–20.

52. Van den Berg CA, van den Bergen B, Van de Kamer JB, et al. Simultaneous B1 + homogenization and specific absorption rate hotspot suppression using a magnetic resonance phased array transmit coil. Magn Reson Med 2007;57(3):577–86.

53. Schneider R, Ritter D, Haueisen J, et al. Novel 2DRF optimization framework for spatially selective RF pulses incorporating B1, B0 and variable density trajectory. In: Proceedings of the 20th scientific meeting, International Society for Magnetic Resonance and Medicine. 2012. p. 1884.

54. Riffel P, Michaely HJ, Morelli JN, et al. Zoomed EPI-DWI of the pancreas using two-dimensional spatially-selective radiofrequency excitation pulses. PLoS One 2014;9(3):e89468.

55. Thierfelder KM, Scherr MK, Notohamiprodjo M, et al. Diffusion-weighted MRI of the prostate: advantages of Zoomed EPI with parallel-transmit-accelerated 2D-selective excitation imaging. Eur Radiol 2014; 24(12):3233–41.

56. Thierfelder KM, Sommer WH, Dietrich O, et al. Parallel-transmit-accelerated spatially-selective excitation MRI for reduced-FOV diffusion-weighted-imaging of the pancreas. Eur J Radiol 2014;83(10):1709–14.

57. Seeger A, Klose U, Bischof F, et al. Zoomed EPI DWI of acute spinal ischemia using a parallel transmission system. Clin Neuroradiol 2014. [Epub ahead of print].

58. Hitz S, Habekost C, Furst S, et al. Systematic comparison of the performance of integrated whole-body PET/MR imaging to conventional PET/CT for 18F-FDG brain imaging in patients examined for suspected dementia. J Nucl Med 2014;55:923–31.

59. Werner P, Barthel H, Drezga A, et al. Current status and future role of brain PET/MRI in clinical and research settings. Eur J Nucl Med Mol Imaging 2015;42(3):512–26.

60. Lee KK, Salamon N. [18F]fluorodeoxyglucose-positron-emission tomography and MR imaging coregistration for presurgical evaluation of medically refractory epilepsy. AJNR Am J Neuroradiol 2009; 30:1811–6.

61. Catana C, Drzezga A, Heiss WD, et al. PET/MRI for neurologic applications. J Nucl Med 2012;53: 1916–25.

62. Garibotto V, Heinzer S, Vulliemoz S, et al. Clinical applications of hybrid PET/MRI in neuroimaging. Clin Nucl Med 2013;38:e13–8.

63. Purz S, Sabri O, Viehweger A, et al. Potential pediatric applications of PET/MR. J Nucl Med 2014; 55(Suppl 2):32S–9S.

64. Dunet V, Maeder P, Nicod-Lalonde M, et al. Combination of MRI and dynamic FET PET for initial glioma grading. Nuklearmedizin 2014;53:155–61.

65. Partovi S, Kohan A, Rubbert C, et al. Review article clinical oncologic applications of PET/MRI: a new horizon. Am J Nucl Med Mol Imaging 2014;4(2):202–12.

66. Schinkel AF, Bax JJ, Poldermans D, et al. Hibernating myocardium: diagnosis and patient outcomes. Curr Probl Cardiol 2007;32(7):375–410.

67. Tillisch J, Brunken R, Marshall R, et al. Reversibility of cardiac wall-motion abnormalities predicted by

positron tomography. N Engl J Med 1986;314(14): 884–8.

68. vom Dahl J, Eitzman DT, al-Aouar ZR, et al. Relation of regional function, perfusion, and metabolism in patients with advanced coronary artery disease undergoing surgical revascularization. Circulation 1994;90(5):2356–66.

69. Naeger DM, Behr SC. PET/MR imaging: current and future applications for cardiovascular disease. Magn Reson Imaging Clin N Am 2015;23:95–103.

70. Schneider S, Batrice A, Rischpler C, et al. Utility of multimodal cardiac imaging with PET/MRI in cardiac sarcoidosis: implications for diagnosis, monitoring and treatment. Eur Heart J 2013; 35(5):312.

71. Campbell P, Stewart GC, Padera RF, et al. Evaluation for cardiac sarcoidosis—uncertainty despite contemporary multi-modality imaging. J Card Fail 2010;16(8):S107.

72. Al-Nabhani KZ, Syed R, Michopoulou S, et al. Qualitative and quantitative comparison of PET/CT and PET/MR imaging in clinical practice. J Nucl Med 2014;55(1):88–94.

73. Pacea L, Nicolai E, Luongoc A, et al. Comparison of whole-body PET/CT and PET/MRI in breast cancer patients: lesion detection and quantitation of 18F-deoxyglucose uptake in lesions and in normal organ tissues. Eur J Radiol 2014;83:289–96.

74. Drzezga A, Souvatzoglou M, Eiber M, et al. First clinical experience with integrated whole-body PET/MR: comparison to PET/CT in patients with oncologic diagnoses. J Nucl Med 2012;53:845–55.

75. Vercher-Conejero JL, Paspulati RM, Kohan A, et al. Imaging pancreatic pathology with PET/MRI: a pictorial essay. Annual Meeting of the Radiological Society of North America. Chicago, December 1-6, 2013.

Index

Note: Page numbers of article titles are in **boldface** type.

Moving?

Make sure your subscription moves with you!

To notify us of your new address, find your **Clinics Account Number** (located on your mailing label above your name), and contact customer service at:

Email: journalscustomerservice-usa@elsevier.com

800-654-2452 (subscribers in the U.S. & Canada)
314-447-8871 (subscribers outside of the U.S. & Canada)

Fax number: 314-447-8029

Elsevier Health Sciences Division
Subscription Customer Service
3251 Riverport Lane
Maryland Heights, MO 63043

ELSEVIER

Printed and bound by CPI Group (UK) Ltd, Croydon, CR0 4YY

03/10/2024

01040376-0019